FATTY LIVER DIET COOKBOOK

400+ HEALTHY AND FLAVORFUL RECIPES TO PREVENT AND REVERSE THE FATTY LIVER DISEASE AND QUICKLY BURN STUBBORN FAT

Contents

Introduction 12

Chapter 1: Understanding your liver 13
Locating Your Liver 14
Liver Functions 14

Chapter 2: Fatty liver disease 15
Liver failure 15
Liver Cancer 15
Alcoholic Liver Disease (ALD) 15
Poor or un-balanced diet. 15
Acute Viral Hepatitis: 16
N.A.F.L.D - Non-Alcoholic Fatty Liver Disease ... 16
Autoimmune Hepatitis 16

Chapter 3: How Fatty Liver Develop 18
Possible risk factors 18
Symptoms and diagnosis of fatty liver 18

Chapter 4: Breakfast Recipes 20
Raspberry Pudding 20
Walnuts Yogurt Mix 20
Mediterranean Egg-feta Scramble 20
Spiced Chickpeas Bowls 21
Orzo And Veggie Bowls 21
Vanilla Oats 22
Mushroom-egg Casserole 22
Bacon Veggies Combo 22
Brown Rice Salad 23
Olive And Milk Bread 23
Breakfast Tostadas 24
Chicken Souvlaki 24
Tahini Pine Nuts Toast 25
Eggs And Veggies 25
Chili Scramble 26
Pear Oatmeal 26
Olive Frittata 27
Mediterranean Egg Casserole 27
Milk Scones 28
Herbed Eggs And Mushroom Mix 28
Cherry Berry Bulgur Bowl 29

Baked Curried Apple Oatmeal Cups 30
Pineapple, Macha & Beet Chia Pudding 30
Coconut & Strawberry Smoothie Bowl 31
Farro Salad 31
Chili Avocado Scramble 31
Tapioca Pudding 32
Feta And Eggs Mix 32
Banana pancakes 32
Nectarine pancakes 33
Pancakes 33
Peaches muffins 33
Lemon muffins 34
Blueberry muffins 34
Kumquat muffins 34
Chocolate muffins 35
Muffins 35
Omelette 36
Carrot omelette 36
Onion omelette 36
Broccoli omelette 37
Beets omelette 37
Breakfast Beans (ful Mudammas) 37
Seeds And Lentils Oats 38
Couscous With Artichokes, Sun-dried Tomatoes And Feta 38
Cinnamon Roll Oats 39
Spinach Wrap 39
Chicken Liver 40
Avocado Spread 40
Eggplant rollatini 40
Asparagus with egg 41
Deviled eggs 41
Spicy cucumbers 41
Red Pepper And Artichoke Frittata 42
Stuffed Figs 42
Keto Egg Fast Snickerdoodle Crepes 43

Cauliflower Hash Brown Breakfast Bowl...43
Pumpkin Coconut Oatmeal 44
Bacon, Vegetable And Parmesan Combo....44
Toasted Crostini 45
Heavenly Egg Bake With Blackberry 45
Quick Cream Of Wheat 46
Herbed Spinach Frittata......46
Ham Spinach Ballet......47
Banana Quinoa 47
Quinoa And Potato Bowl 47
Almond Cream Cheese Bake 48
Slow-cooked Peppers Frittata 48
Peanut Butter and Cacao Breakfast Quinoa 49
Pasta with Indian Lentils 49
Vegetable Buckwheat Pasta......50
Pan-Seared Salmon Salad with Snow Peas & Grapefruit 50
Cleansing Vegetable Broth......51
Barbecued Spiced Tuna with Avocado-Mango Salsa 51
Low Carb Berry Salad with Citrus Dressing 52
Tasty Lime Cilantro Cauliflower Rice......52
Citrus Chicken with Delicious Cold Soup ...53
Pan-Fried Chicken with Oregano-Orange Chimichurri & Arugula Salad......53
Cauliflower Couscous Salad 54
Ultimate Liver Detox Soup 54
Brown Rice and Grilled Chicken Salad 55
Superfood Liver Cleansing Soup 55
Toxin Flush & Detox Salad 56
Grilled Chicken Salad......56
Chicken Stir Fry with Red Onions & Cabbage 57
Green Salad with Herbs......57
Chilled Green Goddess Soup 58
Detox Soup 58

Pumpkin Muffins......59
Spiced French Toast......59
Passionfruit, Cranberry & Coconut Yoghurt Chia Parfait 60
Veggie Omelet......60
Overnight Superfood Parfait 61
Crunchy Peach, Cranberry and Flax Meal Super Bowl......61
Gluten Free Pancakes 62
Detox Porridge 62
Avocado Crab Omelet 62
Buckwheat Pancakes 63
Apple Oatmeal 63
Raspberry Overnight Porridge......64
Cheesy Scrambled Eggs with Fresh Herbs .64
Turkey and Spinach Scramble on Melba Toast 65
Vegetable Omelet 65
Mexican Style Burritos 66

Chapter 5: Snack Recipes 66
Rosemary Cauliflower Dip 66
Light & Creamy Garlic Hummus 67
Style Nachos Recipe 67
Baked Goat Cheese Caprese Salad 68
Grilled Shrimp Kabobs 69
Red Pepper Tapenade 69
Lemon Swordfish 70
Paprika Salmon And Green Beans 70
Cucumber-basil Salsa On Halibut Pouches 70
Sardine Meatballs 71
Basil Tilapia 72
Honey Halibut......72
Stuffed Mackerel 73
Healthy Carrot & Shrimp......73
Tomato Cod Mix 73
Garlic Mussels......74
Mahi Mahi And Pomegranate Sauce 74

Honey Balsamic Salmon	75
Sage Salmon Fillet	75
Seafood Stew Cioppino	75
Shrimp And Lemon Sauce	76
Feta Tomato Sea Bass	76
Salmon And Broccoli	77
Halibut And Quinoa Mix	77
Crab Stew	78
Crazy Saganaki Shrimp	78
Grilled Tuna	79
Rosemary Salmon	79
Easy Seafood French Stew	80
Avocado Dip	80
Feta And Roasted Red Pepper Bruschetta	81
Meat-filled Phyllo (samboosek)	81
Tasty Black Bean Dip	82
Zucchini Cakes	82
Parsley Nachos	83
Plum Wraps	83
Parmesan Chips	83
Chicken Bites	84
Chicken Kale Wraps	84
Savory Pita Chips	85
Artichoke Skewers	85
Kidney Bean Spread	85
Polenta Cups Recipe	86
Tomato Triangles	86
Chili Mango And Watermelon Salsa	87
Tomato Olive Salsa	87
Lavash Chips	87
Homemade Salsa	88
Stuffed Zucchinis	88
Yogurt Dip	89
Popcorn-pine Nut Mix	89
Scallions Dip	89
Date Balls	90
Lavash Roll Ups	90
Chickpeas And Eggplant Bowls	91
Vinegar Beet Bites	91
Baked Sweet-potato Fries	91
Cucumber Rolls	92
Jalapeno Chickpea Hummus	92
Healthy Spinach Dip	93
Marinated Cheese	93
Za'atar Fries	93
Tuna Salad	94
Cheese Rolls	94
Olive, Pepperoni, And Mozzarella Bites	95
Eggplant Dip	95
Roasted Chickpeas	95
Pita Chips	96
Kale Chips	96
Blueberry Granola Bars	97
Veggie Balls	97
Oatmeal Cookies	97
Deviled Avocado Eggs	98
Berry & Veggie Gazpacho	98
Healthy Guacamole	99
Healthy Poached Trout	99
Creamy Curry Salmon	100
Cod And Cabbage	100
Pecan Salmon Fillets	100
Shrimp And Mushrooms Mix	101
Leeks And Calamari Mix	101
Cod With Lentils	101
Honey Garlic Shrimp	102
Pepper Salmon Skewers	102
Orange Salsa	103
Raw Broccoli Poppers	103
Candied Ginger	104
Chia Crackers	104
Orange-Spiced Pumpkin Hummus	105

Superfood Spiced Apricot-Sesame Bliss Balls 105

Crunchy Veggie Chips 105

Superfood Raw Bars 106

Trail Mix 106

Avocado & Pea Dip with Carrots 106

Carrot Chips 107

Spiced Spinach Bites 107

Ginger Tahini Dip with Veggies 107

Spiced Toasted Almonds & Seed Mix 108

Lime Pea Guacamole 108

Chili-lime Cucumber, Jicama, & Apple Sticks 108

Savory Trail Mix 109

Raw Turmeric Cashew Nut & Coconut Balls 109

Homemade Nutella 109

Wheat Crackers 109

Potato Chips 110

Rosemary & Garlic Kale Chips 110

Collard Greens and Tomatoes 111

Blueberry Cauliflower 111

Roasted Asparagus 112

Asparagus Frittata 112

Roasted Radishes 112

Radish Hash Browns 113

Strawberry Frozen Yogurt 113

Walnut & Spiced Apple Tonic 114

Basil & Walnut Pesto 114

Honey Chili Nuts 114

Mozzarella Cauliflower Bars 115

Grape, Celery & Parsley Reviver 115

Roasted Red Endive With Caper Butter ... 116

Zucchini Pepper Chips 116

Apple Chips 117

Carrot Chips 117

Chapter 6: Lunch Recipes 119

Tilapia with Avocado & Red Onion 119

Berries and Grilled Calamari 119

Cajun Garlic Shrimp Noodle Bowl 120

Tarragon Cod Fillets 120

Chicken And White Bean 121

Quinoa & Black Bean Stuffed Sweet Potatoes 121

Feta, Eggplant And Sausage Penne 122

Bell Peppers 'n Tomato-chickpea Rice 123

Lipsmacking Chicken Tetrazzini 123

Spaghetti In Lemon Avocado White Sauce 124

Kidney Beans And Beet Salad 124

Filling Macaroni Soup 125

Simple Penne Anti-pasto 125

Squash And Eggplant Casserole 126

Blue Cheese And Grains Salad 127

Creamy Artichoke Lasagna 127

Brown Rice Pilaf With Butternut Squash . 128

Cranberry And Roasted Squash Delight ... 129

Spanish Rice Casserole With Cheesy Beef 129

Kidney Bean And Parsley-lemon Salad 130

Italian White Bean Soup 130

Mexican Quinoa Bake 131

Citrus Quinoa & Chickpea Salad 131

Chickpea Salad Moroccan Style 132

Garlicky Peas And Clams On Veggie Spiral 132

Leek, Bacon And Pea Risotto 133

Chickpea Fried Eggplant Salad 133

Turkey And Quinoa Stuffed Peppers 134

Pastitsio An Italian Dish 135

Spiced Eggplant Stew 135

Shrimp Soup 136

Halloumi, Grape Tomato And Zucchini Skewers With Spinach-basil Oil 136

Beef Bourguignon 137

Flank Steak	137
Spiced Grilled Flank Steak	138
Pan Roasted Chicken With Olives And Lemon	138
Creamy Salmon Soup	138
Grilled Salmon With Cucumber Dill Sauce	139
Grilled Basil-lemon Tofu Burgers	139
Creamy Green Pea Pasta	140
Meat Cakes	140
Herbed Roasted Cod	141
Mushroom Soup	141
Salmon Parmesan Gratin	142
Chicken Souvlaki 2	142
Rosemary Roasted New Potatoes	143
Artichoke Feta Penne	143
Grilled Chicken And Rustic Mustard Cream	143
Balsamic Steak With Feta, Tomato, And Basil	144
Fried Chicken With Tzatziki Sauce	145
Green smoothie bowl	145
Sweet cream cheese breakfast	145
Avocado boat with salsa	146
Vegetable ribbon noodles with chicken breast fillet	146
Zucchini and mozzarella casserole	147
Oven vegetables with salmon fillet	148
Smoked Salmon and Watercress Salad	148
Salmon and Corn Salad	148
Stuffed Eggplants	149
Mushroom Pilaf	149
Cream Cheese Artichoke Mix	150
Caramelized Shallot Steaks	150
Carrot And Potato Soup	151
Macedonian Greens And Cheese Pie	151
Chicken Stuffed Peppers	152
Turkey Fritters And Sauce	153
Garlic Clove Roasted Chicken	153
Chickpeas, Spinach And Arugula Bowl	153
Tuna Sandwiches	154
Cream Cheese Tart	155
Cherry Tomato Caper Chicken	155
Shrimp Pancakes	156
Herbed Chicken Stew	156
Spiced Seared Scallops With Lemon Relish	157
White Bean Soup	157
Coriander Pork And Chickpeas Stew	157
Crispy Pollock And Gazpacho	158
Falafel	158
Prosciutto Balls	159
Chicken Skillet	160
Salmon Bowls	160
Cod and Mushrooms Mix	161
Salmon Panatela	161
Blackened Fish Tacos with Slaw	162
Red Cabbage Tilapia Taco Bowl	162
Sicilian-Style Zoodle Spaghetti	162
Sour Cream Salmon with Parmesan	163
Vegetable Buckwheat Pasta	163
Pan-Seared Salmon Salad with Snow Peas & Grapefruit	164
Cleansing Vegetable Broth	164
Barbecued Spiced Tuna with Avocado-Mango Salsa	165
Low Carb Berry Salad with Citrus Dressing	166
Tasty Lime Cilantro Cauliflower Rice	166
Citrus Chicken with Delicious Cold Soup	166
Pan-Fried Chicken with Oregano-Orange Chimichurri & Arugula Salad	167
Cauliflower Couscous Salad	167
Ultimate Liver Detox Soup	168
Brown Rice and Grilled Chicken Salad	168
Superfood Liver Cleansing Soup	169

Toxin Flush & Detox Salad 169

Grilled Chicken Salad.................................170

Chicken Stir Fry with Red Onions & Cabbage 170

Green Salad w/ Herbs................................171

Chilled Green Goddess Soup 171

Chicken Avocado Wrap 172

Broccoli and Brown Rice Pasta Shells with Garlic 172

Chicken with Potatoes Olives & Sprouts ..173

Garlic Mushroom Chicken..........................173

Grilled Chicken 174

Roasted Tomato And Chicken Pasta 174

Oat Risotto With Mushrooms, Kale, And Chicken 175

Turkey with Leeks and Radishes 175

Easy Mozzarella & Pesto Chicken Casserole 176

Chapter 7: Dinner Recipes 177

Chicken And Butter Sauce..........................177

Turkey And Cranberry Sauce 177

Coriander And Coconut Chicken 177

Chicken Pilaf 178

Chicken And Black Beans..........................178

Coconut Chicken.......................................179

Ginger Chicken Drumsticks 179

Parmesan Chicken 180

Pomegranate Chicken 180

Chicken With Artichokes And Beans 180

Chicken Pie 181

Chicken And Semolina Meatballs..............181

Lemon Chicken Mix...................................182

Turkey And Chickpeas 182

Cardamom Chicken And Apricot Sauce....182

Chicken And Artichokes 183

Buttery Chicken Spread 183

Chicken And Spinach Cakes 184

Cream Cheese Chicken 184

Chicken And Lemongrass Sauce...............185

Spiced Chicken Meatballs 185

Paprika Chicken Wings 185

Chicken And Parsley Sauce 186

Sage Turkey Mix..186

Chipotle Turkey And Tomatoes 187

Curry Chicken, Artichokes And Olives......187

Roasted Chicken.......................................188

Rosemary Cauliflower Rolls 188

Delicious Lemon Chicken Salad 189

Healthy Chicken Orzo 189

Lemon Garlic Chicken...............................190

Steamed Chicken with Mushroom and Ginger 190

Chicken Breast & Zucchini Linguine.........191

Detox Salad with Grilled White Fish 191

Chicken & Veggies with Toasted Walnuts 192

Lemon-Pepper Tuna Bake 192

Chicken Meatballs with Stir-Fried Greens 193

Sesame Chicken with Black Rice, Broccoli & Snap Peas 193

Clean Eating Lemon Grilled Tuna & Avocado Vegetable Salad 194

Lemon & Garlic Barbecued Ocean Trout with Green Salad 194

Gingery Lemon Roasted Chicken with Steamed Greens......................................195

Grilled Chicken with Rainbow Salad Bowl 195

Pepper Chicken and Lettuce Wraps..........196

Chicken Lettuce Wraps.............................196

Pan-Seared Tuna with Crunchy Cabbage Slaw & Toasted 196

Macadamias 196

Brazilian Inspired Shrimp Stew 197

Pan-Seared Tuna Salad with Snow Peas & Grapefruit 197

Chicken Cacciatore 198
Fennel Wild Rice Risotto................199
Wild Rice Prawn Salad 199
Fragrant Asian Hotpot...................199
Chicken Fry with Peanut Sauce 200
Stewed Chicken Greek Style 201
Hot Pork Meatballs 201
Beef And Zucchini Skillet 202
Greek Chicken Stew 202
Meatloaf 203
Tasty Lamb Ribs 203
Peas And Ham Thick Soup 204
Bell Peppers On Chicken Breasts...........204
Yummy Turkey Meatballs...................205
Garlic Caper Beef Roast...................205
Olive Oil Drenched Lemon Chicken 206
Beef Spread...................206
Pork Chops And Relish 207
Tasty Beef Goulash 207
Beef And Grape Sauce...................208
Lamb And Tomato Sauce...................208
Shrimp Fried 'Rice' 209
Toasted Sardines with Parsley...................209
Tuscan Bean Stew 210
Vegetable Lover's Chicken Soup 210
Lemony Lamb And Potatoes 211
Cumin Lamb Mix 211
Almond Lamb Chops...................211
Pork And Figs Mix 212
Lamb Chops 212
Chicken Quinoa Pilaf 212
Greek Styled Lamb Chops 213
Bulgur And Chicken Skillet 213
Kibbeh With Yogurt 214
Mustard Chops With Apricot-basil Relish 215
Pork And Peas 215

Paprika And Feta Cheese On Chicken Skillet 216
Jalapeno Beef Chili...................216
Kibbeh In A Pan...................217
Saffron Beef 218
Cayenne Pork 218
Basil And Shrimp Quinoa...................218
Kefta Burgers 219
Beef Dish 219
Tasty Beef Stew 220
Pork And Sage Couscous 220
Chicken Burgers With Brussel Sprouts Slaw 221
Sautéed Cabbage...................221
Sautéed Cauliflower Delight 221
Simple Sautéed Spinach 222

Chapter 8: Drinks Recipes and Smoothie Recipes *223*
Clean Liver Green Juice 223
Green Tea Purifying Smoothie 223
PP cleansing smoothie 223
Blue Breeze shake 223
Coconut breezy shake dose 224
Triple C shake...................224
Buttery banana shake 224
Fats burning & water based smoothies ...225
Grapefruit smoothie with cinnamon........225
BB Citric Blast smoothie 225
Lemon and garlic smoothie 225
Smoothie with ginger and cucumber 226
Oatmeal blast with fruit...................226
White bean smoothie to burn fats 226
Meal replacement smoothie with banana 226
Coconut cherry smoothie...................227
Grapes and peach smoothie 227
Twin berry smoothie...................227
Light fiber smoothie 228

Creamy milk smoothie as meal replacement 228
Melon and nuts smoothie..................228
Peach and kiwi smoothie 228
Carrot drink.......................................229
Watermelon drink 229
Muskmelon juice 229
Beetroot & parsley smoothie.............229
Ginger melon juice 230
Papaya juice......................................230
Red capsicum juice 230
Blueberry smoothie 230
Cashew boost smoothie 231
Heavy metal cleansing smoothie 231
Power detox smoothie.......................231
Detox action super green smoothie..........231
Kale batch detox smoothie 232
Smoothie with a spirit 232
Alkaline green bliss smoothie 232
Soothing smoothie for stomach 232
Smooth root green cleansing smoothie....233
Glory smoothie 233
Smoothie for detoxification 233
Strawberry nutty smoothie 233
Berries Almond shake.......................234
Fresh Ginger Lemonade 234
Citrus Mocktail 234
Tropical Green Tea 235
Pumpkin Vanilla Cappuccino 235
Iced Coffee..236
Old Spice Ginger Tea........................236
Pumpkin Ginger Latte 236
Ginger Citrus Liver Detox Drink......237
Ginger, Pineapple & Kale Detox Juice.......237
Beet Citrus Cleanser 237
Super Detox Green Juice...................238

Refreshing Carrot Detoxifier 238
Super Cleanser Juice 239
Ginger, Pineapple & Cabbage Detoxifier..239
Chilled Toxin Flush Detox Drink 239
Liver Detox Juice 240
Ginger Radish Zinger 240
Ginger Pineapple Drink....................241
Detoxifying Turmeric Tea.................241
Lemon Ginger Detox Juice................242
Ginger Pineapple Detox Drink 242
Chilled Ginger Citrus Drink 242
Healthy Vacation Peach Drink.........243
Easy Pumpkin Spice Latte 243
Pineapple, Watermelon Smoothie ...244
Ginger Honey Lemonade..................244
Perfect "Shamrock" Shake 244
Green Pumpkin Spice Smoothie.......245
Summer OatBerry Smoothie............245
Sweet Berry Banana Yogurt Smoothie.....245
Banana Apple Smoothie 245
Eastertide Nectarine Smoothie 246
Ginger Citrus Liver Detox Drink......246
Beet Citrus Cleanser 246
Super Detox Green Juice..................247
Super Green Detox Juice..................247
Ginger, Apple & Kale Detox Juice ...247
Refreshing Carrot Detoxifier 247
Super Cleanser Juice 248
Ginger, Apple & Cabbage Detoxifier 248
Ultimate Toxin Flush Shot................248
Detoxifying Vegetable Juice 249
Hot Golden Elixir..............................249
Ultimate Liver Detox Juice 249
Charcoal Black Lemonade................249
Magical Liver Elixir 250
Chilled Toxin Flush Detox Drink 250

Liver Detox Juice 250
Ginger Radish Zinger 251
Ginger Apple Drink 251
Detoxifying Turmeric Tea 251
Lemon Ginger Detox Juice 251
Ginger Apple Detox Drink 252
Chilled Ginger Citrus Drink 252
Simple Lemon Herb Chicken 252
Grilled Lemon Chicken 253

Chapter 9: Salad Recipes and soups 254

Pumpkin Cream Soup 254
Zucchini Noodles Soup 254
Chicken Oatmeal Soup 255
Celery Cream Soup 255
Cauliflower Soup 256
Buckwheat Soup 256
Spring Greens Salad 256
Tuna Salad 257
Fish Salad 257
Grilled Tomatoes Soup 258
Salmon Salad 258
Arugula Salad with Shallot 259
Watercress Salad 259
Pumpkin Cream Soup 259
Zucchini Noodles Soup 260
Grilled Tomatoes Soup 260
Sliced Mushrooms Salad 261
Tender Green Beans Salad 261
Crispy Fennel Salad 262
Red Beet Feta Salad 262
Cheesy Potato Mash 262
Provencal Summer Salad 263
Sunflower Seeds And Arugula Garden Salad 263
Ginger Pumpkin Mash 263
Yogurt Peppers Mix 264

Lemony Carrots 264
Roasted Vegetable Salad 264
Chicken Kale Soup 265
Mozzarella Pasta Mix 265
Quinoa Salad 266
Couscous And Toasted Almonds 266
Spanish Tomato Salad 266
Chickpeas And Beets Mix 267
Roasted Bell Pepper Salad With Anchovy Dressing 267
Warm Shrimp And Arugula Salad 267
Cheesy Tomato Salad 268
Garlic Cucumber Mix 268
Cucumber Salad Japanese Style 268
Cheesy Keto Zucchini Soup 269
Grilled Salmon Summer Salad 269
Dill Beets Salad 270
Green Couscous With Broad Beans, Pistachio, And Dill 270
Bell Peppers Salad 270
Thyme Corn And Cheese Mix 271
Garden Salad With Oranges And Olives ... 271
Smoked Salmon Lentil Salad 272
Salmon & Arugula Salad 272
Keto Bbq Chicken Pizza Soup 272
Mediterranean Garden Salad 273
Buttery Millet 274
Delicata Squash Soup 274
Parsley Couscous And Cherries Salad 274
Mint Quinoa 275
Spicy Halibut Tomato Soup 275
Chicken salad 276
Farro salad 276
Carrot salad 276
Beets Steamed Edamame Salad 277
Avocado Cilantro Chunky Salsa 277
Potatoes Mixed Vegetables 277

- Toasted Mango Pepitas Kale Salad 278
- Chickpea And Parsley Pumpkin Salad......279
- White Bean Cherry Tomatoes Cucumber Salad 279
- Arugula Cucumber Tuna Salad..................279
- Springtime Chicken Berries Salad 280
- Toaster Almond Spiralized Beet Salad.....280
- Apple Leeks Mascarpone Soup..................281
- Aminos Mushroom Soup 281
- Detox-Liver Arugula And Broccoli Soup ..282
- Unique Lentil with KaleSoup 282
- Pasta Veggies Minestrone Soup 283
- Pear Red Pepper Soup 283
- Low Heat Chicken Provençal 284
- Danny's Tortellini Soup..............................284
- Wellness Parsnip Soup 284
- Feel Good Chicken Soup 285
- Pork Soup..285
- Curry Soup 286
- Yellow Onion Soup 286
- Garlic Soup 287

Chapter 10: Desserts 288
- Coconut Rhubarb Cream 288
- Honey-Cinnamon Grilled Plums...............288
- Raspberry Walnut Sorbet 288
- Chocolate Almond Pudding 289
- Figs with Honey-Chocolate Sauce 289
- Lemon Ricotta Peaches 290
- Rhubarb Compote 290
- Vanilla Pumpkin Pudding 290
- Chocolate Truffles 291
- Grilled Pineapple Strips 291
- Chocolate Chip Banana Muffin Top Cookies 292
- Lemon Cookies 292
- Peanut Butter Chocolate Chip Blondies ...293
- Ginger Snaps...293
- Strawberries and Cream Cheese Crepes ..294
- Apple & Berry Cobbler 294
- Cream Cheese Cake 295
- Nutmeg Lemon Pudding............................296
- Yogurt Panna Cotta With Fresh Berries ...296
- Flourless Chocolate Cake 296
- Strawberry And Avocado Medley 297
- Creamy Mint Strawberry Mix 297
- Creamy Pie 297
- Watermelon Ice Cream...............................298
- Hazelnut Pudding.......................................298
- Cheesecakes..299
- Melon Cucumber Smoothie.......................299
- Fruit Medley...300
- White Wine Grapefruit Poached Peaches 300
- Cinnamon Stuffed Peaches........................300
- Eggless Farina Cake (namoura) 301
- Mixed Berry Sorbet.....................................301
- Almonds And Oats Pudding 302
- Banana And Berries Trifle 302
- Chocolate Rice 303
- Lemon And Semolina Cookies 303
- Strawberry Sorbet 304
- Halva (halawa) 304
- Semolina Cake 304
- Shredded Phyllo And Sweet Cheese Pie (knafe)..305
- Lemon Pear Compote 305
- Cinnamon Pear Jam 306
- Apple And Walnut Salad...........................306
- Banana Kale Smoothie................................306
- Phyllo Custard Pockets (shaabiyat)..........307
- Chocolate Baklava.......................................307
- Apricot Rosemary Muffins 308
- Blueberry Yogurt Mousse 308

Pistachio Cheesecake 309

Almond Citrus Muffins 309

Mediterranean Bread Pudding (aish El Saraya) 310

Cinnamon Apple Rice Pudding 310

Custard-filled Pancakes (atayef) 311

Pomegranate Granita With Lychee 311

Lime Grapes And Apples 312

Mediterranean Baked Apples 312

Honey Cream 312

Dragon Fruit, Pear, And Spinach Salad 313

Kataifi 313

Walnuts Kataifi 314

Cinnamon Tea 314

Biscotti 315

Tiny Orange Cardamom Cookies 315

Mixed Fruit Bowl 316

Spinach & Fruit Treat 316

Cherry Ice Cream 316

Bean & Walnut Mousse 317

Egg Custard 318

Apple Crisp 318

Peach Crumble 319

Black Bean Brownies 319

Chickpeas Almond Fudge 320

Mixed Dried Fruit Oatmeal Cookies 320

Cinnamon Sugar Apple Cake 321

Peanut Butter Oatmeal Chocolate Chip Cookies 321

Peach Crumble Muffins 322

Cinnamon Baked Apples with Walnuts 323

Conclusion *324*

Introduction

Fatty liver can disturb the primary capacity of the liver, which is to eliminate poisons from your body. The liver is the second biggest organ, and it channels the blood and utilizes drugs and different synthetic substances. Nonetheless, abundance liquor utilization and ailments like diabetes type 2, insulin opposition, hereditary sickness, and an inactive way of life can keep the body from processing the glucose appropriately. Thusly, overabundance glucose can be put away in the liver as fat.

If you have already been diagnosed with fatty liver or not, now is the best time to take stock of your health. Start avoiding salty foods, opt for fresh produce whenever possible, workout more often and eliminate alcohol or at least cut back on your alcohol consumption. If you stop putting undue stress on your liver now you may prevent acquiring fatty liver in the future. If you already have fatty liver, follow the suggestions shared in this book to improve and heal your liver.

This Book contains a curated list of what we believe to be the best recipes to reduce fatty liver which cover a variety of cooking methods, flavors, and tastes. All different categories of foods are represented such as your beef, pork, pasta, chicken, fish bacon, shrimp , and among others.

Chapter 1: Understanding your liver

Your liver is the only organ in your body that can completely regenerate and heal itself over time. In fact, because of this miraculous ability, the liver is also the only organ that can be partially transplanted from a living donor – and then both the donor and recipients liver will regrow to full size.

That's not all though, even if up to 75% of your liver were removed, the miraculous organ would regrow to be fully functional in just 10 days.

That's a good thing too, because while you can get dialysis for damaged kidneys or a pacemaker to correct the beating of your heart. There is still no widespread mechanical or technological support options for liver function.

Your liver is an amazing, miraculous, and hard-working organ, but the more you know about how it works, where it is, and what it does, the better you understand how to keep it healthy.

Locating Your Liver

Your liver is actually the largest internal organ in your body. It is about the size of a football, and it sits mostly in the upper right quadrant of your abdomen – between the diaphragm and the stomach.

Your liver is made up of two lobes, each of which are divided into eight segments. These segments are made up of thousands of small lobules, and all of those are connected by a vast network of ducts. All of those ducts are interconnected to form the common hepatic duct, which is the channel that transports bile out of the liver once it has finished its work of cleaning up toxins from your blood.

The liver also receives and transports blood by several major blood vessels, including the hepatic portal vein and the hepatic arteries.

Much of the liver's almost magical abilities is because of the incredibly unique type of cells it is made of. These cells, known as hepatocytes, make up about 80% of the liver by mass. They are the cells that synthesize and store proteins, transform carbohydrates for storage, detoxify, excrete and modify substances in the blood, and create cholesterol, bile, and other chemicals and compounds our bodies need to function.

Since your liver does so many things for you, we thought that an excellent place to start would be to look at some of the more important functions this remarkable organ performs.

Liver Functions

Located at the top right quadrant of the body, the liver is responsible for a wide array of functions, including but not limited to the following:

- The liver produces bile which in turn is responsible for the breakdown of fat as well as the removal of waste as it moves through the small intestine.
- It helps with the production of proteins that move fat throughout the body, allowing for the distribution of energy.
- It acts as a strainer, managing to get rid of drugs, alcohol, and other harmful materials from the body
- It manages to regulate clotting of the blood as well as store glucose and release them if the body needs the energy.
- It manages to collect ammonia that harms the body and essentially excrete it through the urine.
- It manages to help the immune system by removing bacteria from the system
- It helps prevent jaundice or the yellowing of the eyes and teeth, usually from accumulated bilirubin.
- It also produces proteins associated with blood plasma and stores iron.

Simply put, the liver helps the kidney make sure that your body removes all harmful chemicals even as it makes use of vitamins and minerals to keep all vital organs healthy and thriving.

Without a properly functioning liver, your kidney would not be able to handle all the strain and it would essentially shut down, leading to inevitable death.

Chapter 2: Fatty liver disease

There are a variety of illnesses that can affect the liver, including, but not limited to:

Liver failure

When you have liver failure, it means that your liver has lost most, if not all, of its liver function a serious condition that requires emergency medical attention. The first symptoms you are going to notice are diarrhea, extreme nausea, fatigue and a loss of appetite. Because these symptoms are common to many other ailments that your body could be suffering from, it can be really difficult to know that your liver is actually failing.

However as liver failure becomes more and more advanced, the symptoms continue advancing too and the patient may start getting very disoriented and confused and unusually sleepy. If unattended to, there is a very high risk of coma or in the worst-case scenario, death. Doctors will try to save any part of the liver that is still working and if this is impossible the other option will be a transplant.

In an event of a liver failure due to cirrhosis, it means that the patient's liver has been gradually getting sicker and failing over time, possibly for a number of years and is referred to as chronic liver failure or End Stage Liver Disease. Although very rare, liver failure could also be caused by malnutrition. Acute liver failure is when liver failure is very sudden, occurring in as little as two days and is usually cause by a medication overdose or a severe case of poisoning.

Liver Cancer

Cancer that originates in the liver is referred to as primary liver cancer. Hepatitis B and cirrhosis are the two leading risk factors of primary liver cancer. However, it is important to note that cancer in the liver can progress at any stage of liver disease and that's why regular routine checkups are very important as they make it possible to catch cancer, if any, at a very early stage that's removable before it progresses to the entire liver.

Alcoholic Liver Disease (ALD)

If you are a heavy drinker or have been drinking alcohol excessively, this is the first stage of injury to your liver due to buildup of fatty deposits. If proper care is taken and you stay away from alcohol, this can be completely reversed. As per the studies, only 20% of people with alcohol related fatty liver go on to develop inflammation (alcoholic hepatitis) and eventually cirrhosis.

People who have been drinking alcohol excessively and has alcoholic liver damage have been found most of the times malnourished or undernourished which means their body lacks in nutrients that it requires to function properly. This lack of nourishment could be due to several factors, some common ones are:

If you are not eating well and just drinking, you are asking your body to work hard to process alcohol. Alcohol has no nutritional value but requires a lot of energy for the body to process it.

Poor or un-balanced diet.

Loss of appetite due to heavy drinking. If you are drinking as well as smoking, the condition will become worse. Smoking is known for suppressing hunger.

Poor absorption of food nutrients as the liver is less able to produce bile to aid digestion.

You could be under nourished even if you are overweight. It all depends on what and how you eat. If you eat well and still becoming overweight, get yourself checked, if not already. This condition could be due to fluid retention.

You should be prescribed Vitamins B if you have been drinking excessively or at harmful levels. People with alcoholic liver disease generally lack the vitamin called thiamin, which is a vitamin B that helps the body to convert carbohydrates into energy. Consult your doctor or dietitian if this has not been prescribed.

Acute Viral Hepatitis:

People who have an acute hepatitis, also known as short-term hepatitis, caused by a virus like hepatitis, should continue to eat a normal diet. In some cases, it is found that patients lose some weight in this condition. In a situation like this a patient may need extra nutrition to prevent unplanned weight loss. A high energy and high protein diet are recommended for such patients. A dietitian can advise on this.

N.A.F.L.D - Non-Alcoholic Fatty Liver Disease

As the name suggests, non-alcoholic fatty liver disease is a condition when there is a fat buildup in the liver cells even if the patient does not drink alcohol excessively. At the initial stages, the fat deposits may not trigger any symptoms, but it has been found that in some cases, this may progress to inflammation called Nonalcoholic Steatohepatitis (NASH) which further can lead to scarring of the tissues in the liver and even cirrhosis.

People may still develop a fatty liver without excessive consumption of alcohol. There could be several factor or reasons of developing a fatty liver. Your likelihood of developing fatty liver conditions is higher if:

- Have diabetes.
- Are obese or overweight
- An insulin resistance body where your body does not respond to insulin as it should.
- Have high blood cholesterol.

You may be advised to make some changes to your diet and lifestyle, if you have been diagnosed with non-alcoholic fatty liver disease. These diet and lifestyle changes include:

- Eating a lot of vegetables and fruits.
- Eating slow-release starchy foods, such as potatoes and bread.
- Doing regular exercise such as walking, jogging or swimming.
- Reduce or stop the consumption of alcohol.
- Avoiding refined sugars and saturated fats which are commonly found in chocolate, cakes and biscuits.

It is also recommended to maintain a healthy weight for your age and build. If you have diabetes, it is suggested to work with your doctor to keep your blood sugar levels under good control. Consult your doctor if you have issues with high blood cholesterol levels or if you are insulin resistant.

Chronic Viral Hepatitis

If you suffer from a long term hepatitis infection caused by a virus such as hepatitis B or hepatitis C and lasts for more than six to seven months, the condition is called a Chronic Viral Hepatitis. In such a condition, it is recommended to eat a normal well-balanced diet. Fasting due to any reasons is not recommended at all if you have chronic liver disease.

It is highly recommended to maintain an appropriate weight as per your height and build because it has been found in studies that more weight can increase and speed up the damages caused by hepatitis C and can slow down the recovery.

Some studies show that some people have conditions like poor appetite, nausea, vomiting and unintentional loss of weight during the treatment with anti-viral agents. If all or any of these conditions lasts for more than a few days, you must consult a doctor immediately.

Autoimmune Hepatitis

Autoimmune hepatitis is also categorized as a chronic liver disease. It involves liver damage and inflammation due to an attack on the normal components and cells by the immune system. In a condition like this, sometimes, patients are prescribed steroids. In some cases, patients prescribed steroids find that their appetite increases over time and they gradually start gaining weight.

If you are suffering from autoimmune hepatitis and on steroids and have symptoms like increase in appetite and weight gain, it is still important and recommended to eat a well-balanced diet. If you are on steroids for a long time, it is important that you have been prescribed vitamin D and calcium by your doctor.

If, however, you start gaining more weight and it does not seem to slow down, you should try to reduce foods high in calories such as:

- Sugar
- Cakes
- Fried food
- Pies and crisps
- Biscuits
- Chocolate
- Sweets
- Pasties

It is also recommended that you use low fat milk and spreads and eat more fruit and vegetables. If it still increases, you must consult your doctor or dietician immediately.

Chapter 3: How Fatty Liver Develop

The days when fatty liver disease was attributed solely to high alcohol consumption are long gone. Alcoholic fatty liver is caused by the breakdown product acetaldehyde. The human body gets along well with this substance in smaller quantities and breaks it down again within several hours. If you regularly add large amounts of alcohol to the body, liver tissue will break down over time, as the acetaldehyde cannot be broken down quickly enough by the liver. At the same time, there is a lack of oxygen, which influences the fat metabolism in such a way that small droplets of fat are stored in the liver. If the small droplets flow together to form larger units, they impair the function of the liver cells and the entire metabolism is disturbed.

In the case of non-alcoholic fatty liver, fat droplets also form in the liver, but these cannot be attributed to the degradation substance acetaldehyde. The exact causes are not yet known. However, a combination of various possible underlying diseases, an unfavorable diet and obesity are suspected, which lead to a metabolic disorder. Insulin resistance is relatedparticularly closely to the development of fatty liver. This is considered a preliminary stage of diabetes and ensures that the body's cells are insensitive to the hormone insulin. This leads to an increased release of free fatty acids, which are not sufficiently broken down by the body and then transported to the liver. As a result, droplets of fat also form in the liver, which from a certain degree, can restrict the function of the liver cells and thereby burden the liver.

Note: Insulin resistance not only favors fatty liver, but fatty liver also the development of insulin resistance and diabetes. The liver cells make fat, they produce certain proteins, which in turn limit the effectiveness of the body's own insulin. However,the good news here is as soon as the fat deposits in the liver recede, in most cases the insulin resistance improves at the same time.

If you have been diagnosed with fatty liver, you are not alone. Today, this type of fatty liver is the most common cause of liver disease.

Possible risk factors

In addition to insulin resistance, the following causes, among others, are also considered risk factors for the development of fatty liver:

- Diabetes mellitus
- Lipid metabolism disorders
- Obesity
- Malnutrition (especially insufficient intake of protein)
- high sugar consumption
- increased belly fat
- Sedentary lifestyle
- Autoimmune diseases
- certain drugs and pollutants
- Genetic factors
- high age

Some doctors today speak of non-alcoholic fatty liver disease as a general metabolic disorder, which in many cases is associated with several diseases such as diabetes, increased obesity or high cholesterol levels. The consequence is not only a restriction in liver function and an increased risk of developing liver inflammation and liver cancer but above all cardiovascular diseases such as high blood pressure, heart attack or stroke. However, especially at the beginning of the diagnosis and a low degree of fatty liver disease, these consequences rarely occur and you can still do a lot to alleviate or even cure the fatty liver by changing your lifestyle.

Symptoms and diagnosis of fatty liver

Most people with fatty liver disease have either no symptoms at all or very specific digestive problems. Overall, the main symptoms of fatty liver include:

- Sensation of pressure in the right upper abdomen
- Bloating
- Reduction in performance
- Difficulty concentrating

Only at an advanced stage does nausea, vomiting and actual pain occur in the liver area in the right upper abdomen. If the liver function is already significantly restricted, the eyes and skin can also turn yellow.

If you suffer from one or more of these complaints, we recommend a visit to your family doctor. They will first ask you about your symptoms and perform an initial physical examination. Enlargement of the liver can already be detected when palpating, but can have other causes besides fatty liver. For this reason, a laboratory diagnostic determination of the liver values in the blood is usually carried out afterwards. Here it can occasionally happen that the liver values are in the normal range and yet there is a functional impairment of the organ or vice versa. For this reason, your family doctor will make an appointment for an ultrasound with you afterwards. Here it can be seen quite well whether and to what extent the fat storage in the liver has already progressed. As soon as the stored fats make up more than five percent of the weight of the liver, it is called a fatty liver (the weight of a healthy liver is between 1500 and 2000 grams in an adult). In some cases with severe symptoms or unclear findings, your doctor will refer you to a specialist who will take a small sample of the liver in order to determine the condition of the liver cells more precisely.

Chapter 4: Breakfast Recipes

Raspberry Pudding

Preparation time: 10 minutes

Cooking time: 30 minutes

Servings: 2

Ingredients:

½ cup raspberries

2 teaspoons maple syrup

1 ½ cup Plain yogurt

¼ teaspoon ground cardamom

1/3 cup Chia seeds, dried

Directions:

Mix up together Plain yogurt with maple syrup and ground cardamom.

Add Chia seeds. Stir it gently.

Put the yogurt in the serving glasses and top with the raspberries.

Refrigerate the breakfast for at least 30 minutes or overnight.

Nutrition: calories 303, fat 11.2, fiber 11.8, carbs 33.2, protein 15.5

Walnuts Yogurt Mix

Preparation time: 10 minutes

Cooking time: 0 minutes

Servings: 6

Ingredients:

2 and ½ cups Greek yogurt

1 and ½ cups walnuts, chopped

1 teaspoon vanilla extract

¾ cup honey

2 teaspoons cinnamon powder

Directions:

In a bowl, combine the yogurt with the walnuts and the rest of the ingredients, toss, divide into smaller bowls and keep in the fridge for 10 minutes before serving for breakfast.

Nutrition: calories 388, fat 24.6, fiber 2.9, carbs 39.1, protein 10.2

Mediterranean Egg-feta Scramble

Preparation time: 10 minutes

Cooking time: 20 minutes

Servings: 4

Ingredients:

6 eggs

3/4 cup crumbled feta cheese

2 tablespoons green onions, minced

2 tablespoons red peppers, roasted, diced

1/4 teaspoon kosher salt

1/4 teaspoon garlic powder

1/4 cup Greek yogurt

1/2 teaspoon dry oregano

1/2 teaspoon dry basil

1 teaspoon olive oil

A few cracks freshly ground black pepper

Warm whole-wheat tortillas, optional

Directions:

Preheat a skillet over medium heat.

In a bowl, whisk the eggs, the sour cream, basil, oregano, garlic powder, salt, and pepper. Gently add the feta.

When the skillet is hot, add the olive oil and then the egg mixture; allow the egg mix to set then scrape the bottom of the pan to let the uncooked egg to cook. Stir in the red peppers and the green onions. Continue cooking until the eggs mixture is cooked to your preferred doneness. Serve immediately.

If desired, sprinkle with extra feta and then wrap the scrambled eggs in tortillas.

Nutrition: :260 Cal, 16 g total fat (8 g sat. fat), 350 mg chol., 750 mg sodium, 190 mg pot., 12 g carb.,>1 g fiber, 2 g sugar, 16 g protein.

Spiced Chickpeas Bowls

Preparation time: 10 minutes

Cooking time: 30 minutes

Servings: 4

Ingredients:

15 ounces canned chickpeas, drained and rinsed

¼ teaspoon cardamom, ground

½ teaspoon cinnamon powder

1 and ½ teaspoons turmeric powder

1 teaspoon coriander, ground

1 tablespoon olive oil

A pinch of salt and black pepper

¾ cup Greek yogurt

½ cup green olives, pitted and halved

½ cup cherry tomatoes, halved

1 cucumber, sliced

Directions:

Spread the chickpeas on a lined baking sheet, add the cardamom, cinnamon, turmeric, coriander, the oil, salt and pepper, toss and bake at 375 degrees F for 30 minutes.

In a bowl, combine the roasted chickpeas with the rest of the ingredients, toss and serve for breakfast.

Nutrition: calories 519, fat 34.5, fiber 13.3, carbs 49.8, protein 12

Orzo And Veggie Bowls

Preparation time: 10 minutes

Cooking time: 0 minutes

Servings: 4

Ingredients:

2 and ½ cups whole-wheat orzo, cooked

14 ounces canned cannellini beans, drained and rinsed

1 yellow bell pepper, cubed

1 green bell pepper, cubed

A pinch of salt and black pepper

3 tomatoes, cubed

1 red onion, chopped

1 cup mint, chopped

2 cups feta cheese, crumbled

2 tablespoons olive oil

¼ cup lemon juice

1 tablespoon lemon zest, grated

1 cucumber, cubed

1 and ¼ cup kalamata olives, pitted and sliced

3 garlic cloves, minced

Directions:

In a salad bowl, combine the orzo with the beans, bell peppers and the rest of the ingredients, toss, divide the mix between plates and serve for breakfast.

Nutrition: calories 411, fat 17, fiber 13, carbs 51, protein 14

Vanilla Oats

Preparation time: 10 minutes

Cooking time: 10 minutes

Servings: 4

Ingredients:

½ cup rolled oats

1 cup milk

1 teaspoon vanilla extract

1 teaspoon ground cinnamon

2 teaspoon honey

2 tablespoons Plain yogurt

1 teaspoon butter

Directions:

Pour milk in the saucepan and bring it to boil.

Add rolled oats and stir well.

Close the lid and simmer the oats for 5 minutes over the medium heat. The cooked oats will absorb all milk.

Then add butter and stir the oats well.

In the separated bowl, whisk together Plain yogurt with honey, cinnamon, and vanilla extract.

Transfer the cooked oats in the serving bowls.

Top the oats with the yogurt mixture in the shape of the wheel.

Nutrition: calories 243, fat 20.2, fiber 1, carbs 2.8, protein 13.3

Mushroom-egg Casserole

Preparation time: 10 minutes

Cooking time: 30 minutes

Servings: 3

Ingredients:

½ cup mushrooms, chopped

½ yellow onion, diced

4 eggs, beaten

1 tablespoon coconut flakes

½ teaspoon chili pepper

1 oz Cheddar cheese, shredded

1 teaspoon canola oil

Directions:

Pour canola oil in the skillet and preheat well.

Add mushrooms and onion and roast for 5-8 minutes or until the vegetables are light brown.

Transfer the cooked vegetables in the casserole mold.

Add coconut flakes, chili pepper, and Cheddar cheese.

Then add eggs and stir well.

Bake the casserole for 15 minutes at 360F.

Nutrition: Calories 152, fat 11.1, fiber 0.7, carbs 3, protein 10.4

Bacon Veggies Combo

Preparation time: 10 minutes

Cooking time: 35 minutes

Servings: 4

Ingredients:

½ green bell pepper, seeded and chopped

2 bacon slices

¼ cup Parmesan Cheese

½ tablespoon mayonnaise

1 scallion, chopped

Directions:

Preheat the oven to 375 degrees F and grease a baking dish.

Place bacon slices on the baking dish and top with mayonnaise, bell peppers, scallions and Parmesan Cheese.

Transfer in the oven and bake for about 25 minutes.

Dish out to serve immediately or refrigerate for about 2 days wrapped in a plastic sheet for meal preparation ping.

Nutrition: Calories: 197 Fat: 13.8g Carbohydrates: 4.7g Protein: 14.3g Sugar: 1.9g Sodium: 662mg

Brown Rice Salad

Preparation time: 10 minutes

Cooking time: 0 minutes

Servings: 4

Ingredients:

9 ounces brown rice, cooked

7 cups baby arugula

15 ounces canned garbanzo beans, drained and rinsed

4 ounces feta cheese, crumbled

¾ cup basil, chopped

A pinch of salt and black pepper

2 tablespoons lemon juice

¼ teaspoon lemon zest, grated

¼ cup olive oil

Directions:

In a salad bowl, combine the brown rice with the arugula, the beans and the rest of the ingredients, toss and serve cold for breakfast.

Nutrition: calories 473, fat 22, fiber 7, carbs 53, protein 13

Olive And Milk Bread

Preparation time: 10 minutes

Cooking time: 50 minutes

Servings: 6

Ingredients:

1 cup black olives, pitted, chopped

1 tablespoon olive oil

½ teaspoon fresh yeast

½ cup milk, preheated

½ teaspoon salt

1 teaspoon baking powder

2 cup wheat flour, whole grain

2 eggs, beaten

1 teaspoon butter, melted

1 teaspoon sugar

Directions:

In the big bowl combine together fresh yeast, sugar, and milk. Stir it until yeast is dissolved.

Then add salt, baking powder, butter, and eggs. Stir the dough mixture until homogenous and add 1 cup of wheat flour. Mix it up until smooth.

Add olives and remaining flour. Knead the non-sticky dough.

Transfer the dough into the non-sticky dough mold.

Bake the bread for 50 minutes at 350 F.

Check if the bread is cooked with the help of the toothpick. Is it is dry, the bread is cooked.

Remove the bread from the oven and let it chill for 10-15 minutes.

Remove it from the loaf mold and slice.

Nutrition: :calories 238, fat 7.7, fiber 1.9, carbs 35.5, protein 7.2

Breakfast Tostadas

Preparation time: 10 minutes

Cooking time: 30 minutes

Servings: 6

Ingredients:

½ white onion, diced

1 tomato, chopped

1 cucumber, chopped

1 tablespoon fresh cilantro, chopped

½ jalapeno pepper, chopped

1 tablespoon lime juice

6 corn tortillas

1 tablespoon canola oil

2 oz Cheddar cheese, shredded

½ cup white beans, canned, drained

6 eggs

½ teaspoon butter

½ teaspoon Sea salt

Directions:

Make Pico de Galo: in the salad bowl combine together diced white onion, tomato, cucumber, fresh cilantro, and jalapeno pepper.

Then add lime juice and a ½ tablespoon of canola oil. Mix up the mixture well. Pico de Galo is cooked.

After this, preheat the oven to 390F.

Line the tray with baking paper.

Arrange the corn tortillas on the baking paper and brush with remaining canola oil from both sides.

Bake the tortillas for 10 minutes or until they start to be crunchy.

Chill the cooked crunchy tortillas well.

Meanwhile, toss the butter in the skillet.

Crack the eggs in the melted butter and sprinkle them with sea salt.

Fry the eggs until the egg whites become white (cooked). Approximately for 3-5 minutes over the medium heat.

After this, mash the beans until you get puree texture.

Spread the bean puree on the corn tortillas.

Add fried eggs.

Then top the eggs with Pico de Galo and shredded Cheddar cheese.

Nutrition: Calories 246, fat 11.1, fiber 4.7, carbs 24.5, protein 13.7

Chicken Souvlaki

Preparation time: 10 minutes

Cooking time: 2 minutes

Servings: 4

Ingredients:

4 pieces (6-inch) pitas, cut into halves

2 cups roasted chicken breast skinless, boneless, and sliced

1/4 cup red onion, thinly sliced

1/2 teaspoon dried oregano

1/2 cup Greek yogurt, plain

1/2 cup plum tomato, chopped

1/2 cup cucumber, peeled, chopped

1/2 cup (2 ounces) feta cheese, crumbled

1 tablespoon olive oil, extra-virgin, divided

1 tablespoon fresh dill, chopped

1 cup iceberg lettuce, shredded

1 1/4 teaspoons minced garlic, bottled, divided

Directions:

In a small mixing bowl, combine the yogurt, cheese, 1 teaspoon of the olive oil, and 1/4 teaspoon of the garlic until well mixed.

In a large skillet, heat the remaining olive oil over medium-high heat. Add the remaining 1 teaspoon garlic and the oregano; sauté for 20 seconds.

Add the chicken; cook for about 2 minutes or until the chicken are heated through.

Put 1/4 cup chicken into each pita halves. Top with 2 tablespoons yogurt mix, 2 tablespoons lettuce,1 tablespoon tomato, and 1 tablespoon cucumber. Divide the onion between the pita halves.

Nutrition: :414 Cal, 13.7 g total fat (6.4 g sat. fat, 1.4 g poly. Fat, 4.7 g mono), 81 mg chol., 595 mg sodium, 38 g carb.,2 g fiber, 32.3 g protein.

Tahini Pine Nuts Toast

Preparation time: 10 minutes

Cooking time: 0 minutes

Servings: 4

Ingredients:

2 whole wheat bread slices, toasted

1 teaspoon water

1 tablespoon tahini paste

2 teaspoons feta cheese, crumbled

Juice of ½ lemon

2 teaspoons pine nuts

A pinch of black pepper

Directions:

In a bowl, mix the tahini with the water and the lemon juice, whisk really well and spread over the toasted bread slices.

Top each serving with the remaining ingredients and serve for breakfast.

Nutrition: calories 142, fat 7.6, fiber 2.7, carbs 13.7, protein 5.8

Eggs And Veggies

Preparation time: 10 minutes

Cooking time: 10 minutes

Servings: 4

Ingredients:

2 tomatoes, chopped

2 eggs, beaten

1 bell pepper, chopped

1 teaspoon tomato paste

¼ cup of water

1 teaspoon butter

½ white onion, diced

½ teaspoon chili flakes

1/3 teaspoon sea salt

Directions:

Put butter in the pan and melt it.

Add bell pepper and cook it for 3 minutes over the medium heat. Stir it from time to time.

After this, add diced onion and cook it for 2 minutes more.

Stir the vegetables and add tomatoes.

Cook them for 5 minutes over the medium-low heat.

Then add water and tomato paste. Stir well.

Add beaten eggs, chili flakes, and sea salt.

Stir well and cook menemen for 4 minutes over the medium-low heat.

The cooked meal should be half runny.

Nutrition: :calories 67, fat 3.4, fiber 1.5, carbs 6.4, protein 3.8

Chili Scramble

Preparation time: 10 minutes

Cooking time: 13 minutes

Servings: 4

Ingredients:

3 tomatoes

4 eggs

¼ teaspoon of sea salt

½ chili pepper, chopped

1 tablespoon butter

1 cup water, for cooking

Directions:

Pour water in the saucepan and bring it to boil.

Then remove water from the heat and add tomatoes.

Let the tomatoes stay in the hot water for 2-3 minutes.

After this, remove the tomatoes from water and peel them.

Place butter in the pan and melt it.

Add chopped chili pepper and fry it for 3 minutes over the medium heat.

Then chop the peeled tomatoes and add into the chili peppers.

Cook the vegetables for 5 minutes over the medium heat. Stir them from time to time.

After this, add sea salt and crack then eggs.

Stir (scramble) the eggs well with the help of the fork and cook them for 3 minutes over the medium heat.

Nutrition: :calories 105, fat 7.4, fiber 1.1, carbs 4, protein 6.4

Pear Oatmeal

Preparation time: 10 minutes

Cooking time: 20 minutes

Servings: 4

Ingredients:

1 cup oatmeal

1/3 cup milk

1 pear, chopped

1 teaspoon vanilla extract

1 tablespoon Splenda

1 teaspoon butter

½ teaspoon ground cinnamon

1 egg, beaten

Directions:

In the big bowl mix up together oatmeal, milk, egg, vanilla extract, Splenda, and ground cinnamon.

Melt butter and add it in the oatmeal mixture.

Then add chopped pear and stir it well.

Transfer the oatmeal mixture in the casserole mold and flatten gently. Cover it with the foil and secure edges.

Bake the oatmeal for 25 minutes at 350F.

Nutrition: :calories 151, fat 3.9, fiber 3.3, carbs 23.6, protein 4.9

Olive Frittata

Preparation time: 10 minutes

Cooking time: 15 minutes

Servings: 5

Ingredients:

9 large eggs, lightly beaten

8 kalamata olives, pitted, chopped

1/4 cup olive oil

1/3 cup parmesan cheese, freshly grated

1/3 cup fresh basil, thinly sliced

1/2 teaspoon salt

1/2 teaspoon pepper

1/2 cup onion, chopped

1 sweet red pepper, diced

1 medium zucchini, cut to 1/2-inch cubes

1 package (4 ounce) feta cheese, crumbled

Directions:

In a 10-inch oven-proof skillet, heat the olive oil until hot. Add the olives, zucchini, red pepper, and the onions, constantly stirring, until the vegetables are tender.

Ina bowl, mix the eggs, feta cheese, basil, salt, and pepper; pour in the skillet with vegetables. Adjust heat to medium-low, cover, and cook for about 10-12 minutes, or until the egg mixture is almost set.

Remove from the heat and sprinkle with the parmesan cheese. Transfer to the broiler.

With oven door partially open, broil 5 1/2 from the source of heat for about 2-3 minutes or until the top is golden. Cut into wedges.

Nutrition: :288.5 Cal, 22.8 g total fat (7.8 g sat. fat), 301 mg chol., 656 mg sodium, 5.6 g carb.,1.2 g fiber,3.3g sugar, 15.2 g protein.

Mediterranean Egg Casserole

Preparation time: 10 minutes

Cooking time: 50 minutes

Servings: 4

Ingredients:

1 1/2 cups (6 ounces) feta cheese, crumbled

1 jar (6 ounces) marinated artichoke hearts, drained well, coarsely chopped

10 eggs

2 cups milk, low-fat

2 cups fresh baby spinach, packed, coarsely chopped

6 cups whole-wheat baguette, cut into 1-inch cubes

1 tablespoon garlic (about 4 cloves), finely chopped

1 tablespoon olive oil, extra-virgin

1/2 cup red bell pepper, chopped

1/2 cup Parmesan cheese, shredded

1/2 teaspoon pepper

1/2 teaspoon red pepper flakes

1/2 teaspoon salt

1/3 cup kalamata olives, pitted, halved

1/4 cup red onion, chopped

1/4 cup tomatoes (sun-dried) in oil, drained, chopped

Directions:

Preheat oven to 350F.

Grease a 9x13-inch baking dish with olive oil cooking spray.

In an 8-inch non-stick pan over medium heat, heat the olive oil. Add the onions, garlic, and bell pepper; cook for about 3 minutes, frequently stirring, until slightly softened. Add the spinach; cook for about 1 minute or until starting to wilt.

Layer half of the baguette cubes in the preparation ared baking dish, then 1 cup of the eta, 1/4 cup Parmesan, the bell pepper mix, artichokes, the olives, and the tomatoes. Top with the remaining baguette cubes and then with the remaining 1/2 cup of feta.

In a large mixing bowl, whisk the eggs and the low-fat milk together. Beat in the pepper, salt and the pepper. Pour the mix over the bread layer in the baking dish, slightly pressing down. Sprinkle with the remaining 1/4 cup Parmesan.

Bake for about 40-45 minutes, or until the center is set and the top is golden brown. Before serving, let stand for 15 minutes.

Nutrition: :360 Cal, 21 g total fat (9 g sat. fat), 270 mg chol., 880 mg sodium, 24 g carb.,3 g fiber,7 g sugar, 20 g protein.

Milk Scones

Preparation time: 10 minutes

Cooking time: 10 minutes

Servings: 4

Ingredients:

½ cup wheat flour, whole grain

1 teaspoon baking powder

1 tablespoon butter, melted

1 teaspoon vanilla extract

1 egg, beaten

¾ teaspoon salt

3 tablespoons milk

1 teaspoon vanilla sugar

Directions:

In the mixing bowl combine together wheat flour, baking powder, butter, vanilla extract, and egg. Add salt and knead the soft and non-sticky dough. Add more flour if needed.

Then make the log from the dough and cut it into the triangles.

Line the tray with baking paper.

Arrange the dough triangles on the baking paper and transfer in the preheat to the 360F oven.

Cook the scones for 10 minutes or until they are light brown.

After this, chill the scones and brush with milk and sprinkle with vanilla sugar.

Nutrition:calories 112, fat 4.4, fiber 0.5, carbs 14.3, protein 3.4

Herbed Eggs And Mushroom Mix

Preparation time: 10 minutes

Cooking time: 20 minutes

Servings: 4

Ingredients:

1 red onion, chopped

1 bell pepper, chopped

1 tablespoon tomato paste

1/3 cup water

½ teaspoon of sea salt

1 tablespoon butter

1 cup cremini mushrooms, chopped

1 tablespoon fresh parsley

1 tablespoon fresh dill

1 teaspoon dried thyme

½ teaspoon dried oregano

½ teaspoon paprika

½ teaspoon chili flakes

½ teaspoon garlic powder

4 eggs

Directions:

Toss butter in the pan and melt it.

Then add chopped mushrooms and bell pepper.

Roast the vegetables for 5 minutes over the medium heat.

After this, add red onion and stir well.

Sprinkle the ingredients with garlic powder, chili flakes, dried oregano, and dried thyme. Mix up well

After this, add tomato paste and water.

Mix up the mixture until it is homogenous.

Then add fresh parsley and dill.

Cook the mixture for 5 minutes over the medium-high heat with the closed lid.

After this, stir the mixture with the help of the spatula well.

Crack the eggs over the mixture and close the lid.

Cook shakshuka for 10 minutes over the low heat.

Nutrition: :calories 123, fat 7.5, fiber 1.7, carbs 7.8, protein 7.

Cherry Berry Bulgur Bowl

Preparation Time: 15 minutes

Cooking Time: 15 minutes

Servings: 4

Ingredients:

1 cup medium-grind bulgur

2 cups water

Pinch salt

1 cup halved and pitted cherries or 1 cup canned cherries, drained

½ cup raspberries

½ cup blackberries

1 tablespoon cherry jam

2 cups plain whole-milk yogurt

Directions:

Mix the bulgur, water, and salt in a medium saucepan. Do this in a medium heat. Bring to a boil.

Reduce the heat to low and simmer, partially covered, for 12 to 15 minutes or until the bulgur is almost tender. Cover, and let stand for 5 minutes to finish cooking do this after removing the pan from the heat.

While the bulgur is cooking, combine the raspberries and blackberries in a medium bowl. Stir the cherry jam into the fruit.

When the bulgur is tender, divide among four bowls. Top each bowl with ½ cup of yogurt and an equal amount of the berry mixture and serve.

Nutrition:

Calories: 242;

Total fat: 6g;

Saturated fat: 3g;

Sodium: 85mg;

Phosphorus: 237mg;

Potassium: 438mg;

Carbohydrates: 44g;

Fiber: 7g;

Protein: 9g;

Sugar: 13g

Baked Curried Apple Oatmeal Cups

Preparation Time: 10 minutes

Cooking Time: 20 minutes

Servings: 6

Ingredients:

3½ cups old-fashioned oats

3 tablespoons brown sugar

2 teaspoons of your preferred curry powder

⅛ teaspoon salt

1 cup unsweetened almond milk

1 cup unsweetened applesauce

1 teaspoon vanilla

½ cup chopped walnuts

Directions:

Preheat the oven to 375°F. Then spray a 12-cup muffin tin with baking spray then set aside.

Combine the oats, brown sugar, curry powder, and salt, and mix in a medium bowl.

Mix together the milk, applesauce, and vanilla in a small bowl,

Stir the liquid ingredients into the dry ingredients and mix until just combined. Stir in the walnuts.

Using a scant ⅓ cup for each divide the mixture among the muffin cups.

Bake this for 18 to 20 minutes until the oatmeal is firm. Serve.

Nutrition: calories 243, fat 20.2, fiber 1, carbs 2.8, protein 13.3

Pineapple, Macha & Beet Chia Pudding

Preparation time: 10 minutes

Cooking time: 0 minutes

Servings: 4

Ingredients:

1 cup chia seeds

1 teaspoon raw honey

2 cups almond milk

1 teaspoon matcha green tea powder

2 tablespoons fresh beetroot juice

1 whole pineapple

1 cup freshly squeezed lemon juice

1 knob of fresh ginger

Toasted almonds and figs to serve

Directions:

Green Chia pudding layer:

Add another half each of chia seeds, raw honey, almond milk, and matcha green tea powder to the blender and until very smooth; transfer to a bowl.

Beetroot layer: blend together beetroot and ginger with the remaining chia seeds, raw honey, vanilla, and coconut milk until very smooth; transfer to a separate bowl. In a food processor, puree the fresh pineapple until fine.

To assemble, layer the chia pudding in the bottom of serving glasses, followed by the pureed pineapple and then the beetroot layer. Top with figs and toasted almonds for a crunchy finish.

Coconut & Strawberry Smoothie Bowl

Preparation time: 10 minutes

Cooking time: 0 minutes

Servings: 4

Ingredients:

2 cups fresh strawberries

2 cups fresh spinach

1 cup coconut water

1 ripe banana

2 tablespoons raw pumpkin seeds

2 tablespoons chia seeds

½ cup coconut flakes, toasted

Directions:

In a blender, blend together almond milk, banana, and spinach until very smooth and creamy; add in strawberries and pulse to combine well.

Divide the smooth among serving bowls and top each serving with fresh strawberries, pumpkin seeds, chia seeds and toasted coconut flakes.

Enjoy!

Farro Salad

Preparation time: 10 minutes

Cooking time: 4 minutes

Servings: 2

Ingredients:

1 tablespoon olive oil

A pinch of salt and black pepper

1 bunch baby spinach, chopped

1 avocado, pitted, peeled and chopped

1 garlic clove, minced

2 cups farro, already cooked

½ cup cherry tomatoes, cubed

Directions:

Heat up a pan with the oil over medium heat, add the spinach, and the rest of the ingredients, toss, cook for 4 minutes, divide into bowls and serve.

Nutrition: calories 157, fat 13.7, fiber 5.5, carbs 8.6, protein 3.6

Chili Avocado Scramble

Preparation time: 10 minutes

Cooking time: 10 minutes

Servings: 4

Ingredients:

4 eggs, beaten

1 white onion, diced

1 tablespoon avocado oil

1 avocado, finely chopped

½ teaspoon chili flakes

1 oz Cheddar cheese, shredded

½ teaspoon salt

1 tablespoon fresh parsley

Directions:

Pour avocado oil in the skillet and bring it to boil.

Then add diced onion and roast it until it is light brown.

Meanwhile, mix up together chili flakes, beaten eggs, and salt.

Pour the egg mixture over the cooked onion and cook the mixture for 1 minute over the medium heat.

After this, scramble the eggs well with the help of the fork or spatula. Cook the eggs until they are solid but soft.

After this, add chopped avocado and shredded cheese.

Stir the scramble well and transfer in the serving plates.

Sprinkle the meal with fresh parsley.

Nutrition: :calories 236, fat 20.1, fiber 4, carbs 7.4, protein 8.6

Tapioca Pudding

Preparation time: 10 minutes

Cooking time: 15 minutes

Servings: 3

Ingredients:

¼ cup pearl tapioca

¼ cup maple syrup

2 cups almond milk

½ cup coconut flesh, shredded

1 and ½ teaspoon lemon juice

Directions:

In a pan, combine the milk with the tapioca and the rest of the ingredients, bring to a simmer over medium heat, and cook for 15 minutes.

Divide the mix into bowls, cool it down and serve for breakfast.

Nutrition: calories 361, fat 28.5, fiber 2.7, carbs 28.3, protein 2.8

Feta And Eggs Mix

Preparation time: 10 minutes

Cooking time: 5 minutes

Servings: 4

Ingredients:

4 eggs, beaten

½ teaspoon ground black pepper

2 oz Feta, scrambled

½ teaspoon salt

1 teaspoon butter

1 teaspoon fresh parsley, chopped

Directions:

Melt butter in the skillet and add beaten eggs.

Then add parsley, salt, and scrambled eggs. Cook the eggs for 1 minute over the high heat.

Add ground black pepper and scramble eggs with the help of the fork.

Cook the eggs for 3 minutes over the medium-high heat.

Nutrition: :calories 110, fat 8.4, fiber 0.1, carbs 1.1, protein 7.6

Banana pancakes

Preparation time: 10 minutes

Cooking time: 20 minutes

Servings: 4

Ingredients

1 cup whole wheat flour

¼ tsp baking soda

¼ tsp baking powder

1 cup mashed banana

2 eggs

1 cup milk

Directions

In a bowl combine all ingredients together and mix well

In a skillet heat olive oil

Pour ¼ of the batter and cook each pancake for 1-2 minutes per side

When ready remove from heat and serve

Nutrition:7g carbs 14g fat 15g protein 210 Calories

Nectarine pancakes

Preparation time: 10 minutes

Cooking time: 30 minutes

Servings: 4

Ingredients

1 cup whole wheat flour

¼ tsp baking soda

¼ tsp baking powder

1 cup nectarines

2 eggs

1 cup milk

Directions

In a bowl combine all ingredients together and mix well

In a skillet heat olive oil

Pour ¼ of the batter and cook each pancake for 1-2 minutes per side

When ready remove from heat and serve

Nutrition:7g carbs 14g fat 15g protein 210 Calories

Pancakes

Preparation time: 10 minutes

Cooking time: 30 minutes

Servings: 4

Ingredients

1 cup whole wheat flour

¼ tsp baking soda

¼ tsp baking powder

2 eggs

1 cup milk

Directions

In a bowl combine all ingredients together and mix well

In a skillet heat olive oil

Pour ¼ of the batter and cook each pancake for 1-2 minutes per side

When ready remove from heat and serve

Nutrition:2g carbs 6g fat 10g protein 100 Calories

Peaches muffins

Preparation time: 10 minutes

Cooking time: 30 minutes

Servings: 4

Ingredients

2 eggs

1 tablespoon olive oil

1 cup milk

2 cups whole wheat flour

1 tsp baking soda

¼ tsp baking soda

1 cup peaches

1 tsp cinnamon

¼ cup molasses

Directions

In a bowl combine all wet ingredients

In another bowl combine all dry ingredients

Combine wet and dry ingredients together

Pour mixture into 8-12 preparation ared muffin cups, fill 2/3 of the cups

Bake for 18-20 minutes at 375 F, when ready remove and serve

Nutrition:2g carbs 6g fat 10g protein 100 Calories

Lemon muffins

Preparation time: 10 minutes

Cooking time: 30 minutes

Servings: 4

Ingredients

2 eggs

1 tablespoon olive oil

1 cup milk

2 cups whole wheat flour

1 tsp baking soda

¼ tsp baking soda

1 tsp cinnamon

1 cup lemon slices

Directions

In a bowl combine all wet ingredients

In another bowl combine all dry ingredients

Combine wet and dry ingredients together

Pour mixture into 8-12 preparation ared muffin cups, fill 2/3 of the cups

Bake for 18-20 minutes at 375 F

When ready remove from the oven and serve

Nutrition:2g carbs 6g fat 10g protein 100 Calories

Blueberry muffins

Preparation time: 10 minutes

Cooking time: 30 minutes

Servings: 4

Ingredients

2 eggs

1 tablespoon olive oil

1 cup milk

2 cups whole wheat flour

1 tsp baking soda

¼ tsp baking soda

1 tsp cinnamon

1 cup blueberries

Directions

In a bowl combine all wet ingredients

In another bowl combine all dry ingredients

Combine wet and dry ingredients together

Fold in blueberries and mix well

Pour mixture into 8-12 preparation ared muffin cups, fill 2/3 of the cups

Bake for 18-20 minutes at 375 F, when ready remove and serve

Nutrition:2g carbs 6g fat 10g protein 100 Calories

Kumquat muffins

Preparation time: 10 minutes

Cooking time: 30 minutes

Servings: 4

Ingredients

2 eggs

1 tablespoon olive oil

1 cup milk

2 cups whole wheat flour

1 tsp baking soda

¼ tsp baking soda

1 tsp cinnamon

1 cup kumquat

Directions

In a bowl combine all wet ingredients

In another bowl combine all dry ingredients

Combine wet and dry ingredients together

Pour mixture into 8-12 preparation ared muffin cups, fill 2/3 of the cups

Bake for 18-20 minutes at 375 F

When ready remove from the oven and serve

Nutrition:2g carbs 6g fat 10g protein 100 Calories

Chocolate muffins

Preparation time: 10 minutes

Cooking time: 30 minutes

Servings: 7

Ingredients

2 eggs

1 tablespoon olive oil

1 cup milk

2 cups whole wheat flour

1 tsp baking soda

¼ tsp baking soda

1 tsp cinnamon

1 cup chocolate chips

Directions

In a bowl combine all dry ingredients

In another bowl combine all dry ingredients

Combine wet and dry ingredients together

Fold in chocolate chips and mix well

Pour mixture into 8-12 preparation ared muffin cups, fill 2/3 of the cups

Bake for 18-20 minutes at 375 F, when ready remove and serve

Nutrition:2g carbs 6g fat 10g protein 100 Calories

Muffins

Preparation time: 10 minutes

Cooking time: 20 minutes

Servings: 4

Ingredients

2 eggs

1 tablespoon olive oil

1 cup milk

2 cups whole wheat flour

1 tsp baking soda

¼ tsp baking soda

1 tsp cinnamon

Directions

In a bowl combine all wet ingredients

In another bowl combine all dry ingredients

Combine wet and dry ingredients together

Pour mixture into 8-12 preparation ared muffin cups, fill 2/3 of the cups

Bake for 18-20 minutes at 375 F

When ready remove from the oven and serve

Nutrition: 2g carbs 6g fat 10g protein 100 Calories

Omelette

Preparation time: 10 minutes

Cooking time: 15 minutes

Servings: 4

Ingredients

2 eggs

¼ tsp salt

¼ tsp black pepper

1 tablespoon olive oil

¼ cup cheese

¼ tsp basil

Directions

In a bowl combine all ingredients together and mix well

In a skillet heat olive oil and pour the egg mixture

Cook for 1-2 minutes per side

When ready remove omelette from the skillet and serve

Nutrition: 2g carbs 6g fat 10g protein 100 Calories

Carrot omelette

Preparation time: 10 minutes

Cooking time: 20 minutes

Servings: 4

Ingredients

2 eggs

¼ tsp salt

¼ tsp black pepper

1 tablespoon olive oil

¼ cup cheese

¼ tsp basil

1 cup carrot

Directions

In a bowl combine all ingredients together and mix well

In a skillet heat olive oil and pour the egg mixture

Cook for 1-2 minutes per side

When ready remove omelette from the skillet and serve

Nutrition: 50g carbs 11g fat 10g protein 320 Calories

Onion omelette

Preparation time: 10 minutes

Cooking time: 10 minutes

Servings: 1

Ingredients

2 eggs

¼ tsp salt

¼ tsp black pepper

1 tablespoon olive oil

¼ cup cheese

¼ tsp basil

1 cup red onion

Directions

In a bowl combine all ingredients together and mix well

In a skillet heat olive oil and pour the egg mixture

Cook for 1-2 minutes per side

When ready remove omelette from the skillet and serve

Nutrition:50g carbs 11g fat 10g protein 320 Calories

Broccoli omelette

Preparation time: 10 minutes

Cooking time: 10 minutes

Servings: 1

Ingredients

2 eggs

¼ tsp salt

¼ tsp black pepper

1 tablespoon olive oil

¼ cup cheese

¼ tsp basil

1 cup broccoli

Directions

In a bowl combine all ingredients together and mix well

In a skillet heat olive oil and pour the egg mixture

Cook for 1-2 minutes per side

When ready remove omelette from the skillet and serve

Nutrition:50g carbs 11g fat 10g protein 320 Calories

Beets omelette

Preparation time: 10 minutes

Cooking time: 10 minutes

Servings: 1

Ingredients

2 eggs

¼ tsp salt

¼ tsp black pepper

1 tablespoon olive oil

¼ cup cheese

¼ tsp basil

1 cup beets

Directions

In a bowl combine all ingredients together and mix well

In a skillet heat olive oil and pour the egg mixture

Cook for 1-2 minutes per side

When ready remove omelette from the skillet and serve

Nutrition:50g carbs 11g fat 10g protein 320 Calories

Breakfast Beans (ful Mudammas)

Preparation time: 10 minutes

Cooking time: 10 minutes

Servings: 1

Ingredients:

1 (15-oz.) can chickpeas, rinsed and drained

1 (15-oz.) can fava beans, rinsed and drained

1 cup water

1 TB. minced garlic

1 tsp. salt

1/2 cup fresh lemon juice

1/2 tsp. cayenne

1/2 cup fresh parsley, chopped

1 large tomato, diced

3 medium radishes, sliced

1/4 cup extra-virgin olive oil

Directions:

In a 2-quart pot over medium-low heat, combine chickpeas, fava beans, and water. Simmer for 10 minutes.

Pour bean mixture into a large bowl, and add garlic, salt, and lemon juice. Stir and smash half of beans with the back of a wooden spoon.

Sprinkle cayenne over beans, and evenly distribute parsley, tomatoes, and radishes over top. Drizzle with extra-virgin olive oil, and serve warm or at room temperature.

Nutrition: 35g carbs 30g fat 20g protein 460 Calories

Seeds And Lentils Oats

Preparation time: 10 minutes

Cooking time: 50 minutes

Servings: 4

Ingredients:

½ cup red lentils

¼ cup pumpkin seeds, toasted

2 teaspoons olive oil

¼ cup rolled oats

¼ cup coconut flesh, shredded

1 tablespoon honey

1 tablespoon orange zest, grated

1 cup Greek yogurt

1 cup blackberries

Directions:

Spread the lentils on a baking sheet lined with parchment paper, introduce in the oven and roast at 370 degrees F for 30 minutes.

Add the rest of the ingredients except the yogurt and the berries, toss and bake at 370 degrees F for 20 minutes more.

Transfer this to a bowl, add the rest of the ingredients, toss, divide into smaller bowls and serve for breakfast.

Nutrition: calories 204, fat 7.1, fiber 10.4, carbs 27.6, protein 9.5

Couscous With Artichokes, Sun-dried Tomatoes And Feta

Preparation time: 10 minutes

Cooking time: 20 minutes

Servings: 46

Ingredients:

3 cups chicken breast, cooked, chopped

2 1/3 cups water, divided

2 jars (6-ounces each) marinated artichoke hearts, undrained

1/4 teaspoon black pepper, freshly ground

1/2 cup tomatoes, sun-dried

1/2 cup (2 ounces) feta cheese, crumbled

1 cup flat-leaf parsley, fresh, chopped

1 3/4 cups whole-wheat Israeli couscous, uncooked

1 can (14 1/2 ounces) vegetable broth

Directions:

In a microwavable bowl, combine 2 cups of the water and the tomatoes. Microwave on HIGH for about 3 minutes or until the water boils. When water is boiling, remove from the microwave, cover, and let stand for about 3 minutes or until the tomatoes are soft; drain, chop, and set aside.

In a large saucepan, place the vegetable broth and the remaining 1/3 cup of water; bring to boil. Stir in the couscous, cover, reduce heat, and simmer for about 8 minutes or until tender. Remove the pan from the heat; add the tomatoes and the remaining ingredients. Stir to combine.

Nutrition: :419 Cal, 14.1 g total fat (3.9 g sat. fat, 0.8 g poly. Fat, 1.4 g mono), 64 mg chol.,677 mg sodium, 42.5 g carb.,2.6 g fiber, 30.2 g protein.

Cinnamon Roll Oats

Preparation time: 10 minutes

Cooking time: 10 minutes

Servings: 4

Ingredients:

½ cup rolled oats

1 cup milk

1 teaspoon vanilla extract

1 teaspoon ground cinnamon

2 teaspoon honey

2 tablespoons Plain yogurt

1 teaspoon butter

Directions:

Pour milk in the saucepan and bring it to boil.

Add rolled oats and stir well.

Close the lid and simmer the oats for 5 minutes over the medium heat. The cooked oats will absorb all milk.

Then add butter and stir the oats well.

In the separated bowl, whisk together Plain yogurt with honey, cinnamon, and vanilla extract.

Transfer the cooked oats in the serving bowls.

Top the oats with the yogurt mixture in the shape of the wheel.

Nutrition: Calories 243, fat 20.2, fiber 1, carbs 2.8, protein 13.3

Spinach Wrap

Preparation time: 10 minutes

Cooking time: 10 minutes

Servings: 4

Ingredients:

4 pieces (10-inch) spinach wraps (or whole wheat tortilla or sun-dried tomato wraps)

1 pound chicken tenders

1 cup cucumber, chopped

3 tablespoons extra-virgin olive oil

1 medium tomato, chopped

1/3 cup couscous, whole-wheat

2 teaspoons garlic, minced

1/4 teaspoon salt, divided

1/4 teaspoon freshly ground pepper

1/4 cup lemon juice

1/2 cup water

1/2 cup fresh mint, chopped

1 cup fresh parsley, chopped

Directions:

In a small saucepan, pour the water and bring to a boil. Stir in the couscous, remove pan from heat, cover, and allow to stand for 5 minutes, then fluff using a fork; set aside.

Meanwhile, in a small mixing bowl, combine the mint, parsley, oil, lemon juice, garlic, 1/8 teaspoon of the salt, and the pepper.

In a medium mixing bowl, toss the chicken with the 1 tablespoon of the mint mixture and the remaining 1/8 teaspoon of salt.

Place the chicken mixture into a large non-stick skillet; cook for about 3-5 minutes each side, or until heated through. Remove from the skillet, allow to cool enough to handle, and cut into bite-sized pieces.

Stir the remaining mint mixture, the cucumber, and the tomato into the couscous.

Spread about 3/4 cup of the couscous mix onto each wrap and divide the chicken between the wraps, roll like a burrito, tucking the sides in to hold to secure the ingredients in. Cut in halves and serve.

Nutrition: :479 Cal, 17 g total fat (3 g sat. fat, 11 g mono), 67 mg chol., 653 mg sodium, 382 pot., 49 g carb.,5 g fiber, 15 g protein.

Chicken Liver

Preparation time: 10 minutes

Cooking time: 10 minutes

Servings: 4

Ingredients:

2 lb. chicken liver

3 TB. extra-virgin olive oil

3 TB. minced garlic

1 tsp. salt

1/2 tsp. ground black pepper

1 cup fresh cilantro, finely chopped

1/4 cup fresh lemon juice

Directions:

Cut chicken livers in half, rinse well, and pat dry with paper towels.

Preheat a large skillet over medium heat. Add extra-virgin olive oil and garlic, and cook for 2 minutes.

Add chicken liver and salt, and cook, tossing gently, for 5 minutes. Remove the skillet from heat, and spoon liver onto a plate.

Add black pepper, cilantro, and lemon juice. Lightly toss, and serve warm.

Nutrition:35g carbs 30g fat 20g protein 460 Calories

Avocado Spread

Preparation time: 10 minutes

Cooking time: 0 minutes

Servings: 8

Ingredients:

2 avocados, peeled, pitted and roughly chopped

1 tablespoon sun-dried tomatoes, chopped

2 tablespoons lemon juice

3 tablespoons cherry tomatoes, chopped

¼ cup red onion, chopped

1 teaspoon oregano, dried

2 tablespoons parsley, chopped

4 kalamata olives, pitted and chopped

A pinch of salt and black pepper

Directions:

Put the avocados in a bowl and mash with a fork.

Add the rest of the ingredients, stir to combine and serve as a morning spread.

Nutrition: calories 110, fat 10, fiber 3.8, carbs 5.7, protein 1.2

Eggplant rollatini

Preparation time: 10 minutes

Cooking time: 25 minutes

Servings: 4

Ingredients

1 eggplant

12 oz. ricotta cheese

2 oz. mozzarella cheese

1 can tomatoes

¼ tsp salt

2 tablespoons seasoning

Directions

Lay the eggplant on a baking sheet

Roast at 350 F for 12-15 minutes

In a bowl combine mozzarella, seasoning, tomatoes, ricotta cheese and salt

Add cheese mixture to the eggplant and roll

Place the rolls into a baking dish and bake for another 10-12 minutes

When ready remove from the oven and serve

Nutrition:35g carbs 30g fat 20g protein 460 Calories

Asparagus with egg

Preparation time: 10 minutes

Cooking time: 20 minutes

Servings: 4

Ingredients

1 lb. asparagus

4-5 pieces prosciutto

¼ tsp salt

2 eggs

Directions

Trim the asparagus and season with salt

Wrap each asparagus pieces with prosciutto

Place the wrapped asparagus in a baking dish

Bake at 375 F for 22-25 minutes

When ready remove from the oven and serve

Nutrition:35g carbs 30g fat 20g protein 460 Calories

Deviled eggs

Preparation time: 10 minutes

Cooking time: 20 minutes

Servings: 8

Ingredients

8 eggs

½ cup Greek Yogurt

1 tablespoon mustard

1 tsp smoked paprika

1 tablespoon green onions

Directions

In a saucepan add the eggs and bring to a boil

Cover and boil for 10-15 minutes

When ready slice the eggs in half and remove the yolks

In a bowl combine remaining ingredients and mix well

Spoon 1 tablespoon of the mixture into each egg

Garnish with green onions and serve

Nutrition:35g carbs 30g fat 20g protein 460 Calories

Spicy cucumbers

Preparation time: 10 minutes

Cooking time: 20 minutes

Servings: 7

Ingredients

2 cucumbers

1 cup Greek yogurt

1 garlic clove

1 tsp paprika

1 tsp dill

1 tsp chili powder

Directions

In a bowl combine all ingredients together except cucumbers

Cut the cucumbers into rounds and scoot out the inside

Fill each cucumber with the spicy mixture

When ready sprinkle paprika and serve

Nutrition:3g carbs 10g fat 12g protein 165 Calories

Red Pepper And Artichoke Frittata

Preparation time: 10 minutes

Cooking time: 15 minutes

Servings: 2

Ingredients:

4 large eggs

1 can (14-ounce) artichoke hearts, rinsed, coarsely chopped

1 medium red bell pepper, diced

1 teaspoon dried oregano

1/4 cup Parmesan cheese, freshly grated

1/4 teaspoon red pepper, crushed

1/4 teaspoon salt, or to taste

2 garlic cloves, minced

2 teaspoons extra-virgin olive oil, divided

Freshly ground pepper, to taste

Directions:

In a 10-inch non-stick skillet, heat 1 teaspoon of the olive oil over medium heat. Add the bell pepper; cook for about 2 minutes or until tender. Add the garlic and the red pepper; cook for about 30 seconds, stirring. Transfer the mixture to a plate and wipe the skillet clean.

In a medium mixing bowl, whisk the eggs. Stir in the artichokes, cheese, the bell pepper mixture, and season with salt and pepper.

Place an over rack 4 inches from the source of heat; preheat broiler.

Brush the skillet with the remaining 1 teaspoon olive oil and heat over medium heat. Pour the egg mixture into the skillet and tilt to evenly distribute. Reduce the heat to medium low; cook for about 3-4 minutes, lifting the edges to allow the uncooked egg to flow underneath, until the bottom of the frittata is light golden.

Transfer the pan into the broiler, cook for about 1 1/2-2 1/2 minutes, or until the top is set.

Slide into a platter; cut into wedges and serve.

Nutrition: :305 Cal, 18 g total fat (6 g sat. fat, 8 g mono), 432 mg chol., 734 mg sodium, 1639 mg pot., 18 g carb.,8 g fiber, 21 g protein.

Stuffed Figs

Preparation time: 10 minutes

Cooking time: 15 minutes

Servings: 2

Ingredients:

7 oz fresh figs

1 tablespoon cream cheese

½ teaspoon walnuts, chopped

4 bacon slices

¼ teaspoon paprika

¼ teaspoon salt

½ teaspoon canola oil

½ teaspoon honey

Directions:

Make the crosswise cuts in every fig.

In the shallow bowl mix up together cream cheese, walnuts, paprika, and salt.

Fill the figs with cream cheese mixture and wrap in the bacon.

Secure the fruits with toothpicks and sprinkle with honey.

Line the baking tray with baking paper.

Place the preparation ared figs in the tray and sprinkle them with olive oil gently.

Bake the figs for 15 minutes at 350F.

Nutrition: Calories 299, fat 19.4, fiber 2.3, carbs 16.7, protein 15.2

Keto Egg Fast Snickerdoodle Crepes

Preparation time: 10 minutes

Cooking time: 15 minutes

Servings: 2

Ingredients:

5 oz cream cheese, softened

6 eggs

1 teaspoon cinnamon

Butter, for frying

1 tablespoon Swerve

2 tablespoons granulated Swerve

8 tablespoons butter, softened

1 tablespoon cinnamon

Directions:

For the crepes: Put all the ingredients together in a blender except the butter and process until smooth.

Heat butter on medium heat in a non-stick pan and pour some batter in the pan.

Cook for about 2 minutes, then flip and cook for 2 more minutes.

Repeat with the remaining mixture.

Mix Swerve, butter and cinnamon in a small bowl until combined.

Spread this mixture onto the centre of the crepe and serve rolled up.

Nutrition: Calories: 543 Carbs: 8g Fats: 51.6g Proteins: 15.7g Sodium: 455mg Sugar: 0.9g

Cauliflower Hash Brown Breakfast Bowl

Preparation time: 10 minutes

Cooking time: 30 minutes

Servings: 2

Ingredients:

1 tablespoon lemon juice

1 egg

1 avocado

1 teaspoon garlic powder

2 tablespoons extra virgin olive oil

2 oz mushrooms, sliced

½ green onion, chopped

¼ cup salsa

¾ cup cauliflower rice

½ small handful baby spinach

Salt and black pepper, to taste

Directions:

Mash together avocado, lemon juice, garlic powder, salt and black pepper in a small bowl.

Whisk eggs, salt and black pepper in a bowl and keep aside.

Heat half of olive oil over medium heat in a skillet and add mushrooms.

Sauté for about 3 minutes and season with garlic powder, salt, and pepper.

Sauté for about 2 minutes and dish out in a bowl.

Add rest of the olive oil and add cauliflower, garlic powder, salt and pepper.

Sauté for about 5 minutes and dish out.

Return the mushrooms to the skillet and add green onions and baby spinach.

Sauté for about 30 seconds and add whisked eggs.

Sauté for about 1 minute and scoop on the sautéed cauliflower hash browns.

Top with salsa and mashed avocado and serve.

Nutrition: Calories: 400 Carbs: 15.8g Fats: 36.7g Proteins: 8g Sodium: 288mg Sugar: 4.2g

Pumpkin Coconut Oatmeal

Preparation time: 10 minutes

Cooking time: 13 minutes

Servings: 6

Ingredients:

2 cups oatmeal

1 cup of coconut milk

1 cup milk

1 teaspoon Pumpkin pie spices

2 tablespoons pumpkin puree

1 tablespoon Honey

½ teaspoon butter

Directions:

Pour coconut milk and milk in the saucepan. Add butter and bring the liquid to boil.

Add oatmeal, stir well with the help of a spoon and close the lid.

Simmer the oatmeal for 7 minutes over the medium heat.

Meanwhile, mix up together honey, pumpkin pie spices, and pumpkin puree.

When the oatmeal is cooked, add pumpkin puree mixture and stir well.

Transfer the cooked breakfast in the serving plates.

Nutrition: :calories 232, fat 12.5, fiber 3.8, carbs 26.2, protein 5.9

Bacon, Vegetable And Parmesan Combo

Preparation time: 10 minutes

Cooking time: 30 minutes

Servings: 2

Ingredients:

2 slices of bacon, thick-cut

½ tbsp mayonnaise

½ of medium green bell pepper, deseeded, chopped

1 scallion, chopped

¼ cup grated Parmesan cheese

1 tbsp olive oil

Directions:

Switch on the oven, then set its temperature to 375°F and let it preheat.

Meanwhile, take a baking dish, grease it with oil, and add slices of bacon in it.

Spread mayonnaise on top of the bacon, then top with bell peppers and scallions, sprinkle with Parmesan cheese and bake for about 25 minutes until cooked thoroughly.

When done, take out the baking dish and serve immediately.

For meal preparation ping, wrap bacon in a plastic sheet and refrigerate for up to 2 days.

When ready to eat, reheat bacon in the microwave and then serve.

Nutrition: Calories 197, Total Fat 13.8g, Total Carbs 4.7g, Protein 14.3g, Sugar 1.9g, Sodium 662mg

Toasted Crostini

Preparation time: 10 minutes

Cooking time: 15 minutes

Servings: 4

Ingredients:

12 slices (1/3-inch thick) whole-wheat baguette, toasted

Coarse salt and freshly ground pepper

For the spread:

1 can chickpeas (15 1/2 ounces), drained, rinsed

1/4 cup olive oil, extra-virgin

1 tablespoon lemon juice, freshly squeezed

1 small clove garlic, minced

2 tablespoons olive oil, extra-virgin, divided

2 tablespoons celery, finely diced, plus celery leaves for garnish

8 large green olives, pitted, cut into 1/8-inch slivers

Directions:

In a food processor, combine the spread ingredients and season with salt and pepper; set aside.

In a small mixing bowl, combine 1 tablespoon of olive oil and the remaining ingredients. Season with salt and pepper. Set aside.

Divide the spread between the toasted baguette slices, top with the relish. Drizzle the remaining1 tablespoon of olive oil over each and season with pepper. If desired, garnish with the celery leaves. Serve immediately.

Nutrition: :603 Cal, 3.7 g total fat (3.7 g sat. fat), 0 mg chol., 781 mg sodium, 483 mg pot, 79.2 g carb.,9.6 g fiber,6.8 g sugar, 19.1 g protein.

Heavenly Egg Bake With Blackberry

Preparation time: 10 minutes

Cooking time: 15 minutes

Servings: 4

Ingredients:

Chopped rosemary

1 tsp lime zest

½ tsp salt

¼ tsp vanilla extract, unsweetened

1 tsp grated ginger

3 tbsp coconut flour

1 tbsp unsalted butter

5 organic eggs

1 tbsp olive oil

½ cup fresh blackberries

Black pepper to taste

Directions:

Switch on the oven, then set its temperature to 350°F and let it preheat.

Meanwhile, place all the ingredients in a blender, reserving the berries and pulse for 2 to 3 minutes until well blended and smooth.

Take four silicon muffin cups, grease them with oil, evenly distribute the blended batter in the cups, top with black pepper and bake for 15 minutes until cooked through and the top has golden brown.

When done, let blueberry egg bake cool in the muffin cups for 5 minutes, then take them out, cool them on a wire rack and then serve.

For meal preparation ping, wrap each egg bake with aluminum foil and freeze for up to 3 days.

When ready to eat, reheat blueberry egg bake in the microwave and then serve.

Nutrition: Calories 144, Total Fat 10g, Total Carbs 2g, Protein 8.5g

Quick Cream Of Wheat

Preparation time: 10 minutes

Cooking time: 12 minutes

Servings: 1

Ingredients:

4 cups whole milk

1/2 cup farina

1/2 tsp. salt

3 TB. sugar

3 TB. butter

3 TB. pine nuts

Directions:

In a large saucepan over medium heat, bring whole milk to a simmer, and cook for about 4 minutes. Do not allow milk to scorch.

Whisk in farina, salt, and sugar, and bring to a slight boil. Cook for 2 minutes, reduce heat to low, and cook for 3 more minutes. Stay close to the pan to ensure it doesn't boil over.

Pour mixture into 4 bowls, and let cool for 5 minutes.

Meanwhile, in a small pan over low heat, cook butter and pine nuts for about 3 minutes or until pine nuts are lightly toasted.

Evenly spoon butter and pine nuts over each bowl, and serve warm.

Nutrition:3g carbs 10g fat 12g protein 165 Calories

Herbed Spinach Frittata

Preparation time: 10 minutes

Cooking time: 20 minutes

Servings: 4

Ingredients:

5 eggs, beaten

1 cup fresh spinach

2 oz Parmesan, grated

1/3 cup cherry tomatoes

½ teaspoon dried oregano

1 teaspoon dried thyme

1 teaspoon olive oil

Directions:

Chop the spinach into the tiny pieces and or use a blender.

Then combine together chopped spinach with eggs, dried oregano and thyme.

Add Parmesan and stir frittata mixture with the help of the fork.

Brush the springform pan with olive oil and pour the egg mixture inside.

Cut the cherry tomatoes into the halves and place them over the egg mixture.

Preheat the oven to 360F.

Bake the frittata for 20 minutes or until it is solid.

Chill the cooked breakfast till the room temperature and slice into the servings.

Nutrition: :calories 140, fat 9.8, fiber 0.5, carbs 2.1, protein 11.9

Ham Spinach Ballet

Preparation time: 10 minutes

Cooking time: 40 minutes

Servings: 4

Ingredients:

4 teaspoons cream

¾ pound fresh baby spinach

7-ounce ham, sliced

Salt and black pepper, to taste

1 tablespoon unsalted butter, melted

Directions:

Preheat the oven to 360 degrees F. and grease 2 ramekins with butter.

Put butter and spinach in a skillet and cook for about 3 minutes.

Add cooked spinach in the ramekins and top with ham slices, cream, salt and black pepper.

Bake for about 25 minutes and dish out to serve hot.

For meal preparation ping, you can refrigerate this ham spinach ballet for about 3 days wrapped in a foil.

Nutrition: Calories: 188 Fat: 12.5g Carbohydrates: 4.9g Protein: 14.6g Sugar: 0.3g Sodium: 1098mg

Banana Quinoa

Preparation time: 10 minutes

Cooking time: 12 minutes

Servings: 4

Ingredients:

1 cup quinoa

2 cup milk

1 teaspoon vanilla extract

1 teaspoon honey

2 bananas, sliced

¼ teaspoon ground cinnamon

Directions:

Pour milk in the saucepan and add quinoa.

Close the lid and cook it over the medium heat for 12 minutes or until quinoa will absorb all liquid.

Then chill the quinoa for 10-15 minutes and place in the serving mason jars.

Add honey, vanilla extract, and ground cinnamon.

Stir well.

Top quinoa with banana and stir it before serving.

Nutrition: Calories 279, fat 5.3, fiber 4.6, carbs 48.4, protein 10.7

Quinoa And Potato Bowl

Preparation time: 10 minutes

Cooking time: 20 minutes

Servings: 4

Ingredients:

1 sweet potato, peeled, chopped

1 tablespoon olive oil

½ teaspoon chili flakes

½ teaspoon salt

1 cup quinoa

2 cups of water

1 teaspoon butter

1 tablespoon fresh cilantro, chopped

Directions:

Line the baking tray with parchment.

Arrange the chopped sweet potato in the tray and sprinkle it with chili flakes, salt, and olive oil.

Bake the sweet potato for 20 minutes at 355F.

Meanwhile, pour water in the saucepan.

Add quinoa and cook it over the medium heat for 7 minutes or until quinoa will absorb all liquid.

Add butter in the cooked quinoa and stir well.

Transfer it in the bowls, add baked sweet potato and chopped cilantro.

Nutrition: :calories 221, fat 7.1, fiber 3.9, carbs 33.2, protein 6.6

Almond Cream Cheese Bake

Preparation time: 10 minutes

Cooking time: 60 minutes

Servings: 4

Ingredients:

1 cup cream cheese

4 tablespoons honey

1 oz almonds, chopped

½ teaspoon vanilla extract

3 eggs, beaten

1 tablespoon semolina

Directions:

Put beaten eggs in the mixing bowl.

Add cream cheese, semolina, and vanilla extract.

Blend the mixture with the help of the hand mixer until it is fluffy.

After this, add chopped almonds and mix up the mass well.

Transfer the cream cheese mash in the non-sticky baking mold.

Flatten the surface of the cream cheese mash well.

Preheat the oven to 325F.

Cook the breakfast for 2 hours.

The meal is cooked when the surface of the mash is light brown.

Chill the cream cheese mash little and sprinkle with honey.

Nutrition: :calories 352, fat 27.1, fiber 1, carbs 22.6, protein 10.4

Slow-cooked Peppers Frittata

Preparation time: 10 minutes

Cooking time: 60 minutes

Servings: 4

Ingredients:

½ cup almond milk

8 eggs, whisked

Salt and black pepper to the taste

1 teaspoon oregano, dried

1 and ½ cups roasted peppers, chopped

½ cup red onion, chopped

4 cups baby arugula

1 cup goat cheese, crumbled

Cooking spray

Directions:

In a bowl, combine the eggs with salt, pepper and the oregano and whisk.

Grease your slow cooker with the cooking spray, arrange the peppers and the remaining ingredients inside and pour the eggs mixture over them.

Put the lid on and cook on Low for 3 hours.

Divide the frittata between plates and serve.

Nutrition: calories 259, fat 20.2, fiber 1, carbs 4.4, protein 16.3

Peanut Butter and Cacao Breakfast Quinoa

Preparation Time: 5 minutes

Cooking Time: 10 minutes

Servings: 1

Ingredients:

1/3 cup quinoa flakes

1/2 cup unsweetened nondairy milk,

1/2 cup of water

1/8 cup raw cacao powder

One tablespoon natural creamy peanut butter

1/8 teaspoon ground cinnamon

One banana, mashed

Fresh berries of choice, for serving

Chopped nuts of choice, for serving

Directions:

Using an 8-quart pot over medium-high heat, stir together the quinoa flakes, milk, water, cacao powder, peanut butter, and cinnamon. Cook and stir it until the mixture begins to simmer. Turn the heat to medium-low and cook for 3 to 5 minutes, stirring frequently.

Stir in the bananas and cook until hot.

Serve topped with fresh berries, nuts, and a splash of milk.

Nutrition:

Calories: 471

Fat: 16g

Protein: 18g

Carbohydrates: 69g

Fiber: 16g

Pasta with Indian Lentils

Preparation Time: 5 minutes

Cooking Time: 0 minutes

Servings: 6

Ingredients:

¼-½ cup fresh cilantro (chopped)

3 cups water

2 small dry red peppers (whole)

1 teaspoon turmeric

1 teaspoon ground cumin

2-3 cloves garlic (minced)

1 can diced tomatoes (w/juice)

1 large onion (chopped)

½ cup dry lentils (rinsed)

½ cup orzo or tiny pasta

Directions:

Combine all ingredients in the skillet except for the cilantro then boil on medium-high heat.

Ensure to cover and slightly reduce heat to medium-low and simmer until pasta is tender for about 35 minutes.

Afterwards, take out the chili peppers then add cilantro and top it with low-fat sour cream.

Nutrition:

Calories: 175;

Carbs: 40g;

Protein: 3g;

Fats: 2g;

Phosphorus: 139mg;

Potassium: 513mg;

Sodium: 61mg

Vegetable Buckwheat Pasta

Preparation time: 6 minutes

Cooking time: 10 minutes

Servings: 4

Ingredients:

4 tablespoons coconut oil

500g buckwheat pasta

2 garlic cloves, diced

1 medium white onion, cut into rings

3 carrots, sliced

1 head broccoli

1 red bell pepper, chopped into strips

3 medium tomatoes, diced

1 teaspoon vegetable broth

1 tablespoon fresh lemon juice

1 teaspoon oregano

A pinch of Sea salt

A pinch of pepper

Directions:

Chop al the veggies read to cook. Cook buckwheat pasta in boiling salt water. In a separate pot, boil broccoli in boiling salt water.

Meanwhile, heat two tablespoons of oil in a pan and sauté garlic and onion until fragrant and translucent. Remove from pan and set aside.

Heat the remaining oil in the same pan and cook veggies for a few minutes until tender. Add broccoli and onions to the pan and stir in broth, lemon juice, oregano, salt and pepper.

Stir to mix well and serve the veggie mix over the buckwheat pasta.

Nutrition:3g carbs 10g fat 12g protein 165 Calories

Pan-Seared Salmon Salad with Snow Peas & Grapefruit

Preparation time: 10 minutes

Cooking time: 0 minutes

Servings: 4

Ingredients:

4 (100g) skin-on salmon fillets

1/8 teaspoon sea salt

2 teaspoons extra virgin olive oil

4 cups arugula

8 leaves Boston lettuce, washed and dried

1 cup snow peas, cooked

2 avocados, diced

For Grapefruit-Dill Dressing:

1/4 cup grapefruit juice

1/4 cup extra virgin olive oil

1 teaspoon raw honey

1 tablespoon Dijon mustard

1 tablespoon chopped fresh dill

2 garlic cloves, minced

1/2 teaspoon pepper

Directions:

Sprinkle fish with about 1/8 teaspoon salt and cook in 2 teaspoons of olive oil over medium heat for about 4 minutes per side or until golden.

In a small bowl, whisk together al dressing ingredients and set aside. Divide arugula and lettuce among four serving plates.

Divide lettuce and arugula among 4 plates and add the remaining salad ingredients; top each with seared fish and drizzle with dressing. Enjoy!

Nutrition:3g carbs 10g fat 12g protein 165 Calories

Cleansing Vegetable Broth

Preparation time: 10 minutes

Cooking time: 20 minutes

Servings: 4

Ingredients:

1/4 cup water

2 cloves garlic, minced

1/2 cup chopped red onion

1 tablespoon minced fresh ginger

1 cup chopped tomatoes

1 small head of broccoli, chopped into florets

3 medium carrots, diced

3 celery stalks, diced

1/8 teaspoon cayenne pepper

1/4 teaspoon cinnamon

1 teaspoon turmeric

Sea salt and pepper

6 cups vegetable broth

¼ cup fresh lemon juice

1 cup chopped purple cabbage

2 cups chopped kale

Directions:

Boil ¼ cup of water in a large pot; add garlic and onion and sauté for about 2 minutes, stirring.

Stir in ginger, tomatoes, broccoli, carrots and celery and cook for about 3 minutes. Stir in spices.

Add in vegetable broth and bring the mixture to a boil; lower heat and simmer for about 15 minutes or until veggies are tender.

Stir in lemon juice, cabbage and kale and cook for about 2 minutes or until kale is wilted. Adjust the seasoning and serve hot.

Nutrition:3g carbs 10g fat 12g protein 165 Calories

Barbecued Spiced Tuna with Avocado-Mango Salsa

Preparation time: 10 minutes

Cooking time: 10 minutes

Servings: 3

Ingredients:

4 (120g each) skinless tuna fillets

1 teaspoon dried oregano

1 teaspoon onion powder

1 teaspoon ground paprika

1 teaspoon ground coriander

1 teaspoon ground cumin

1 tablespoon olive oil

Thinly shaved fennel

Baby rocket leaves

Avocado-Mango Salsa:

1/2 red onion, chopped

1 cucumber, chopped

1 avocado, diced

1 mango, diced

1 long red chilli, chopped

2 tablespoons lime juice

1/2 cup chopped coriander

Directions:

In a bowl, mix together onion powder, paprika, coriander, cumin, and oil until well combined; add in tuna and turn until well coated; sprinkle with salt and pepper.

Preheat the BBQ grill on medium high and grill the fish for about 3 minutes per side or until cooked to your liking. Wrap in foil and let set for at least 5 minutes.

In the meantime, in a bowl, mix together avocado, mango, red onion, cucumber, chili, coriander, and fresh lime juice until well combined.

Divide fennel and rocket on serving plates and top each with the grilled tuna and mango-avocado salsa. Serve right away.

Nutrition:3g carbs 10g fat 12g protein 165 Calories

Low Carb Berry Salad with Citrus Dressing

Preparation time: 10 minutes

Cooking time: 0 minutes

Servings: 4

Ingredients:

Salad:

¼ cup blueberries

½ cup chopped strawberries

1 cup mixed greens (kale and chard)

2 cups baby spinach

2 chopped green onions

½ cup chopped avocado

1 shredded carrots

Citrus Dressing:

1 tablespoon extra-virgin olive oil

2 tablespoons apple cider vinegar

¼ cup fresh orange juice

5 strawberries chopped

Directions:

In a blender, blend together all dressing ingredients until very smooth; set aside.

Combine all salad ingredients in a large bowl; drizzle with dressing and toss to coat well before serving.

Nutrition:3g carbs 10g fat 12g protein 165 Calories

Tasty Lime Cilantro Cauliflower Rice

Preparation time: 10 minutes

Cooking time: 20 minutes

Servings: 4

Ingredients:

1 head cauliflower, rinsed

1 tablespoon extra-virgin olive oil

2 garlic cloves, minced

2 scallions, chopped

½ teaspoon sea salt

Pinch of pepper

4 tablespoons fresh lime juice

1/4 cup chopped fresh cilantro

Directions:

Chop cauliflower into florets and transfer to a food processor; pulse into rice texture.

Heat a large skillet over medium heat and add olive oil; sauté garlic and scallions for about 4 minutes or until fragrant and tender.

Increase heat to medium high and stir in cauliflower rice; cook, covered, for about 6 minutes or until cauliflower is crispy on outside and soft inside.

Season with salt and pepper and transfer to a bowl. Toss with freshly squeezed lime juice and cilantro and serve right away.

Nutrition:3g carbs 10g fat 12g protein 165 Calories

Citrus Chicken with Delicious Cold Soup

Preparation time: 10 minutes

Cooking time: 30 minutes

Servings: 3

Ingredients:

2 tablespoons extra-virgin olive oil

500g ounces chicken breast

1 teaspoon fresh rosemary

1 lemon, sliced

1 orange, sliced

For the Cold Soup:

2 tablespoons apple cider vinegar

1/4 cup green pepper, chopped

1/4 cup cucumber, chopped

1/2 cup onion, chopped

3 cloves garlic, minced

1 cup stewed tomatoes

Directions:

Generously coat chicken with extra virgin olive oil and cover with rosemary, lemon and orange slices. Bake in the oven at 350°F for about 30 minutes.

In a blender, blend together all the soup ingredients until very smooth and then serve with chicken and cooked brown rice.

Nutrition:3g carbs 10g fat 12g protein 165 Calories

Pan-Fried Chicken with Oregano-Orange Chimichurri & Arugula Salad

Preparation time: 10 minutes

Cooking time: 5 minutes

Servings: 3

Ingredients:

1 tablespoon orange juice

1 teaspoon orange zest

1 teaspoon dried oregano

1 small garlic clove, grated

2 teaspoon apple cider vinegar

1/2 cup chopped parsley

1 1/2 pound chicken, cut into 4 pieces

1 tablespoon lemon juice

A pinch of pepper

1/4 cup olive oil

4 cups arugula

2 bulbs fennel, shaved

2 tablespoons whole-grain mustard

Directions:

Make chimichurri: In a medium bowl, combine orange zest, oregano and garlic. Mix in vinegar, orange juice and parsley and then slowly whisk in ¼ cup of olive oil until emulsified. Season with black pepper.

Sprinkle the chicken with lemon juice and pepper; heat the remaining olive oil in a large skillet and cook the chicken over medium high heat for about 6 minutes per side or until browned.

Remove from heat and let rest for at least 10 minutes. Toss chicken, greens, and fennel with mustard in a medium bowl; season with salt and pepper.

Serve steak with chimichurri and salad. Enjoy!

Nutrition:3g carbs 10g fat 12g protein 165 Calories

Cauliflower Couscous Salad

Preparation time: 10 minutes

Cooking time: 25 minutes

Servings: 0

Ingredients:

1 large head cauliflower, cut into florets

3-4 green onions, thinly sliced

2 garlic cloves, finely minced

1 jalapeño, seeds and ribs removed, minced

1 cup shredded carrots

1 cup diced celery

1 cup diced cucumber

1 green apple, diced

Juice of 1 lemon

1 tablespoon extra-virgin olive oil

Sea salt

Freshly ground black pepper

Directions:

Using two batches, set your cauliflower to pulse in a food processor until finely chopped.

Transfer to a mixing bowl with the remaining ingredients then gently toss until combined.

Serve and enjoy.

Nutrition:3g carbs 10g fat 12g protein 165 Calories

Ultimate Liver Detox Soup

Preparation time: 10 minutes

Cooking time: 20 minutes

Servings: 5

Ingredients:

2 tablespoons extra-virgin olive oil

1 cup chopped shallot

1 tablespoon grated ginger

2 cloves garlic, minced

4 cups homemade chicken broth

1 medium golden beet, diced

1 large carrot, sliced

1 cup shredded red cabbage

1 cup sliced mushrooms

a handful of pea pods, halved

1 hot chili pepper, sliced

1 cup chopped cauliflower

1 cup chopped broccoli

1 bell pepper, diced

A pinch of cayenne pepper

A pinch of sea salt

1 cup baby spinach

1 cup chopped kale

1 cup grape tomatoes, halved

Directions:

In a large skillet, heat olive oil until hot but not smoky; sauté in shallots, ginger and garlic for about 2 minutes or until tender; stir in broth and bring the mixture to a gentle simmer.

Add in beets and carrots and simmer for about 5 minutes. Stir in hot pepper, cauliflower and broccoli and cook for about 3 minutes. stir in bell pepper, red cabbage, mushrooms, and peas and cook for 1 minute.

Remove from heat and stir in salt and pepper. Stir in leafy greens and tomatoes and cover the pot for about 5 minutes. Serve.

Nutrition:3g carbs 10g fat 12g protein 165 Calories

Brown Rice and Grilled Chicken Salad

Preparation time: 10 minutes

Cooking time: 10 minutes

Servings: 3

Ingredients:

300g grilled chicken breasts

3/4 cup brown rice

1 1/4 cup coconut water

1 teaspoon minced garlic

2 tablespoons teriyaki sauce

1 tablespoon extra-virgin olive oil

2 tablespoons cider vinegar

1 small red onion, chopped

5 radishes, sliced

1 cup broccoli, chopped

Dash of pepper

Directions:

Cook rice in coconut water following package instructions. Remove from heat and let cool completely, and then fluff with a fork.

Whisk together garlic, teriyaki sauce, extra virgin olive oil, and vinegar. Stir in red onion, radishes, broccoli and rice. Season with pepper and stir until well blended. Serve with grilled chicken breasts.

Nutrition:283.6 Calories 11.5g fat 31g carbs 10.9g protein

Superfood Liver Cleansing Soup

Preparation time: 10 minutes

Cooking time: 20 minutes

Servings: 3

Ingredients:

1/4 cup water

2 cloves garlic, minced

1/2 of a red onion, diced

1 tablespoon fresh ginger, peeled and minced

1 cup chopped tomatoes

1 small head of broccoli, florets

3 medium carrots, diced

3 celery stalks, diced

6 cups water

1/4 teaspoon cinnamon

1 teaspoon turmeric

1/8 teaspoon cayenne pepper

Freshly ground black pepper

juice of 1 lemon

1 cup purple cabbage, chopped

2 cups kale, torn in pieces

Directions:

Bring a large pot of water to a gentle boil over medium heat. Add garlic and onion and cook for about 2 minutes, stirring occasionally.

Stir in carrots, broccoli, tomatoes, fresh ginger, celery and cook for another 3 minutes. Stir in cayenne, turmeric, cinnamon, and black pepper.

Add half cup of water to the pot and bring to a gentle boil; lower heat and simmer until the veggies and tender, for about 15 minutes.

Stir in kale, cabbage, and fresh lemon juice during the last 2 minutes of cooking. Serve hot or warm.

Nutrition:283.6 Calories 11.5g fat 31g carbs 10.9g protein

Toxin Flush & Detox Salad

Preparation time: 10 minutes

Cooking time: 0 minutes

Servings: 3

Ingredients:

For the salad:

2 cups broccoli florets

2 cups red cabbage, thinly sliced

2 cups chopped kale

1 cup grated carrot

1 red bell pepper, sliced into strips

2 avocados, diced

1/2 cup chopped parsley

1 cup walnuts

1 tablespoon sesame seeds

For the dressing:

2 teaspoons gluten-free mustard

1 tablespoon freshly grated ginger

1/2 cup fresh lemon juice

1/3 cup grapeseed oil

1 teaspoon raw honey

1/4 teaspoon salt

Directions:

In a blender, blend all the dressing ingredients until well blended; set aside.

In a salad bowl, mix broccoli, cabbage, kale, carrots and bell pepper; pour the dressing over the salad and toss until well coated.

Add diced avocado, parsley, walnuts and sesame seed; toss again to coat and serve.

Nutrition:283.6 Calories 11.5g fat 31g carbs 10.9g protein

Grilled Chicken Salad

Preparation time: 10 minutes

Cooking time: 20 minutes

Servings: 2

Ingredients:

4 cups chopped broccoli

- 1/4 cup extra virgin olive oil
- 1/2 small red onion, thinly sliced
- 1 carrot, coarsely grated
- 4 chicken thighs, skinless
- 1 1/2 tablespoons Cajun seasoning
- 1/4 cup lemon juice
- 1 tablespoon drained baby capers
- 1 lemon, cut into wedges, to serve

Directions:

Drizzle chicken with oil and sprinkle with seasoning; rub to coat well.

Heat your grill to medium heat and grill the chicken for about 8 minutes per side or until cooked through and golden browned on the outside.

In the meantime, place the grated broccoli in a bowl and add in red onion, carrots, capers, lime juice and the remaining oil, salt and pepper; toss to combine well and serve with grilled chicken garnished with lemon wedges.

Nutrition:283.6 Calories 11.5g fat 31g carbs 10.9g protein

Chicken Stir Fry with Red Onions & Cabbage

Preparation time: 10 minutes

Cooking time: 10 minutes

Servings: 3

Ingredients:

- 550g chicken, thinly sliced strips
- 1 tablespoon apple cider wine
- 2 teaspoons balsamic vinegar
- Pinch of sea salt
- pinch of pepper
- 4 tablespoons extra-virgin olive oil
- 1 large yellow onion, thinly chopped
- 1/2 red bell pepper, sliced
- 1/2 green bell pepper, sliced
- 1 tablespoon toasted sesame seeds
- 1 teaspoon crushed red pepper flakes
- 4 cups cabbage
- 1 ½ avocados, diced

Directions:

Place meat in a bowl; stir in rice wine and vinegar, sea salt and pepper. Toss to coat well.

Heat a tablespoon of olive oil in a pan set over medium high heat; add meat and cook for about 2 minutes or until meat is browned; stir for another 2 minutes and then remove from heat.

Heat the remaining oil to the pan and sauté onions for about 2 minutes or until caramelized; stir in pepper and cook for 2 minutes more.

Stir in cabbage and cook for 2 minutes; return meat to pan and stir in sesame seeds and red pepper flakes. Serve hot topped with diced avocado!

Nutrition:283.6 Calories 11.5g fat 31g carbs 10.9g protein

Green Salad with Herbs

Preparation time: 10 minutes

Cooking time: 30 minutes

Servings: 0

Ingredients:

- 1 bunch rocket
- 2 baby cos, outer leaves discarded, roughly chopped

1 curly endive, outer leaves removed, roughly chopped

2 tablespoons chopped parsley

2 tablespoons chopped fresh dill

2 tablespoons snipped chives

1/2 cup extra-virgin olive oil

2 tablespoons fresh lemon juice

Directions:

In a large bowl, mix rocket, cos and endive and herbs.

In another small bowl, whisk together olive oil, fresh lemon juice, salt and pepper until well blended; pour over the salad and toss to coat well. Serve.

Nutrition:283.6 Calories 11.5g fat 31g carbs 10.9g protein

Chilled Green Goddess Soup

Preparation time: 10 minutes

Cooking time: 10 minutes

Servings: 3

Ingredients:

6 cups cucumber

2 stalks celery chopped

1-2 cups water (depending how thin you want it)

2 tablespoons fresh lime juice

1 cup watercress leaves

1 cup rocket leaves

½ cup mashed avocado (roughly 1 avocado)

1 teaspoon wheatgrass power or a mixed green powder, optional

Sea salt to taste

Directions:

Blend all ingredients except the avocado in a blender until a broth forms. Strain the liquid through a cheesecloth or fine sieve. Then return to blender and add the avocado and blend until smooth.

Garnish with a few watercress leaves and cracked black pepper.

Nutrition:283.6 Calories 11.5g fat 31g carbs 10.9g protein

Detox Soup

Preparation time: 5 minutes

Cooking time: 40 minutes

Servings: 3

Ingredients:

4 cloves garlic, crushed

2 medium leeks, chopped

1 serrano pepper, thinly sliced

4 celery stalks, chopped

4 carrots, diced

3 rutabagas, peeled and diced

8 cups water

2 cups pinto beans, cooked with cooking liquids

3 tomatoes, diced

3 zucchini, diced

2 bunches kale, thinly sliced

3 tablespoons lemon juice

Sea salt

Freshly cracked black pepper

Directions:

Heat a pot over medium heat; add garlic, leeks, and serranoes. Cook for about 5 minutes, stirring.

Add celery, carrots, and rutabagas; cook for about 3 minutes more and stir in water, pinto beans, and tomatoes; simmer for about 30 minutes or until the beans are cooked through.

Stir in zucchini and kale, 15 minutes before serving. Remove from heat and stir in lemon juice; season with sea salt and black pepper and serve.

Nutrition:283.6 Calories 11.5g fat 31g carbs 10.9g protein

Pumpkin Muffins

Preparation Time: 15 minutes

Cooking Time: 20 minutes

Servings: 12

Ingredients:

1 cup all-purpose flour

1 cup wheat bran

2 teaspoons Phosphorus Powder

1 cup pumpkin purée

¼ cup honey

¼ cup olive oil

1 egg

1 teaspoon vanilla extract

½ cup cored diced apple

Directions:

Preheat the oven to 400°F.

Line 12 muffin cups with paper liners.

Stir together the flour, wheat bran, and baking powder, mix this in a medium bowl.

In a small bowl, whisk together the pumpkin, honey, olive oil, egg, and vanilla.

Stir the pumpkin mixture into the flour mixture until just combined.

Stir in the diced apple.

Spoon the batter in the muffin cups.

Bake for about 20 minutes, or until a toothpick inserted in the center of a muffin comes out clean.

Nutrition:

Calories: 125;

Total Fat: 5g;

Saturated Fat: 1g;

Cholesterol: 18mg;

Sodium: 8mg;

Carbohydrates: 20g;

Fiber: 3g;

Phosphorus: 120mg;

Potassium: 177mg;

Protein: 2g

Spiced French Toast

Preparation Time: 15 minutes

Cooking Time: 12 minutes

Servings: 4

Ingredients:

4 eggs

½ cup Homemade Rice Milk (here, or use unsweetened store-bought) or almond milk

¼ cup freshly squeezed orange juice

1 teaspoon ground cinnamon

½ teaspoon ground ginger

Pinch ground cloves

1 tablespoon unsalted butter, divided

8 slices white bread

Directions:

Whisk eggs, rice milk, orange juice, cinnamon, ginger, and cloves until well blended in a large bowl.

Melt half the butter in a large skillet. It should be in medium-high heat only.

Dredge four of the bread slices in the egg mixture until well soaked, and place them in the skillet.

Cook the toast until golden brown on both sides, turning once, about 6 minutes total.

Repeat with the remaining butter and bread.

Serve 2 pieces of hot French toast to each person.

Nutrition:

Calories: 236;

Total fat: 11g;

Saturated fat: 4g;

Cholesterol: 220mg;

Sodium: 84mg;

Carbohydrates: 27g;

Fiber: 1g;

Phosphorus: 119mg;

Potassium: 158mg;

Protein: 11g

Passionfruit, Cranberry & Coconut Yoghurt Chia Parfait

Preparation time: 10 minutes

Cooking time: 0 minutes

Servings: 3

Ingredients:

4 tablespoons organic chia seeds

2 cups almond milk

½ teaspoon raw honey

½ teaspoon natural vanilla extract

1 cup organic frozen cranberries

1/2 fresh banana

1/3 cup almond milk

1 tablespoon Lucuma powder

1 tablespoon raw honey

1 cup fresh passionfruit pulp

1 cup coconut yogurt

Directions:

Make the chia base by mixing milk, chia seeds, raw honey and vanilla extract until well combined; let rest for a few minutes.

In a blender, blend together the frozen cranberries, almond milk, banana, lucuma powder and raw honey until very smooth.

To assemble, divide the chia seeds base among the bottom of tall serving glasses; layer with coconut yogurt, passion fruit pulp, and top with cranberry smooth. Serve garnished with fresh fruit and toasted walnuts.

Nutrition:283.6 Calories 11.5g fat 31g carbs 10.9g protein

Veggie Omelet

Preparation time: 10 minutes

Cooking time: 20 minutes

Servings: 3

Ingredients:

3 egg whites

1 egg

1/2 teaspoon extra-virgin olive oil

1/8 teaspoon red pepper flakes

1/8 teaspoon ground nutmeg

1/8 teaspoon garlic powder

A Pinch of salt

1/8 teaspoon ground black pepper

1/2 cup sliced fresh mushrooms

2 tablespoons chopped red bell pepper

1/4 cup chopped green onion

1/2 cup chopped tomato

1 cup chopped fresh spinach

Directions:

In a large bowl, whisk together egg whites, egg, garlic powder, red pepper flakes, nutmeg, salt and pepper until well blended.

Heat olive oil in a skillet over medium heat; add green onion, mushrooms and belle pepper and cook for about 5 minutes or until tender; stir in tomato and egg mixture and cook for about 5 minutes per side or until egg is set. Slice and serve hot.

Nutrition:283.6 Calories 11.5g fat 31g carbs 10.9g protein

Overnight Superfood Parfait

Preparation time: 10 minutes

Cooking time: 0 minutes

Servings: 3

Ingredients:

1 cup almond milk

1 teaspoon spirulina powder

1 teaspoon raw honey

4 tablespoons chia seeds

4 tablespoons Greek yogurt, to serve

1 cup fresh cranberries, to serve

1 cup fresh blueberries

1 cup toasted almonds

Directions:

In a bowl, mix together all the ingredients until well combined; let set for overnight. To serve, add half of the yogurt in a serving glass and top with a third of berries and toasted almonds; repeat the layers until the glass is full. Enjoy!

Nutrition:242 Calories 7g Carbs 19g Fat 12g Protein

Crunchy Peach, Cranberry and Flax Meal Super Bowl

Preparation time: 10 minutes

Cooking time: 0 minutes

Servings: 3

Ingredients:

10 ounces frozen cranberries

10 ounces frozen peaches (or mangoes)

1 cup almond milk

1 cup water

1/4 cup flax meal

1/3 cup chia seeds

1/4 cup raw honey

Toasted walnuts and toasted coconut for serving

Directions:

In a blender, combine water and peaches and blend until very smooth; transfer to a bowl.

Blend almond milk and cranberries until very smooth.

In a serving bowl, mix together the fruit purees and then stir in flax meal, chia seeds, and raw honey until well combined.

Let sit for at least 10 minutes before serving. Serve topped with toasted walnuts and toasted coconut.

Nutrition:242 Calories 7g Carbs 19g Fat 12g Protein

Gluten Free Pancakes

Preparation time: 10 minutes

Cooking time: 15 minutes

Servings: 3

Ingredients:

1 cup almond flour

1/4 cup coconut flour

1/3 cup unsweetened almond milk

3 large eggs

1/4 cup olive oil

1 teaspoon baking powder

1 1/2 teaspoons vanilla extract

1 tablespoon raw honey

1 cup fresh blueberries for serving

Directions:

In a large bowl, whisk together all the ingredients until very smooth. Heat a pan and then add in oil; drop about three tablespoons of batter into the pan and cook for about 2 minutes. flip over and cook for 2 minutes more or until lightly browned on both sides. Repeat with the remaining batter.

Serve topped with fresh blueberries.

Nutrition:242 Calories 7g Carbs 19g Fat 12g Protein

Detox Porridge

Preparation time: 10 minutes

Cooking time: 2 minutes

Servings: 2

Ingredients:

1 cup unsweetened almond milk

2 tablespoons ground golden flax

1/2 cup coconut flour

1 tablespoon coconut oil

1 teaspoon cinnamon

1 cup water

1 tablespoon raw honey

Toasted coconut to serve

Toasted almonds to serve

Directions:

In a microwave safe bowl, stir together all the ingredients until well combined; place in the microwave and heat for 1 minute.

Stir again to mix well and microwave for another 1 minute. Serve right away topped with toasted almonds and toasted coconut.

Nutrition:242 Calories 7g Carbs 19g Fat 12g Protein

Avocado Crab Omelet

Preparation time: 10 minutes

Cooking time: 10 minutes

Servings: 2

Ingredients:

1/4 pound crab meat

4 large free-range eggs, beaten

1/2 medium avocado, diced

1 medium tomato, diced

1 teaspoon olive oil

1/8 teaspoon freshly ground black pepper

A pinch of salt

1 tablespoon freshly chopped cilantro

Directions:

Cook crab in a skillet following the instructions on the packet; chop the cooked crab and set aside.

In a small bowl, toss together avocado, tomato, and cilantro; season with sea salt and pepper and set aside.

In a separate bowl, beat the eggs and set aside.

Set a skillet over medium heat; add olive oil and heat until hot.

Add half of the egg to the skillet and tilt the skillet to cover the bottom. When almost cooked, add crab onto one side of the egg and fold in half. Cook for 1 minute more and top with the avocado-tomato mixture.

Repeat with the remaining ingredients for the second omelet.

Nutrition:242 Calories 7g Carbs 19g Fat 12g Protein

Buckwheat Pancakes

Preparation time: 10 minutes

Cooking time: 15 minutes

Servings: 3

Ingredients:

1/2 cup buckwheat flour

2 ripe bananas

2 tablespoons olive

2 tablespoons water

1 teaspoon ground cinnamon

1 teaspoon vanilla extract

1/2 teaspoon baking soda

2 teaspoons apple cider vinegar

1/4 cup fresh blueberries for serving

Directions:

Preheat your oven to 350 degrees.

Add the ripe banana to a large bowl and mash until smooth; whisk in ground buckwheat flour, water, oil, vanilla, vinegar, cinnamon and baking powder until well combined.

Heat a skillet over medium heat; add in oil and heat until hot but not smoky; add in about a quarter cup of batter and spread to cover the bottom of the pan.

Cook for about 2 minutes and then flip to cook the other side for about 1 minute or until browned.

Serve right away topped with fresh blueberries.

Nutrition: 242 Calories 25g carbs 12g fat 13g protein

Apple Oatmeal

Preparation time: 10 minutes

Cooking time: 8 minutes

Servings: 3

Ingredients:

1/2 tsp ground cinnamon

4 tbsp. fat free vanilla yogurt

1 1/2 cups quick oats

1/4 cup maple syrup

3 cups apple juice

1/4 cup raisins

1/2 cup chopped apple

1/4 cup chopped walnuts

Directions:

Combine your cinnamon and apple juice in a saucepan and allow to boil.

Stir in your raisins, maple syrup, apples and oats.

Switch the heat to low and cook while stirring until most of juice is absorbed. Fold in walnuts, serve and top with yogurt.

Nutrition: 242 Calories 25g carbs 12g fat 13g protein

Raspberry Overnight Porridge

Preparation Time: Overnight

Cooking Time: 0 minute

Servings: 12

Ingredients:

⅓ cup of rolled oats

½ cup almond milk

1 tablespoon of honey

5-6 raspberries, fresh or canned and unsweetened

⅓ cup of rolled oats

½ cup almond milk

1 tablespoon of honey

5-6 raspberries, fresh or canned and unsweetened

Directions:

Combine the oats, almond milk, and honey in a mason jar and place into the fridge for overnight.

Serve the next morning with the raspberries on top.

Nutrition:

Calories: 143.6 kcal

Carbohydrate: 34.62 g

Protein: 3.44 g

Sodium: 77.88 mg

Potassium: 153.25 mg

Phosphorus: 99.3 mg

Dietary Fiber: 7.56 g

Fat: 3.91 g

Cheesy Scrambled Eggs with Fresh Herbs

Preparation Time: 15 minutes

Cooking Time: 10 minutes

Servings: 4

Ingredients:

Eggs – 3

Egg whites – 2

Cream cheese – ½ cup

Unsweetened rice milk – ¼ cup

Chopped scallion – 1 Tablespoon green part only

Chopped fresh tarragon – 1 Tablespoon

Unsalted butter – 2 Tablespoons.

Ground black pepper to taste

Directions:

In a container, mix the eggs, egg whites, cream cheese, rice milk, scallions, and tarragon until mixed and smooth.

Melt the butter in a skillet.

Pour in the egg mix and cook, stirring, for 5 minutes or until the eggs are thick and curds creamy.

Season with pepper and serve.

Nutrition:

Calories: 221

Fat: 19g

Carb: 3g

Phosphorus: 119mg

Potassium: 140mg

Sodium: 193mg

Protein: 8g

Turkey and Spinach Scramble on Melba Toast

Preparation Time: 2 minutes

Cooking Time: 15 minutes

Servings: 2

Ingredients:

Extra virgin olive oil – 1 teaspoon

Raw spinach – 1 cup

Garlic – ½ clove, minced

Nutmeg – 1 teaspoon grated

Cooked and diced turkey breast – 1 cup

Melba toast – 4 slices

Balsamic vinegar – 1 teaspoon

Directions:

Heat a pot over a source of heat and add oil.

Add turkey and heat through for 6 to 8 minutes.

Add spinach, garlic, and nutmeg and stir-fry for 6 minutes more.

Plate up the Melba toast and top with spinach and turkey scramble.

Drizzle with balsamic vinegar and serve.

Nutrition:

Calories: 301

Fat: 19g

Carb: 12g

Phosphorus: 215mg

Potassium: 269mg

Sodium: 360mg

Protein: 19g

Vegetable Omelet

Preparation Time: 15 minutes

Cooking Time: 10 minutes

Servings: 3

Ingredients:

Egg whites – 4

Egg – 1

Chopped fresh parsley – 2 Tablespoons.

Water – 2 Tablespoons.

Olive oil spray

Chopped and boiled red bell pepper – ½ cup

Chopped scallion – ¼ cup, both green and white parts

Ground black pepper

Directions:

Whisk together the egg, egg whites, parsley, and water until well blended. Set aside.

Spray a skillet with olive oil spray and place over medium heat.

Sauté the peppers and scallion for 3 minutes or until softened.

Over the vegetables, you can now pour the egg and cook, swirling the skillet, for 2 minutes or until the edges start to set. Cook until set.

Season with black pepper and serve.

Nutrition:

Calories: 77

Fat: 3g

Carb: 2g

Phosphorus: 67mg

Potassium: 194mg

Sodium: 229mg

Protein: 12g

Mexican Style Burritos

Preparation Time: 5 minutes

Cooking Time: 15 minutes

Servings: 2

Ingredients:

Olive oil – 1 Tablespoon

Corn tortillas – 2

Red onion – ¼ cup, chopped

Red bell peppers – ¼ cup, chopped

Red chili – ½, deseeded and chopped

Eggs – 2

Juice of 1 lime

Cilantro – 1 Tablespoon chopped

Directions:

Turn the broiler to medium heat and place the tortillas underneath for 1 to 2 minutes on each side or until lightly toasted.

Remove and keep the broiler on.

Sauté onion, chili and bell peppers for 5 to 6 minutes or until soft.

Place the eggs on top of the onions and peppers and place skillet under the broiler for 5-6 minutes or until the eggs are cooked.

Serve half the eggs and vegetables on top of each tortilla and sprinkle with cilantro and lime juice to serve.

Nutrition:

Calories: 202

Fat: 13g

Carb: 19g

Phosphorus: 184mg

Potassium: 233mg

Sodium: 77mg

Protein: 9g

Chapter 5: Snack Recipes

Rosemary Cauliflower Dip

Preparation time: 10 minutes

Cooking time: 10 minutes

Servings: 3

Ingredients:

1 lb cauliflower florets

1 tbsp fresh parsley, chopped

1/2 cup heavy cream

1/2 cup vegetable stock

1 tbsp garlic, minced

1 tbsp rosemary, chopped

1 tbsp olive oil

1 onion, chopped

Pepper

Salt

Directions:

Add oil into the inner pot of instant pot and set the pot on sauté mode.

Add onion and sauté for 5 minutes.

Add remaining ingredients except for parsley and heavy cream and stir well.

Seal pot with lid and cook on high for 10 minutes.

Once done, allow to release pressure naturally for 10 minutes then release remaining using quick release. Remove lid.

Add cream and stir well. Blend cauliflower mixture using immersion blender until smooth.

Garnish with parsley and serve.

Nutrition: Calories 128 Fat 9.4 g Carbohydrates 10.4 g Sugar 4 g Protein 3.1 g Cholesterol 21 mg

Light & Creamy Garlic Hummus

Preparation time: 10 minutes

Cooking time: 40 minutes

Servings: 10

Ingredients:

1 1/2 cups dry chickpeas, rinsed

2 1/2 tbsp fresh lemon juice

1 tbsp garlic, minced

1/2 cup tahini

6 cups of water

Pepper

Salt

Directions:

Add water and chickpeas into the instant pot.

Seal pot with a lid and select manual and set timer for 40 minutes.

Once done, allow to release pressure naturally. Remove lid.

Drain chickpeas well and reserved 1/2 cup chickpeas liquid.

Transfer chickpeas, reserved liquid, lemon juice, garlic, tahini, pepper, and salt into the food processor and process until smooth.

Serve and enjoy.

Nutrition: Calories 152 Fat 6.9 g Carbohydrates 17.6 g Sugar 2.8 g Protein 6.6 g Cholesterol 0 mg

Style Nachos Recipe

Preparation time: 10 minutes

Cooking time: 10 minutes

Servings: 3

Ingredients:

6 pieces whole-wheat pita breads

Cooking spray

1/2 teaspoon ground cumin

1/2 teaspoon ground coriander

1/2 teaspoon paprika

1/2 teaspoon pepper

1/2 teaspoons salt

1/2 cup hot water

1/2 teaspoon beef stock concentrate

1 pound ground lamb or beef

2 garlic cloves, minced

1 teaspoon cornstarch

2 medium cucumbers, peeled, seeded, grated

2 cups Greek yogurt, plain

2 tablespoons lemon juice

1/4 teaspoon grated lemon peel

1 teaspoon salt, divided

1/4 teaspoon pepper

1/2 cup pitted Greek olives, sliced

4 green onions, thinly sliced

1/2 cup crumbled feta cheese

2 cups torn romaine lettuce

2 medium tomatoes, seeded and chopped

Directions:

In a colander set over a bowl, toss the cucumbers with 1/2 teaspoon of the salt; let stand for 30 minutes, then squeeze and pat dry. Set aside.

In a small-sized bowl, combine the coriander, cumin, 1/2 teaspoon pepper, paprika, and 1/2 teaspoon salt; set aside.

Cut each pita bread into 8 wedges. Arrange them in a single layer on ungreased baking sheets. Sprits both sides of the wedges with cooking spray. Sprinkle with 3/4 teaspoon of the seasoning mix. Broil 3-4 inches from the heat source for about 3-4 minutes per side, or until golden brown. Transfer to wire racks, let cool.

Whisk hot water and beef stock cube in a 1-cup liquid measuring cup until blended. In a large-sized skillet, cook the lamb, seasoning with the remaining seasoning mix, over medium heat until the meat is no longer pink. Add the garlic; cook for 1 minute. Drain.

Stir in the cornstarch into the broth; mix until smooth. Gradually stir into the skillet; bring to a boil and cook, stirring, for 2 minutes or until thick.

In a small-sized bowl, combine the cucumbers, yogurt, lemon peel, lemon juice, and the remaining salt and 1/4 teaspoon pepper.

Arrange the pita wedges on a serving platter. Layer with the lettuce, lamb mixture, tomatoes, onions, olives, and cheese; serve immediately with the cucumber sauce.

Nutrition: :232 cal, 6.7 g total fat (2.9 g sat. fat), 42 mg chol., 630 mg sodium, 412 mg pot., 24 total carbs., 3.3 g fiber, 4.1 g sugar, 20.2 g protein, 8% vitamin A, 12% vitamin C, 11% calcium, and 15% iron.

Baked Goat Cheese Caprese Salad

Preparation time: 10 minutes

Cooking time: 15 minutes

Servings: 3

Ingredients:

1 (log 4 ounce) fresh goat cheese, halved

1 pinch cayenne pepper, or to taste

16 cherry tomatoes, diagonally cut into halves

2 tablespoons olive oil, divided

3 tablespoons basil chiffonade (thinly sliced fresh basil leaves), divided

Freshly ground black pepper, to taste

Directions:

Preheat the oven to 400F or 200C.

Drizzle about 1 1/2 teaspoons olive oil into the bottom of 2 pieces 6-ounch ramekin. Sprinkle about 1 tablespoon of basil per ramekin.

Place 1 goat half over each ramekin; surround with cherry tomato halves.

Sprinkle with the black pepper and the cayenne. Spread the remaining basil on top of each.

Place the ramekins on a baking sheet. Drizzle each serve with the remaining olive oil; bake for about 15 minutes or until bubbling. Serve warm.

Nutrition: :178 cal., 15.5 g total fat (6.8 sat. fat), 22 mg chol., 152 mg sodium, 4.1 g total carbs., 0.9 g fiber, 0.7 g sugar, and 6.8 g protein.

Grilled Shrimp Kabobs

Preparation time: 10 minutes

Cooking time: 30 minutes

Servings: 4

Ingredients:

1 1/2 cups whole-wheat dry breadcrumbs

1 clove garlic, finely minced or pressed

1 teaspoon dried basil leaves

1/4 cup olive oil

2 pounds shrimp, peeled, deveined, leaving the tails on

2 tablespoons vegetable oil

2 teaspoons dried parsley flakes

Salt and pepper

16 skewers, soaked for at least 20 minutes in water or until ready to use if using wooden

Directions:

Rinse the shrimps and dry.

Put the vegetable and the olive oil in a re-sealable plastic bag; add the shrimp and toss to coat with the oil mixture.

Add the breadcrumbs, parsley, garlic, basil, salt, and pepper; toss to coat with the dry mix.

Seal the bag, refrigerate for 1 hour. Thread the shrimps on the skewers.

Grill on preheated grill for about 2 minutes each side or until golden, making sure not to overcook.

Nutrition: : 502.7 cal., 24.8 g total fat (3.5 sat. fat), 285.8 mg chol., 1581.8 mg sodium, 31.7 g total carbs., 2 g fiber, 2.5 g sugar, and 36.4 g protein.

Red Pepper Tapenade

Preparation time: 10 minutes

Cooking time: 0 minutes

Servings: 3

Ingredients:

7 ounces roasted red peppers, chopped

½ cup parmesan, grated

1/3 cup parsley, chopped

14 ounces canned artichokes, drained and chopped

3 tablespoons olive oil

¼ cup capers, drained

1 and ½ tablespoons lemon juice

2 garlic cloves, minced

Directions:

In your blender, combine the red peppers with the parmesan and the rest of the ingredients and pulse well.

Divide into cups and serve as a snack.

Nutrition: calories 200, fat 5.6, fiber 4.5, carbs 12.4, protein 4.6

Lemon Swordfish

Preparation time: 10 minutes

Cooking time: 30 minutes

Servings: 2

Ingredients:

12 oz swordfish steaks (6 oz every fish steak)

1 teaspoon ground cumin

1 tablespoon lemon juice

¼ teaspoon salt

1 teaspoon olive oil

Directions:

Sprinkle the fish steaks with ground cumin and salt from each side.

Then drizzle the lemon juice over the steaks and massage them gently with the help of the fingertips.

Preheat the grill to 395F.

Bruhs every fish steak with olive oil and place in the grill.

Cook the swordfish for 3 minutes from each side.

Nutrition: :calories 289, fat 1.4, fiber 0.1, carbs 0.6, protein 43.4

Paprika Salmon And Green Beans

Preparation time: 10 minutes

Cooking time: 20 minutes

Servings: 3

Ingredients:

¼ cup olive oil

½ tablespoon onion powder

½ teaspoon bouillon powder

½ teaspoon cayenne pepper

1 tablespoon smoked paprika

1-pound green beans

2 teaspoon minced garlic

3 tablespoon fresh herbs

6 ounces of salmon steak

Salt and pepper to taste

Directions:

Preheat the oven to 400F.

Grease a baking sheet and set aside.

Heat a skillet over medium low heat and add the olive oil. Sauté the garlic, smoked paprika, fresh herbs, cayenne pepper and onion powder. Stir for a minute then let the mixture sit for 5 minutes. Set aside.

Put the salmon steaks in a bowl and add salt and the paprika spice mixture. Rub to coat the salmon well.

Place the salmon on the baking sheet and cook for 18 minutes.

Meanwhile, blanch the green beans in boiling water with salt.

Serve the beans with the salmon.

Nutrition: Calories per Serving: 945.8; Fat: 66.6 g; Protein: 43.5 g; Carbs: 43.1 g

Cucumber-basil Salsa On Halibut Pouches

Preparation time: 10 minutes

Cooking time: 17 minutes

Servings: 4

Ingredients:

1 lime, thinly sliced into 8 pieces

2 cups mustard greens, stems removed

2 tsp olive oil

4 – 5 radishes trimmed and quartered

4 4-oz skinless halibut filets

4 large fresh basil leaves

Cayenne pepper to taste – optional

Pepper and salt to taste

1 ½ cups diced cucumber

1 ½ finely chopped fresh basil leaves

2 tsp fresh lime juice

Pepper and salt to taste

Directions:

Preheat oven to 400oF.

Preparation are parchment papers by making 4 pieces of 15 x 12-inch rectangles. Lengthwise, fold in half and unfold pieces on the table.

Season halibut fillets with pepper, salt and cayenne—if using cayenne.

Just to the right of the fold going lengthwise, place ½ cup of mustard greens. Add a basil leaf on center of mustard greens and topped with 1 lime slice. Around the greens, layer ¼ of the radishes. Drizzle with ½ tsp of oil, season with pepper and salt. Top it with a slice of halibut fillet.

Just as you would make a calzone, fold parchment paper over your filling and crimp the edges of the parchment paper beginning from one end to the other end. To seal the end of the crimped parchment paper, pinch it.

Repeat process to remaining ingredients until you have 4 pieces of parchment papers filled with halibut and greens.

Place pouches in a baking pan and bake in the oven until halibut is flaky, around 15 to 17 minutes.

While waiting for halibut pouches to cook, make your salsa by mixing all salsa ingredients in a medium bowl.

Once halibut is cooked, remove from oven and make a tear on top. Be careful of the steam as it is very hot. Equally divide salsa and spoon ¼ of salsa on top of halibut through the slit you have created.

Serve and enjoy.

Nutrition: Calories per serving: 335.4; Protein: 20.2g; Fat: 16.3g; Carbs: 22.1g

Sardine Meatballs

Preparation time: 10 minutes

Cooking time: 10 minutes

Servings: 3

Ingredients:

11 oz sardines, canned, drained

1/3 cup shallot, chopped

1 teaspoon chili flakes

½ teaspoon salt

2 tablespoon wheat flour, whole grain

1 egg, beaten

1 tablespoon chives, chopped

1 teaspoon olive oil

1 teaspoon butter

Directions:

Put the butter in the skillet and melt it.

Add shallot and cook it until translucent.

After this, transfer the shallot in the mixing bowl.

Add sardines, chili flakes, salt, flour, egg, chives, and mix up until smooth with the help of the fork.

Make the medium size cakes and place them in the skillet.

Add olive oil.

Roast the fish cakes for 3 minutes from each side over the medium heat.

Dry the cooked fish cakes with the paper towel if needed and transfer in the serving plates.

Nutrition: calories 221, fat 12.2, fiber 0.1, carbs 5.4, protein 21.3

Basil Tilapia

Preparation time: 10 minutes

Cooking time: 20 minutes

Servings: 3

Ingredients:

12 oz tilapia fillet

2 oz Parmesan, grated

1 tablespoon olive oil

½ teaspoon ground black pepper

1 cup fresh basil

3 tablespoons avocado oil

1 tablespoon pine nuts

1 garlic clove, peeled

¾ teaspoon white pepper

Directions:

Make pesto sauce: blend the avocado oil, fresh basil, pine nuts, garlic clove, and white pepper until smooth.

After this, cut the tilapia fillet on 3 servings.

Sprinkle every fish serving with olive oil and ground black pepper.

Roast the fillets over the medium heat for 2 minutes from each side.

Meanwhile, line the baking tray with baking paper.

Arrange the roasted tilapia fillets in the tray.

Then top them with pesto and Parmesan.

Bake the fish for 15 minutes at 365F.

Nutrition: :calories 321, fat 17, fiber 1.2, carbs 4.4, protein 37.4

Honey Halibut

Preparation time: 10 minutes

Cooking time: 15 minutes

Servings: 3

Ingredients:

1-pound halibut

1 teaspoon lime zest

½ teaspoon honey

1 teaspoon olive oil

½ teaspoon lime juice

¼ teaspoon salt

¼ teaspoon chili flakes

Directions:

Cut the fish on the sticks and sprinkle with salt and chili flakes.

Whisk together lime zest, honey, olive oil, and lime juice.

Brush the halibut sticks with the honey mixture from each side.

Line the baking tray with baking paper and place the fish inside.

Bake the halibut for 15 minutes at 375F. Flip the fish on another side after 7 minutes of cooking.

Nutrition: :calories 254, fat 19, fiber 0, carbs 0.7, protein 18.8

Stuffed Mackerel

Preparation time: 10 minutes

Cooking time: 30 minutes

Servings: 5

Ingredients:

4 teaspoons capers, drained

1-pound whole mackerel, peeled, trimmed

1 teaspoon garlic powder

½ teaspoon ground coriander

½ teaspoon salt

1 tablespoon lime juice

¼ teaspoon chili flakes

½ white onion, sliced

4 teaspoons butter

3 tablespoons water

Directions:

Rub the fish with salt, garlic powder, and chili flakes.

Then sprinkle it with lime juice.

Line the baking tray with parchment and arrange the fish inside.

Fill the mackerel with capers and butter.

Then sprinkle fish with water.

Cover the fish with foil and secure the edges.

Bake the mackerel for 30 minutes at 365F.

Nutrition: :calories 262, fat 17.5, fiber 0.4, carbs 1.8, protein 25.5

Healthy Carrot & Shrimp

Preparation time: 10 minutes

Cooking time: 30 minutes

Servings: 4

Ingredients:

1 lb shrimp, peeled and deveined

1 tbsp chives, chopped

1 onion, chopped

1 tbsp olive oil

1 cup fish stock

1 cup carrots, sliced

Pepper

Salt

Directions:

Add oil into the inner pot of instant pot and set the pot on sauté mode.

Add onion and sauté for 2 minutes.

Add shrimp and stir well.

Add remaining ingredients and stir well.

Seal pot with lid and cook on high for 4 minutes.

Once done, release pressure using quick release. Remove lid.

Serve and enjoy.

Nutrition: Calories 197 Fat 5.9 g Carbohydrates 7 g Sugar 2.5 g Protein 27.7 g Cholesterol 239 mg

Tomato Cod Mix

Preparation time: 10 minutes

Cooking time: 5 Hours 30 minutes

Servings: 2

Ingredients:

1 teaspoon tomato paste

1 teaspoon garlic, diced

1 white onion, sliced

1 jalapeno pepper, chopped

1/3 cup chicken stock

7 oz Spanish cod fillet

1 teaspoon paprika

1 teaspoon salt

Directions:

Pour chicken stock in the saucepan.

Add tomato paste and mix up the liquid until homogenous.

Add garlic, onion, jalapeno pepper, paprika, and salt.

Bring the liquid to boil and then simmer it.

Chop the cod fillet and add it in the tomato liquid.

Close the lid and simmer the fish for 10 minutes over the low heat.

Serve the fish in the bowls with tomato sauce.

Nutrition: :calories 113, fat 1.2, fiber 1.9, carbs 7.2, protein 18.9

Garlic Mussels

Preparation time: 10 minutes

Cooking time: 10 minutes

Servings: 4

Ingredients:

1-pound mussels

1 chili pepper, chopped

1 cup chicken stock

½ cup milk

1 teaspoon olive oil

1 teaspoon minced garlic

1 teaspoon ground coriander

½ teaspoon salt

1 cup fresh parsley, chopped

4 tablespoons lemon juice

Directions:

Pour milk in the saucepan.

Add chili pepper, chicken stock, olive oil, minced garlic, ground coriander, salt, and lemon juice.

Bring the liquid to boil and add mussels.

Boil the mussel for 4 minutes or until they will open shells.

Then add chopped parsley and mix up the meal well.

Remove it from the heat.

Nutrition: :calories 136, fat 4.7, fiber 0.6, carbs 7.5, protein 15.3

Mahi Mahi And Pomegranate Sauce

Preparation time: 10 minutes

Cooking time: 10 minutes

Servings: 4

Ingredients:

1 and ½ cups chicken stock

1 tablespoon olive oil

4 mahi mahi fillets, boneless

4 tablespoons tahini paste

Juice of 1 lime

Seeds from 1 pomegranate

1 tablespoon parsley, chopped

Directions:

Heat up a pan with the oil over medium-high heat, add the fish and cook for 3 minutes on each side.

Add the rest of the ingredients, flip the fish again, cook for 4 minutes more, divide everything between plates and serve.

Nutrition: calories 224, fat 11.1, fiber 5.5, carbs 16.7, protein 11.4

Honey Balsamic Salmon

Preparation time: 10 minutes

Cooking time: 3 minutes

Servings: 2

Ingredients:

2 salmon fillets

1/4 tsp red pepper flakes

2 tbsp honey

2 tbsp balsamic vinegar

1 cup of water

Pepper

Salt

Directions:

Pour water into the instant pot and place trivet in the pot.

In a small bowl, mix together honey, red pepper flakes, and vinegar.

Brush fish fillets with honey mixture and place on top of the trivet.

Seal pot with lid and cook on high for 3 minutes.

Once done, release pressure using quick release. Remove lid.

Serve and enjoy.

Nutrition: Calories 303 Fat 11 g Carbohydrates 17.6 g Sugar 17.3 g Protein 34.6 g Cholesterol 78 mg

Sage Salmon Fillet

Preparation time: 10 minutes

Cooking time: 30 minutes

Servings: 1

Ingredients:

4 oz salmon fillet

½ teaspoon salt

1 teaspoon sesame oil

½ teaspoon sage

Directions:

Rub the fillet with salt and sage.

Place the fish in the tray and sprinkle it with sesame oil.

Cook the fish for 25 minutes at 365F.

Flip the fish carefully onto another side after 12 minutes of cooking.

Nutrition: :calories 191, fat 11.6, fiber 0.1, carbs 0.2, protein 22

Seafood Stew Cioppino

Preparation time: 10 minutes

Cooking time: 40 minutes

Servings: 6

Ingredients:

¼ cup Italian parsley, chopped

¼ tsp dried basil

¼ tsp dried thyme

½ cup dry white wine like pinot grigio

½ lb. King crab legs, cut at each joint

½ onion, chopped

½ tsp red pepper flakes (adjust to desired spiciness)

1 28-oz can crushed tomatoes

1 lb. mahi mahi, cut into ½-inch cubes

1 lb. raw shrimp

1 tbsp olive oil

2 bay leaves

2 cups clam juice

50 live clams, washed

6 cloves garlic, minced

Pepper and salt to taste

Directions:

On medium fire, place a stockpot and heat oil.

Add onion and for 4 minutes sauté until soft.

Add bay leaves, thyme, basil, red pepper flakes and garlic. Cook for a minute while stirring a bit.

Add clam juice and tomatoes. Once simmering, place fire to medium low and cook for 20 minutes uncovered.

Add white wine and clams. Cover and cook for 5 minutes or until clams have slightly opened.

Stir pot then add fish pieces, crab legs and shrimps. Do not stir soup to maintain the fish's shape. Cook while covered for 4 minutes or until clams are fully opened; fish and shrimps are opaque and cooked.

Season with pepper and salt to taste.

Transfer Cioppino to serving bowls and garnish with parsley before serving.

Nutrition: Calories per Serving: 371; Carbs: 15.5 g; Protein: 62 g; Fat: 6.8 g

Shrimp And Lemon Sauce

Preparation time: 10 minutes

Cooking time: 15 minutes

Servings: 4

Ingredients:

1 pound shrimp, peeled and deveined

1/3 cup lemon juice

4 egg yolks

2 tablespoons olive oil

1 cup chicken stock

Salt and black pepper to the taste

1 cup black olives, pitted and halved

1 tablespoon thyme, chopped

Directions:

In a bowl, mix the lemon juice with the egg yolks and whisk well.

Heat up a pan with the oil over medium heat, add the shrimp and cook for 2 minutes on each side and transfer to a plate.

Heat up a pan with the stock over medium heat, add some of this over the egg yolks and lemon juice mix and whisk well.

Add this over the rest of the stock, also add salt and pepper, whisk well and simmer for 2 minutes.

Add the shrimp and the rest of the ingredients, toss and serve right away.

Nutrition: calories 237, fat 15.3, fiber 4.6, carbs 15.4, protein 7.6

Feta Tomato Sea Bass

Preparation time: 10 minutes

Cooking time: 8 minutes

Servings: 3

Ingredients:

4 sea bass fillets

1 1/2 cups water

1 tbsp olive oil

1 tsp garlic, minced

1 tsp basil, chopped

1 tsp parsley, chopped

1/2 cup feta cheese, crumbled

1 cup can tomatoes, diced

Pepper

Salt

Directions:

Season fish fillets with pepper and salt.

Pour 2 cups of water into the instant pot then place steamer rack in the pot.

Place fish fillets on steamer rack in the pot.

Seal pot with lid and cook on high for 5 minutes.

Once done, release pressure using quick release. Remove lid.

Remove fish fillets from the pot and clean the pot.

Add oil into the inner pot of instant pot and set the pot on sauté mode.

Add garlic and sauté for 1 minute.

Add tomatoes, parsley, and basil and stir well and cook for 1 minute.

Add fish fillets and top with crumbled cheese and cook for a minute.

Serve and enjoy.

Nutrition: Calories 219 Fat 10.1 g Carbohydrates 4 g Sugar 2.8 g Protein 27.1 g Cholesterol 70 mg

Salmon And Broccoli

Preparation time: 10 minutes

Cooking time: 20 minutes

Servings: 3

Ingredients:

2 tablespoons balsamic vinegar

1 broccoli head, florets separated

4 pieces salmon fillets, skinless

1 big red onion, roughly chopped

1 tablespoon olive oil

Sea salt and black pepper to the taste

Directions:

In a baking dish, combine the salmon with the broccoli and the rest of the ingredients, introduce in the oven and bake at 390 degrees F for 20 minutes.

Divide the mix between plates and serve.

Nutrition: calories 302, fat 15.5, fiber 8.5, carbs 18.9, protein 19.8

Halibut And Quinoa Mix

Preparation time: 10 minutes

Cooking time: 30 minutes

Servings: 4

Ingredients:

4 halibut fillets, boneless

2 tablespoons olive oil

1 teaspoon rosemary, dried

2 teaspoons cumin, ground

1 tablespoons coriander, ground

2 teaspoons cinnamon powder

2 teaspoons oregano, dried

A pinch of salt and black pepper

2 cups quinoa, cooked

1 cup cherry tomatoes, halved

1 avocado, peeled, pitted and sliced

1 cucumber, cubed

½ cup black olives, pitted and sliced

Juice of 1 lemon

Directions:

In a bowl, combine the fish with the rosemary, cumin, coriander, cinnamon, oregano, salt and pepper and toss.

Heat up a pan with the oil over medium heat, add the fish, and sear for 2 minutes on each side.

Introduce the pan in the oven and bake the fish at 425 degrees F for 7 minutes.

Meanwhile, in a bowl, mix the quinoa with the remaining ingredients, toss and divide between plates.

Add the fish next to the quinoa mix and serve right away.

Nutrition: calories 364, fat 15.4, fiber 11.2, carbs 56.4, protein 24.5

Crab Stew

Preparation time: 10 minutes

Cooking time: 13 minutes

Servings: 2

Ingredients:

1/2 lb lump crab meat

2 tbsp heavy cream

1 tbsp olive oil

2 cups fish stock

1/2 lb shrimp, shelled and chopped

1 celery stalk, chopped

1/2 tsp garlic, chopped

1/4 onion, chopped

Pepper

Salt

Directions:

Add oil into the inner pot of instant pot and set the pot on sauté mode.

Add onion and sauté for 3 minutes.

Add garlic and sauté for 30 seconds.

Add remaining ingredients except for heavy cream and stir well.

Seal pot with lid and cook on high for 10 minutes.

Once done, release pressure using quick release. Remove lid.

Stir in heavy cream and serve.

Nutrition: Calories 376 Fat 25.5 g Carbohydrates 5.8 g Sugar 0.7 g Protein 48.1 g Cholesterol 326 mg

Crazy Saganaki Shrimp

Preparation time: 10 minutes

Cooking time: 10 minutes

Servings: 4

Ingredients:

¼ tsp salt

½ cup Chardonnay

½ cup crumbled Greek feta cheese

1 medium bulb. fennel, cored and finely chopped

1 small Chile pepper, seeded and minced

1 tbsp extra virgin olive oil

12 jumbo shrimps, peeled and deveined with tails left on

2 tbsp lemon juice, divided

5 scallions sliced thinly

Pepper to taste

Directions:

In medium bowl, mix salt, lemon juice and shrimp.

On medium fire, place a saganaki pan (or large nonstick saucepan) and heat oil.

Sauté Chile pepper, scallions, and fennel for 4 minutes or until starting to brown and is already soft.

Add wine and sauté for another minute.

Place shrimps on top of fennel, cover and cook for 4 minutes or until shrimps are pink.

Remove just the shrimp and transfer to a plate.

Add pepper, feta and 1 tbsp lemon juice to pan and cook for a minute or until cheese begins to melt.

To serve, place cheese and fennel mixture on a serving plate and top with shrimps.

Nutrition: Calories per serving: 310; Protein: 49.7g; Fat: 6.8g; Carbs: 8.4g

Grilled Tuna

Preparation time: 10 minutes

Cooking time: 6 minutes

Servings: 3

Ingredients:

3 tuna fillets

3 teaspoons teriyaki sauce

½ teaspoon minced garlic

1 teaspoon olive oil

Directions:

Whisk together teriyaki sauce, minced garlic, and olive oil.

Bruhs every tuna fillet with teriyaki mixture.

Preheat grill to 390F.

Grill the fish for 3 minutes from each side.

Nutrition: :calories 382, fat 32.6, fiber 0, carbs 1.1, protein 21.4

Rosemary Salmon

Preparation time: 10 minutes

Cooking time: 10 minutes

Servings: 3

Ingredients:

2-pound salmon fillet

2 tablespoons avocado oil

2 teaspoons fresh rosemary, chopped

½ teaspoon minced garlic

½ teaspoon dried cilantro

½ teaspoon salt

1 teaspoon butter

½ teaspoon white pepper

Directions:

Whisk together avocado oil, fresh rosemary, minced garlic, dried cilantro, salt, and white pepper.

Rub the salmon fillet with the rosemary mixture generously and leave fish in the fridge for 20 minutes to marinate.

After this, put butter in the saucepan or big skillet and melt it.

Then put heat on maximum and place a salmon fillet in the hot butter.

Roast it for 1 minute from each side.

After this, preheat grill to 385F and grill the fillet for 8 minutes (for 4 minutes from each side).

Cut the cooked salmon on the servings.

Nutrition: :calories 257, fat 12.8, fiber 0.5, carbs 0.9, protein 35.3

Easy Seafood French Stew

Preparation time: 10 minutes

Cooking time: 45 minutes

Servings: 12

Ingredients:

Pepper and Salt

1/2 lb. littleneck clams

1/2 lb. mussels

1 lb. shrimp, peeled and deveined

1 large lobster

2 lbs. assorted small whole fresh fish, scaled and cleaned

2 tbsp parsley, finely chopped

2 tbsp garlic, chopped

1 cup fennel, julienned

Juice and zest of one orange

3 cups tomatoes, peeled, seeded, and chopped

1 cup leeks, julienned

Pinch of Saffron

1 cup white wine

Water

1 lb. fish bones

2 sprigs thyme

8 peppercorns

1 bay leaf

3 cloves garlic

Salt and pepper

1/2 cup chopped celery

1/2 cup chopped onion

2 tbsp olive oil

Directions:

Do the stew: Heat oil in a large saucepan. Sauté the celery and onions for 3 minutes. Season with pepper and salt. Stir in the garlic and cook for about a minute. Add the thyme, peppercorns, and bay leaves. Stir in the wine, water and fish bones. Let it boil then before reducing to a simmer. Take the pan off the fire and strain broth into another container.

For the Bouillabaisse: Bring the strained broth to a simmer and stir in the parsley, leeks, orange juice, orange zest, garlic, fennel, tomatoes and saffron. Sprinkle with pepper and salt. Stir in the lobsters and fish. Let it simmer for eight minutes before stirring in the clams, mussels and shrimps. For six minutes, allow to cook while covered before seasoning again with pepper and salt.

Assemble in a shallow dish all the seafood and pour the broth over it.

Nutrition: Calories per serving: 348; Carbs: 20.0g; Protein: 31.8g; Fat: 15.2g

Avocado Dip

Preparation time: 10 minutes

Cooking time: 0 minutes

Servings: 8

Ingredients:

½ cup heavy cream

1 green chili pepper, chopped

Salt and pepper to the taste

4 avocados, pitted, peeled and chopped

1 cup cilantro, chopped

¼ cup lime juice

Directions:

In a blender, combine the cream with the avocados and the rest of the ingredients and pulse well.

Divide the mix into bowls and serve cold as a party dip.

Nutrition: calories 200, fat 14.5, fiber 3.8, carbs 8.1, protein 7.6

Feta And Roasted Red Pepper Bruschetta

Preparation time: 10 minutes

Cooking time: 15minutes

Servings: 8

Ingredients:

6 Kalamata olives, pitted, chopped

2 tablespoons green onion, minced

1/4 cup Parmesan cheese, grated, divided

1/4 cup extra-virgin olive oil brushing, or as needed

1/4 cup cherry tomatoes, thinly sliced

1 teaspoon lemon juice

1 tablespoon extra-virgin olive oil

1 tablespoon basil pesto

1 red bell pepper, halved, seeded

1 piece (12 inch) whole-wheat baguette, cut into 1/2-inch thick slices

1 package (4 ounce) feta cheese with basil and sun-dried tomatoes, crumbled

1 clove garlic, minced

Directions:

Preheat the oven broiler. Place the oven rack 6 inches from the source of heat.

Brush both sides of the baguette slices, with the 1/4 cup olive oil. Arrange the bread slices on a baking sheet; toast for about 1 minute each side, carefully watching to avoid burning. Remove the toasted slices, transferring into another baking sheet.

With the cut sides down, place the red peppers in a baking sheet; broil for about 8 to 10 minutes or until the skin is charred and blistered. Transfer the roasted peppers into a bowl; cover with plastic wrap. Let cool, remove the charred skin. Discard skin and chop the roasted peppers.

In a bowl, mix the roasted red peppers, cherry tomatoes, feta cheese, green onion, olives, pesto, 1 tablespoon olive oil, garlic, and lemon juice.

Top each bread with 1 tablespoon of the roasted pepper mix, sprinkle lightly with the Parmesan cheese.

Return the baking sheet with the topped bruschetta; broil for about 1-2 minutes or until the topping is lightly browned.

Nutrition: :73 cal., 4.8 g total fat (1.4 sat. fat), 5 mg chol., 138 mg sodium, 5.3 g total carbs., 0.4 g fiber, 0.6 g sugar, and 2.1 g protein.

Meat-filled Phyllo (samboosek)

Preparation time: 10 minutes

Cooking time: 10 minutes

Servings: 1

Ingredients:

1 lb. ground beef or lamb

1 medium yellow onion, finely chopped

1 TB. seven spices

1 tsp. salt

1 pkg. frozen phyllo dough (12 sheets)

2/3 cup butter, melted

Directions:

In a medium skillet over medium heat, brown beef for 3 minutes, breaking up chunks with a wooden spoon.

Add yellow onion, seven spices, and salt, and cook for 5 to 7 minutes or until beef is browned and onions are translucent. Set aside, and let cool.

Place first sheet of phyllo on your work surface, brush with melted butter, lay second sheet of phyllo on top, and brush with melted butter. Cut sheets into 3-inch-wide strips.

Spoon 2 tablespoons meat filling at end of each strip, and fold end strip to cover meat and form a triangle. Fold pointed end up and over to the opposite end, and you should see a triangle forming. Continue to fold up and then over until you come to the end of strip.

Place phyllo pies on a baking sheet, seal side down, and brush tops with butter. Repeat with remaining phyllo and filling.

Bake for 10 minutes or until golden brown.

Remove from the oven and set aside for 5 minutes before serving warm or at room temperature.

Nutrition: 242 Calories 25g carbs 12g fat 13g protein

Tasty Black Bean Dip

Preparation time: 10 minutes

Cooking time: 18 minutes

Servings: 3

Ingredients:

2 cups dry black beans, soaked overnight and drained

1 1/2 cups cheese, shredded

1 tsp dried oregano

1 1/2 tsp chili powder

2 cups tomatoes, chopped

2 tbsp olive oil

1 1/2 tbsp garlic, minced

1 medium onion, sliced

4 cups vegetable stock

Pepper

Salt

Directions:

Add all ingredients except cheese into the instant pot.

Seal pot with lid and cook on high for 18 minutes.

Once done, allow to release pressure naturally. Remove lid. Drain excess water.

Add cheese and stir until cheese is melted.

Blend bean mixture using an immersion blender until smooth.

Serve and enjoy.

Nutrition: Calories 402 Fat 15.3 g Carbohydrates 46.6 g Sugar 4.4 g Protein 22.2 g Cholesterol 30 mg

Zucchini Cakes

Preparation time: 10 minutes

Cooking time: 10 minutes

Servings: 4

Ingredients:

1 zucchini, grated

¼ carrot, grated

¼ onion, minced

1 teaspoon minced garlic

3 tablespoons coconut flour

1 teaspoon Italian seasonings

1 egg, beaten

1 teaspoon coconut oil

Directions:

In the mixing bowl combine together grated zucchini, carrot, minced onion, and garlic.

Add coconut flour, Italian seasoning, and egg.

Stir the mass until homogenous.

Heat up coconut oil in the skillet.

Place the small zucchini fritters in the hot oil. Make them with the help of the spoon.

Roast the zucchini fritters for 4 minutes from each side.

Nutrition: :calories 65, fat 3.3, fiber 3, carbs 6.3, protein 3.3

Parsley Nachos

Preparation time: 10 minutes

Cooking time: 0 minutes

Servings: 3

Ingredients:

3 oz tortilla chips

¼ cup Greek yogurt

1 tablespoon fresh parsley, chopped

¼ teaspoon minced garlic

2 kalamata olives, chopped

1 teaspoon paprika

¼ teaspoon ground thyme

Directions:

In the mixing bowl mix up together Greek yogurt, parsley, minced garlic, olives, paprika, and thyme.

Then add tortilla chips and mix up gently.

The snack should be served immediately.

Nutrition: :calories 81, fat 1.6, fiber 2.2, carbs 14.1, protein 3.5

Plum Wraps

Preparation time: 10 minutes

Cooking time: 10 minutes

Servings: 3

Ingredients:

4 plums

4 prosciutto slices

¼ teaspoon olive oil

Dirctions:

Preheat the oven to 375F.

Wrap every plum in prosciutto slice and secure with a toothpick (if needed).

Place the wrapped plums in the oven and bake for 10 minutes.

Nutrition: :calories 62, fat 2.2, fiber 0.9, carbs 8, protein 4.3

Parmesan Chips

Preparation time: 10 minutes

Cooking time: 20 minutes

Servings: 4

Ingredients:

1 zucchini

2 oz Parmesan, grated

½ teaspoon paprika

1 teaspoon olive oil

Directions:

Trim zucchini and slice it into the chips with the help of the vegetable slices.

Then mix up together Parmesan and paprika.

Sprinkle the zucchini chips with olive oil.

After this, dip every zucchini slice in the cheese mixture.

Place the zucchini chips in the lined baking tray and bake for 20 minutes at 375F.

Flip the zucchini sliced onto another side after 10 minutes of cooking.

Chill the cooked chips well.

Nutrition: :calories 64, fat 4.3, fiber 0.6, carbs 2.3, protein 5.2

Chicken Bites

Preparation time: 10 minutes

Cooking time: 5 minutes

Servings: 5

Ingredients:

½ cup coconut flakes

8 oz chicken fillet

¼ cup Greek yogurt

1 teaspoon dried dill

1 teaspoon salt

1 teaspoon ground black pepper

1 tablespoon tomato sauce

1 teaspoon honey

4 tablespoons sunflower oil

Directions:

Chop the chicken fillet on the small cubes (popcorn cubes)

Sprinkle them with dried dill, salt, and ground black pepper.

Then add Greek yogurt and stir carefully.

After this, pour sunflower oil in the skillet and heat it up.

Coat chicken cubes in the coconut flakes and roast in the hot oil for 3-4 minutes or until the popcorn cubes are golden brown.

Dry the popcorn chicken with the help of the paper towel.

Make the sweet sauce: whisk together honey and tomato sauce.

Serve the popcorn chicken hot or warm with sweet sauce.

Nutrition: :calories 107, fat 5.2, fiber 0.8, carbs 2.8, protein 12.1

Chicken Kale Wraps

Preparation time: 10 minutes

Cooking time: 10 minutes

Servings: 4

Ingredients:

4 kale leaves

4 oz chicken fillet

½ apple

1 tablespoon butter

¼ teaspoon chili pepper

¾ teaspoon salt

1 tablespoon lemon juice

¾ teaspoon dried thyme

Directions:

Chop the chicken fillet into the small cubes.

Then mix up together chicken with chili pepper and salt.

Heat up butter in the skillet.

Add chicken cubes. Roast them for 4 minutes.

Meanwhile, chop the apple into small cubes and add it in the chicken.

Mix up well.

Sprinkle the ingredients with lemon juice and dried thyme.

Cook them for 5 minutes over the medium-high heat.

Fill the kale leaves with the hot chicken mixture and wrap.

Nutrition: calories 106, fat 5.1, fiber 1.1, carbs 6.3, protein 9

Savory Pita Chips

Preparation time: 10 minutes

Cooking time: 10 minutes

Servings: 1

Ingredients:

3 pitas

1/4 cup extra-virgin olive oil

1/4 cup zaatar

Directions:

Preheat the oven to 450ºF.

Cut pitas into 2-inch pieces, and place in a large bowl.

Drizzle pitas with extra-virgin olive oil, sprinkle with zaatar, and toss to coat.

Spread out pitas on a baking sheet, and bake for 8 to 10 minutes or until lightly browned and crunchy.

Let pita chips cool before removing from the baking sheet. Store in an airtight container for up to 1 month.

Nutrition: 242 Calories 25g carbs 12g fat 13g protein

Artichoke Skewers

Preparation time: 10 minutes

Cooking time: 0 minutes

Servings: 4

Ingredients:

4 prosciutto slices

4 artichoke hearts, canned

4 kalamata olives

4 cherry tomatoes

¼ teaspoon cayenne pepper

¼ teaspoon sunflower oil

Directions:

Skewer prosciutto slices, artichoke hearts, kalamata olives, and cherry tomatoes on the wooden skewers.

Sprinkle antipasto skewers with sunflower oil and cayenne pepper.

Nutrition: :calories 152, fat 3.7, fiber 10.8, carbs 23.2, protein 11.1

Kidney Bean Spread

Preparation time: 10 minutes

Cooking time: 18 minutes

Servings: 3

Ingredients:

1 lb dry kidney beans, soaked overnight and drained

1 tsp garlic, minced

2 tbsp olive oil

1 tbsp fresh lemon juice

1 tbsp paprika

4 cups vegetable stock

1/2 cup onion, chopped

Pepper

Salt

Directions:

Add beans and stock into the instant pot.

Seal pot with lid and cook on high for 18 minutes.

Once done, allow to release pressure naturally. Remove lid.

Drain beans well and reserve 1/2 cup stock.

Transfer beans, reserve stock, and remaining ingredients into the food processor and process until smooth.

Serve and enjoy.

Nutrition: Calories 461 Fat 8.6 g Carbohydrates 73 g Sugar 4 g Protein 26.4 g Cholesterol 0 mg

Polenta Cups Recipe

Preparation time: 10 minutes

Cooking time: 20 minutes

Servings: 3

Ingredients:

1 cup yellow cornmeal

1 garlic clove, minced

1/2 teaspoon fresh thyme, minced or 1/4 teaspoon dried thyme

1/2 teaspoon salt

1/4 cup feta cheese, crumbled

1/4 teaspoon pepper

2 tablespoons fresh basil, chopped

4 cups water

4 plum tomatoes, finely chopped

Directions:

In a heavy, large saucepan, bring the water and the salt to a boil; reduce the heat to a gentle boil. Slowly whisk in the cornmeal; cook, stirring with a wooden spoon for about 15 to 20 minutes, or until the polenta is thick and pulls away cleanly from the sides of the pan. Remove from the heat; stir in the pepper and the thyme.

Grease miniature muffin cups with cooking spray. Spoon a heaping tablespoon of the polenta mixture into each muffin cups.

With the back of a spoon, make an indentation in the center of each; cover and chill until the mixture is set.

Meanwhile, combine the feta cheese, tomatoes, garlic, and basil in a small-sized bowl.

Unmold the chilled polenta cups; place them on an ungreased baking sheet. Tops each indentation with 1 heaping tablespoon of the feta mixture. Broil the cups 4 inches from the heat source for about 5 to 7 minutes, or until heated through.

Nutrition: :26 cal, 1 mg chol., 62 mg sodium, 5 g carbs., 1 g fiber, and 1 g protein.

Tomato Triangles

Preparation time: 10 minutes

Cooking time: 0 minutes

Servings: 6

Ingredients:

6 corn tortillas

1 tablespoon cream cheese

1 tablespoon ricotta cheese

½ teaspoon minced garlic

1 tablespoon fresh dill, chopped

2 tomatoes, sliced

Directions:

Cut every tortilla into 2 triangles.

Then mix up together cream cheese, ricotta cheese, minced garlic, and dill.

Spread 6 triangles with cream cheese mixture.

Then place sliced tomato on them and cover with remaining tortilla triangles.

Nutrition: :calories 71, fat 1.6, fiber 2.1, carbs 12.8, protein 2.3

Chili Mango And Watermelon Salsa

Preparation time: 10 minutes

Cooking time: 0 minutes

Servings: 8

Ingredients:

1 red tomato, chopped

Salt and black pepper to the taste

1 cup watermelon, seedless, peeled and cubed

1 red onion, chopped

2 mangos, peeled and chopped

2 chili peppers, chopped

¼ cup cilantro, chopped

3 tablespoons lime juice

Pita chips for serving

Directions:

In a bowl, mix the tomato with the watermelon, the onion and the rest of the ingredients except the pita chips and toss well.

Divide the mix into small cups and serve with pita chips on the side.

Nutrition: calories 62, fat 4.7, fiber 1.3, carbs 3.9, protein 2.3

Tomato Olive Salsa

Preparation time: 10 minutes

Cooking time: 5 minutes

Servings: 3

Ingredients:

2 cups olives, pitted and chopped

1/4 cup fresh parsley, chopped

1/4 cup fresh basil, chopped

2 tbsp green onion, chopped

1 cup grape tomatoes, halved

1 tbsp olive oil

1 tbsp vinegar

Pepper

Salt

Directions:

Add all ingredients into the inner pot of instant pot and stir well.

Seal pot with lid and cook on high for 5 minutes.

Once done, allow to release pressure naturally for 5 minutes then release remaining using quick release. Remove lid.

Stir well and serve.

Nutrition: Calories 119 Fat 10.8 g Carbohydrates 6.5 g Sugar 1.3 g Protein 1.2 g Cholesterol 0 mg

Lavash Chips

Preparation time: 10 minutes

Cooking time: 30 minutes

Servings: 3

Ingredients:

1 lavash sheet, whole grain

1 tablespoon canola oil

1 teaspoon paprika

½ teaspoon chili pepper

½ teaspoon salt

Directions:

In the shallow bowl whisk together canola oil, paprika, chili pepper, and salt.

Then chop lavash sheet roughly (in the shape of chips).

Sprinkle lavash chips with oil mixture and arrange in the tray to get one thin layer.

Bake the lavash chips for 10 minutes at 365F. Flip them on another side from time to time to avoid burning.

Cool the cooked chips well.

Nutrition: :calories 73, fat 4, fiber 0.7, carbs 8.4, protein 1.6

Homemade Salsa

Preparation time: 10 minutes

Cooking time: 30 minutes

Servings: 8

Ingredients:

12 oz grape tomatoes, halved

1/4 cup fresh cilantro, chopped

1 fresh lime juice

28 oz tomatoes, crushed

1 tbsp garlic, minced

1 green bell pepper, chopped

1 red bell pepper, chopped

2 onions, chopped

6 whole tomatoes

Salt

Directions:

Add whole tomatoes into the instant pot and gently smash the tomatoes.

Add remaining ingredients except cilantro, lime juice, and salt and stir well.

Seal pot with lid and cook on high for 5 minutes.

Once done, allow to release pressure naturally for 10 minutes then release remaining using quick release. Remove lid.

Add cilantro, lime juice, and salt and stir well.

Serve and enjoy.

Nutrition: Calories 146 Fat 1.2 g Carbohydrates 33.2 g Sugar 4 g Protein 6.9 g Cholesterol 0 mg

Stuffed Zucchinis

Preparation time: 10 minutes

Cooking time: 30 minutes

Servings: 6

Ingredients:

6 zucchinis, halved lengthwise and insides scooped out

2 garlic cloves, minced

2 tablespoons oregano, chopped

Juice of 2 lemons

Salt and black pepper to the taste

2 tablespoons olive oil

8 ounces feta cheese, crumbed

Directions:

Arrange the zucchini halves on a baking sheet lined with parchment paper, divide the cheese and the rest of the ingredients in each zucchini half and bake at 450 degrees F for 40 minutes.

Arrange the stuffed zucchinis on a platter and serve as an appetizer.

Nutrition: 242 Calories 25g carbs 12g fat 13g protein

Yogurt Dip

Preparation time: 10 minutes

Cooking time: 0 minutes

Servings: 5

Ingredients:

2 cups Greek yogurt

2 tablespoons pistachios, toasted and chopped

A pinch of salt and white pepper

2 tablespoons mint, chopped

1 tablespoon kalamata olives, pitted and chopped

¼ cup za'atar spice

¼ cup pomegranate seeds

1/3 cup olive oil

Directions:

In a bowl, combine the yogurt with the pistachios and the rest of the ingredients, whisk well, divide into small cups and serve with pita chips on the side.

Nutrition: calories 294, fat 18, fiber 1, carbs 21, protein 10

Popcorn-pine Nut Mix

Preparation time: 10 minutes

Cooking time: 10 minutes

Servings: 3

Ingredients:

1 tablespoon olive oil

1/2 cup pine nuts

1/2 teaspoon Italian seasoning

1/4 cup popcorn, white kernels, popped

1/4 teaspoon salt

2 tablespoons honey

1/2 lemon zest

Directions:

Place the popped corn in a medium bowl.

In a dry pan or skillet over low heat, toast the pine nuts, stirring frequently for about 4 to 5 minutes, until fragrant and some begin to brown; remove from the heat.

Stir the oil in; add honey, the Italian seasoning, the lemon zest, and the salt. Stir to mix and pour over the popcorn; toss the ingredients to coat the popcorn kernels with the honey syrup.

It's alright if most of the nuts sink in the bowl bottom.

Let the mixture sit for about 2 minutes to allow the honey to cool and to get stickier.

Transfer the bowl contents into a Servings: bowl so the nuts are on the top. Gently stir and serve.

Nutrition: :80 cal, 6 g total fat (0.5 g sat. fat), 0 mg chol., 105 mg sodium, 60 mg pot., 5 total carbs., <1 g fiber, 4 g sugar, 2 g protein, 2% vitamin A, 8% vitamin C, 4% calcium, and 4% iron.

Scallions Dip

Preparation time: 10 minutes

Cooking time: 0 minutes

Servings: 8

Ingredients:

6 scallions, chopped

1 garlic clove, minced

3 tablespoons olive oil

Salt and black pepper to the taste

1 tablespoon lemon juice

1 and ½ cups cream cheese, soft

2 ounces prosciutto, cooked and crumbled

Directions:

In a bowl, mix the scallions with the garlic and the rest of the ingredients except the prosciutto and whisk well.

Divide into bowls, sprinkle the prosciutto on top and serve as a party dip.

Nutrition: calories 144, fat 7.7, fiber 1.4, carbs 6.3, protein 5.5

Date Balls

Preparation time: 10 minutes

Cooking time: 5 minutes

Servings: 3

Ingredients:

3 dates, pitted

3 pistachio nuts

½ teaspoon butter, softened, salted

Directions:

Fill dates with butter and pistachio nuts.

Bake the preparation ared dates for 5 minutes at 395F.

Chill the cooked appetizer to the room temperature.

Nutrition: :calories 42, fat 1.8, fiber 0.9, carbs 6.9, protein 0.7

Lavash Roll Ups

Preparation time: 10 minutes

Cooking time: 10 minutes

Servings: 4

Ingredients:

2 lavash wraps (whole-wheat)

1/4 cup roasted red peppers, sliced

1/4 cup black olives, sliced

1/2 cup hummus of choice

1/2 cup grape tomatoes, halved

1 Medium cucumber, sliced

Fresh dill, for garnish

Directions:

Lay out the lavash wraps on a clean surface. Evenly spread hummus over each piece.

Layer the cucumbers across the wraps, about 1/2-inch from each other, leaving about 2-icnh empty space at the bottom of the wrap for rolling purposes.

Place the roasted pepper slices around the cucumbers. Sprinkle with black olives and the tomatoes. Garnish with freshly chopped dill.

Tightly roll each wrap, using the hummus at the end to almost glue the wrap into a roll.

Slice each roll into 4 equal pieces. Secure each piece by sticking a toothpick through the center of each roll slice.

Lay each on a serving bowl or tray; garnish more with fresh dill.

Nutrition: :250 cal, 8 g total fat (0.5 g sat. fat), 0 mg chol., 440 mg sodium, 340 mg pot., 43 total carbs., 40 g fiber, 3 g sugar, 10 g protein, 15% vitamin A, 25% vitamin C, 6% calcium, and 8% iron.

Chickpeas And Eggplant Bowls

Preparation time: 10 minutes

Cooking time: 30 minutes

Servings: 5

Ingredients:

2 eggplants, cut in half lengthwise and cubed

1 red onion, chopped

Juice of 1 lime

1 tablespoon olive oil

28 ounces canned chickpeas, drained and rinsed

1 bunch parsley, chopped

A pinch of salt and black pepper

1 tablespoon balsamic vinegar

Directions:

Spread the eggplant cubes on a baking sheet lined with parchment paper, drizzle half of the oil all over, season with salt and pepper and cook at 425 degrees F for 10 minutes.

Cool the eggplant down, add the rest of the ingredients, toss, divide between appetizer plates and serve.

Nutrition: calories 263, fat 12, fiber 9.3, carbs 15.4, protein 7.5

Vinegar Beet Bites

Preparation time: 10 minutes

Cooking time: 30 minutes

Servings: 4

Ingredients:

2 beets, sliced

A pinch of sea salt and black pepper

1/3 cup balsamic vinegar

1 cup olive oil

Directions:

Spread the beet slices on a baking sheet lined with parchment paper, add the rest of the ingredients, toss and bake at 350 degrees F for 30 minutes.

Serve the beet bites cold as a snack.

Nutrition: calories 199, fat 5.4, fiber 3.5, carbs 8.5, protein 3.5

Baked Sweet-potato Fries

Preparation time: 10 minutes

Cooking time: 20 minutes

Servings: 6

Ingredients:

1 1/2 teaspoons dried oregano

1 teaspoon dried thyme

1 teaspoon garlic powder

1/2 teaspoon salt

2 large sweet potatoes (about 2 pounds), skins on, scrubbed, cut into 1/2-inch thick 4-inch long sticks

3 large egg whites (a scant 1/2 cup)

Vegetable oil, for the parchment

For the Mediterranean spice:

Oregano

Thyme

Garlic

Directions:

Place all of the Mediterranean spice ingredients in a small food processor or a spice grinder; briefly grind or process to blend.

Place the oven racks in the middle and upper position; preheat the oven to 450F.

Line 2 baking sheets with parchment paper; rub the paper with the oil.

Put the potatoes in a microwavable container, cover, and microwave for 2 minutes. Stir gently, cover, and microwave for about 1-2 minutes more or until the pieces are pliable; let rest for about 5 minutes covered. Pour into a platter.

In a large-sized bowl, whisk the eggs until frothy. Add the spice mix and whisk again to blend.

Working in batches, toss the sweet potatoes in the seasoned egg whites letting the excess liquid drip back into the bowl. Arrange the coated potatoes in a single layer on the preparation ared baking sheets.

Bake for 10 minutes; flip the pieces over using a spatula. Rotate the baking sheets from back to front and one to the other; bake for about 15 minutes or until dark golden brown. Serve immediately.

Nutrition: :100 cal., 4 g total fat (0 g sat. fat), 0 mg chol., 60 mg sodium, 230 mg pot., 12 g total carbs., 2 g fiber, 2 g sugar, 3 g protein, 150% vitamin A, 2% vitamin C, 4% calcium, and 6% iron.

Cucumber Rolls

Preparation time: 10 minutes

Cooking time: 0 minutes

Servings: 3

Ingredients:

1 big cucumber, sliced lengthwise

1 tablespoon parsley, chopped

8 ounces canned tuna, drained and mashed

Salt and black pepper to the taste

1 teaspoon lime juice

Directions:

Arrange cucumber slices on a working surface, divide the rest of the ingredients, and roll.

Arrange all the rolls on a platter and serve as an appetizer.

Nutrition: calories 200, fat 6, fiber 3.4, carbs 7.6, protein 3.5

Jalapeno Chickpea Hummus

Preparation time: 10 minutes

Cooking time: 20 minutes

Servings: 3

Ingredients:

1 cup dry chickpeas, soaked overnight and drained

1 tsp ground cumin

1/4 cup jalapenos, diced

1/2 cup fresh cilantro

1 tbsp tahini

1/2 cup olive oil

Pepper

Salt

Directions:

Add chickpeas into the instant pot and cover with vegetable stock.

Seal pot with lid and cook on high for 25 minutes.

Once done, allow to release pressure naturally. Remove lid.

Drain chickpeas well and transfer into the food processor along with remaining ingredients and process until smooth.

Serve and enjoy.

Nutrition: Calories 425 Fat 30.4 g Carbohydrates 31.8 g Sugar 5.6 g Protein 10.5 g Cholesterol 0 mg

Healthy Spinach Dip

Preparation time: 10 minutes

Cooking time: 8 minutes

Servings: 4

Ingredients:

14 oz spinach

2 tbsp fresh lime juice

1 tbsp garlic, minced

2 tbsp olive oil

2 tbsp coconut cream

Pepper

Salt

Directions:

Add all ingredients except coconut cream into the instant pot and stir well.

Seal pot with lid and cook on low pressure for 8 minutes.

Once done, allow to release pressure naturally for 5 minutes then release remaining using quick release. Remove lid.

Add coconut cream and stir well and blend spinach mixture using a blender until smooth.

Serve and enjoy.

Nutrition: Calories 109 Fat 9.2 g Carbohydrates 6.6 g Sugar 1.1 g Protein 3.2 g Cholesterol 0 mg

Marinated Cheese

Preparation time: 10 minutes

Cooking time: 10 minutes

Servings: 3

Ingredients:

8 ounces cream cheese

6 sprigs fresh thyme

3 sprigs fresh rosemary

2 garlic cloves, sliced

1/2 cup sun-dried tomato vinaigrette dressing

1 teaspoon black pepper

1 lemon peel, cut into thin strips

Directions:

Cut the cream cheese into 36 cubes. Place on a serving tray.

Combine the remaining ingredients together.

Pour the dressing over the cheese; toss lightly.

Refrigerate for at least 1 hour to marinate.

Nutrition: :44 cal., 4.3 g total fat (2.4 sat. fat), 13.9 mg chol., 40.6 mg sodium, 0.7 g total carbs., 0 g fiber, 0.4 g sugar, and 0.8 g protein.

Za'atar Fries

Preparation time: 10 minutes

Cooking time: 35 minutes

Servings: 3

Ingredients:

1 teaspoon Za'atar spices

3 sweet potatoes

1 tablespoon dried dill

1 teaspoon salt

3 teaspoons sunflower oil

½ teaspoon paprika

Directions:

Pour water in the crockpot. Peel the sweet potatoes and cut them into the fries.

Line the baking tray with parchment.

Place the layer of the sweet potato in the tray.

Sprinkle the vegetables with dried dill, salt, and paprika.

Then sprinkle sweet potatoes with Za'atar and mix up well with the help of the fingertips.

Sprinkle the sweet potato fries with sunflower oil.

Preheat the oven to 375F.

Bake the sweet potato fries for 35 minutes. Stir the fries every 10 minutes.

Nutrition: :calories 28, fat 2.9, fiber 0.2, carbs 0.6, protein 0.2

Tuna Salad

Preparation time: 10 minutes

Cooking time: 30 minutes

Servings: 6

Ingredients:

1 can (5 ounce) albacore tuna, solid white

1 to 2 tablespoons mayo or Greek yogurt

1 whole-wheat crackers (I used sleeve Ritz®)

1/4 cup chickpeas, rinsed, drained (or preferred white beans)

1/4 cup Kalamata olives, quartered

1/4 cup roughly chopped marinated artichoke hearts

Directions:

Flake the tuna out of the can into medium-sized bowl.

Add the chickpeas, olives, and artichoke hearts; toss to combine.

Add mayo or Greek yogurt according to your taste; stir until well combined.

Spoon the salad mixture onto crackers; serve.

Nutrition: :130 cal., 5 g total fat (0.5 g sat. fat), 25 mg chol., 240 mg sodium, 240 mg pot., 8 g total carbs., 1 g fiber, <1 g sugar, 12 g protein, 2% vitamin A, 2% vitamin C, 4% calcium, and 6% iron.

Cheese Rolls

Preparation time: 10 minutes

Cooking time: 5 minutes

Servings: 1

Ingredients:

1 cup ackawi cheese

1 cup shredded mozzarella cheese

2 TB. fresh parsley, finely chopped

1 large egg

1/2 tsp. ground black pepper

1 large egg yolk, beaten

2 TB. water

1 pkg. egg roll dough (20 count)

4 TB. extra-virgin olive oil

Directions:

In a large bowl, combine ackawi cheese, mozzarella cheese, parsley, egg, and black pepper.

In a small bowl, whisk together egg yolk and water.

Lay out 1 egg roll, place 2 tablespoons cheese mixture at one corner of egg roll, and brush opposite corner with egg yolk mixture.

Fold over side of egg roll, with cheese, to the middle. Fold in left and right sides, and complete rolling egg roll, using egg-brushed side to seal. Set aside, seal side down, and repeat with remaining egg rolls and cheese mixture.

In a skillet over low heat, heat 2 tablespoons extra-virgin olive oil. Add up to 4 cheese rolls, seal side down, and cook for 1 or 2 minutes per side or until browned. Repeat with remaining 2 tablespoons extra-virgin olive oil and egg rolls.

Serve warm.

Nutrition: 242 Calories 25g carbs 12g fat 13g protein

Olive, Pepperoni, And Mozzarella Bites

Preparation time: 10 minutes

Cooking time: 30 minutes

Servings: 2

Ingredients:

1 pound block Mozzarella cheese

1 package pepperoni

1 can whole medium black olives

Directions:

Slice the block of mozzarella cheese into 1/2x1/2-inch cubes. Drain the olives from the liquid.

With a toothpick, skewer the olive, pushing it 1/3 way up the toothpick.

Fold a pepperoni into half or quarters and skewer after the olive.

Finally, skewer a mozzarella cheese, not pushing all the way through the cube, about only half way through. Repeat with the remaining olives, pepperoni, and mozzarella cubes.

Nutrition: :75 cal., 5.6 g total fat (2.5 g sat. fat), 14 mg chol., 221 mg sodium, 16 mg pot., 0.8 g total carbs., 0 g fiber, 0 g sugar, 5.6 g protein, 3% vitamin A, 0% vitamin C, 11% calcium, and 1% iron.

Eggplant Dip

Preparation time: 10 minutes

Cooking time: 40 minutes

Servings: 3

Ingredients:

1 eggplant, poked with a fork

2 tablespoons tahini paste

2 tablespoons lemon juice

2 garlic cloves, minced

1 tablespoon olive oil

Salt and black pepper to the taste

1 tablespoon parsley, chopped

Directions:

Put the eggplant in a roasting pan, bake at 400 degrees F for 40 minutes, cool down, peel and transfer to your food processor.

Add the rest of the ingredients except the parsley, pulse well, divide into small bowls and serve as an appetizer with the parsley sprinkled on top.

Nutrition: calories 121, fat 4.3, fiber 1, carbs 1.4, protein 4.3

Roasted Chickpeas

Preparation time: 10 minutes

Cooking time: 30 minutes

Servings: 3

Ingredients

1 C. cooked chickpeas

1 small garlic clove, minced

½ tsp. dried oregano, crushed

1/8 tsp. ground cumin

1/8 tsp. smoked paprika

Pinch of cayenne pepper

Salt, to taste

½ tbsp. olive oil

Directions

Preheat the oven to 400 degrees F. Grease a large baking sheet.

Place chickpeas in the preparation ared baking sheet in a single layer.

Roast for about 30 minutes, stirring the after every 10 minutes.

Meanwhile, in a small mixing bowl, mix together garlic, thyme and spices.

Remove the baking sheet from oven.

Add the garlic mixture and oil and toss to coat well.

Roast for about 10-15 minutes more.

Now, turn the oven off but keep the baking sheet in oven for about 10 minutes.

Nutrition: 242 Calories 25g carbs 12g fat 13g protein

Pita Chips

Preparation time: 10 minutes

Cooking time: 30 minutes

Servings: 3

Ingredients

6 whole wheat pitas, cut each into 8 wedges

2 tsp. olive oil

Red chili powder, to taste

Garlic powder, to taste

Pinch of salt

Directions

Preheat the oven to 400 degrees F.

In the bottom of a large baking sheet, place the pita wedges.

Brush the both sides of each with oil and sprinkle with chili powder, garlic powder and salt.

Now, arrange the pita wedges in a single layer.

Bake for about 8 minutes or until golden brown.

Serve with your favorite dip.

Nutrition: 242 Calories 25g carbs 12g fat 13g protein

Kale Chips

Preparation time: 10 minutes

Cooking time: 5 minutes

Servings: 3

Ingredients

1 lb. fresh kale leaves, stemmed and torn

¼ tsp. cayenne pepper

Salt, to taste

1 tbs. olive oil

Directions

Preheat the oven to 350 degrees F. Line a large baking sheet with a parchment paper.

Place the kale pieces onto preparation ared baking sheet in a single layer.

Sprinkle the kale with cayenne and salt and drizzle with oil.

Bake for about 10-15 minutes.

Nutrition: 242 Calories 25g carbs 12g fat 13g protein

Blueberry Granola Bars

Preparation time: 10 minutes

Cooking time: 10 minutes

Servings: 3

Ingredients

½ C. rolled oats

2 tbsp. flaxseeds

1 tbsp. sunflower seeds

1 tbsp. walnuts, chopped

2 tbsp. raisins

¾ C. fresh blueberries

1 banana, peeled and mashed

2 tbsp. dates, pitted and chopped finely

1 tbsp. fresh pomegranate juice

Directions

Preheat your oven to 350 degrees F. Lightly, grease an 8-inch baking dish.

In a large bowl, add all ingredients and mix until well combined.

Place the mixture into preparation ared baking dish evenly and with the back of a spoon, smooth the surface.

Bake for about 25 minutes.

Remove from oven and keep onto a wire rack to cool.

With a sharp knife, cut into desired size bars and serve.

Nutrition: 448 Calories 27g fat 41g carbs 15g protein

Veggie Balls

Preparation time: 10 minutes

Cooking time: 30 minutes

Servings: 3

Ingredients

2 medium sweet potatoes, peeled and cubed into ½-inch size

2 tbsp. unsweetened coconut milk

1 C. fresh kale leaves, trimmed and chopped

1 medium shallot, chopped finely

1 tsp. ground cumin

½ tsp. granulated garlic

¼ tsp. ground turmeric

Salt and freshly ground black pepper, to taste

Ground flax seeds, as required

Directions

Preheat the oven to 400 degrees F. Line a baking sheet with parchment paper.

In a pan of water, arrange a steamer basket.

Place the sweet potato in steamer basket and steam for about 10-15 minutes.

In a large bowl, place the sweet potato with the coconut milk and mash well.

Add remaining ingredients except flax seeds and mix till well combined.

Make about 1½-2-inch balls from the mixture.

Arrange the balls onto preparation ared baking sheet in a single layer and sprinkle with flax seeds.

Bake for about 20-25 minutes.

Nutrition: 448 Calories 27g fat 41g carbs 15g protein

Oatmeal Cookies

Preparation time: 10 minutes

Cooking time: 30 minutes

Servings: 3

Ingredients

¾ C. whole wheat flour

1 C. instant oats

1½ tsp. organic baking powder

1½ tsp. ground cinnamon

1/8 tsp. salt

1 large organic egg, room temperature

½ C. organic honey

2 tbsp. coconut oil, melted

1 tsp. organic vanilla extract

1 C. red apple, cored and chopped finely

Directions

In a large bowl, mix together flour, oats, baking powder, cinnamon and salt.

In another bowl, add remaining ingredients except apple and beat until well combined.

Add the flour mixture and mix until just combined.

Gently, fold in the apple.

Refrigerate for about 30 minutes.

Preheat the oven to 325 degrees F. Line a large baking sheet with parchment paper.

Place about 2 tbsp. of the mixture onto the preparation ared baking sheet in the shape of small mounds.

With the back of a spoon, flatten each cookie slightly

Bake for about 13-15 minutes.

Cool on the pan for 10 minutes before turning out onto a wire rack.

Remove from oven and keep onto a wire rack to cool for about 5 minutes.

Carefully invert the cookies onto the wire rack to cool completely before serving.

Nutrition: 448 Calories 27g fat 41g carbs 15g protein

Deviled Avocado Eggs

Preparation time: 10 minutes

Cooking time: 30 minutes

Servings: 3

Ingredients

6 large organic eggs

1 medium avocado, peeled, pitted and chopped

2 tsp. fresh lime juice

Salt, to taste

Cayenne pepper, to taste

Directions

In a pan of water, add eggs and cook for about 15-20 minutes.

Drain and keep aside to cool completely.

Peel the eggs and with a sharp knife, slice them in half vertically.

Scoop out the yolks.

In a bowl, add half of egg yolks, avocado, lime juice and salt and with a fork, mash until well combined.

Scoop the avocado mixture in the egg halves evenly.

Serve with the sprinkling of cayenne pepper.

Nutrition: 448 Calories 27g fat 41g carbs 15g protein

Berry & Veggie Gazpacho

Preparation time: 10 minutes

Cooking time: 30 minutes

Servings: 3

Ingredients

1½ lb. fresh strawberries, hulled and sliced

½ C. red bell pepper, seeded and chopped

1 small cucumber, peeled, seeded and chopped

¼ C. onion, chopped

¼ C. fresh basil leaves

1 small garlic clove, chopped

¼ of small jalapeño pepper, seeded and chopped

1 tbsp. olive oil

3 tbsp. balsamic vinegar

Directions

In a high-speed blender, add all ingredients and pulse until smooth.

Transfer the gazpacho into a large bowl.

Cover and refrigerate to chill completely before serving.

Nutrition: 448 Calories 27g fat 41g carbs 15g protein

Healthy Guacamole

Preparation time: 10 minutes

Cooking time: 30 minutes

Servings: 3

Ingredients

2 medium ripe avocados, peeled, pitted and chopped

1 small red onion, chopped

1 garlic clove, minced

1 Serrano pepper, seeded and chopped

1 tomato, seeded and chopped

2 tbsp. fresh cilantro leaves, chopped

1 tbsp. fresh lime juice

Salt, to taste

Directions

In a large bowl, add avocado and with a fork, mash it completely.

Add remaining all ingredients and gently stir to combine.

Serve immediately.

Nutrition: 448 Calories 27g fat 41g carbs 15g protein

Healthy Poached Trout

Preparation time: 10 minutes

Cooking time: 10 minutes

Servings: 2

Ingredients:

1 8-oz boneless, skin on trout fillet

2 cups chicken broth or water

2 leeks, halved

6-8 slices lemon

salt and pepper to taste

Directions:

On medium fire, place a large nonstick skillet and arrange leeks and lemons on pan in a layer. Cover with soup stock or water and bring to a simmer.

Meanwhile, season trout on both sides with pepper and salt. Place trout on simmering pan of water. Cover and cook until trout is flaky, around 8 minutes.

In a serving platter, spoon leek and lemons on bottom of plate, top with trout and spoon sauce into plate. Serve and enjoy.

Nutrition: Calories per serving: 360.2; Protein: 13.8g; Fat: 7.5g; Carbs: 51.5g

Creamy Curry Salmon

Preparation time: 10 minutes

Cooking time: 30 minutes

Servings: 2

Ingredients:

2 salmon fillets, boneless and cubed

1 tablespoon olive oil

1 tablespoon basil, chopped

Sea salt and black pepper to the taste

1 cup Greek yogurt

2 teaspoons curry powder

1 garlic clove, minced

½ teaspoon mint, chopped

Directions:

Heat up a pan with the oil over medium-high heat, add the salmon and cook for 3 minutes.

Add the rest of the ingredients, toss, cook for 15 minutes more, divide between plates and serve.

Nutrition: calories 284, fat 14.1, fiber 8.5, carbs 26.7, protein 31.4

Cod And Cabbage

Preparation time: 10 minutes

Cooking time: 15 minutes

Servings: 4

Ingredients:

3 cups green cabbage, shredded

1 sweet onion, sliced

A pinch of salt and black pepper

½ cup feta cheese, crumbled

4 teaspoons olive oil

4 cod fillets, boneless

¼ cup green olives, pitted and chopped

Directions:

Grease a roasting pan with the oil, add the fish, the cabbage and the rest of the ingredients, introduce in the pan and cook at 450 degrees F for 15 minutes.

Divide the mix between plates and serve.

Nutrition: calories 270, fat 10, fiber 3, carbs 12, protein 31

Pecan Salmon Fillets

Preparation time: 10 minutes

Cooking time: 30 minutes

Servings: 6

Ingredients:

3 tablespoons olive oil

3 tablespoons mustard

5 teaspoons honey

1 cup pecans, chopped

6 salmon fillets, boneless

1 tablespoon lemon juice

3 teaspoons parsley, chopped

Salt and pepper to the taste

Directions:

In a bowl, mix the oil with the mustard and honey and whisk well.

Put the pecans and the parsley in another bowl.

Season the salmon fillets with salt and pepper, arrange them on a baking sheet lined with parchment paper, brush with the honey and mustard mix and top with the pecans mix.

Introduce in the oven at 400 degrees F, bake for 15 minutes, divide between plates, drizzle the lemon juice on top and serve.

Nutrition: calories 282, fat 15.5, fiber 8.5, carbs 20.9, protein 16.8

Shrimp And Mushrooms Mix

Preparation time: 10 minutes

Cooking time: 30 minutes

Servings: 4

Ingredients:

1 pound shrimp, peeled and deveined

2 green onions, sliced

½ pound white mushrooms, sliced

2 tablespoons balsamic vinegar

2 tablespoons sesame seeds, toasted

2 teaspoons ginger, minced

2 teaspoons garlic, minced

3 tablespoons olive oil

2 tablespoons dill, chopped

Directions:

Heat up a pan with the oil over medium-high heat, add the green onions and the garlic and sauté for 2 minutes.

Add the rest of the ingredients except the shrimp and cook for 6 minutes more.

Add the shrimp, cook for 4 minutes, divide everything between plates and serve.

Nutrition: calories 245, fat 8.5, fiber 45.8, carbs 11.8, protein 17.7

Leeks And Calamari Mix

Preparation time: 10 minutes

Cooking time: 15 minutes

Servings: 6

Ingredients:

2 tablespoon avocado oil

2 leeks, chopped

1 red onion, chopped

Salt and black to the taste

1 pound calamari rings

1 tablespoon parsley, chopped

1 tablespoon chives, chopped

2 tablespoons tomato paste

Directions:

Heat up a pan with the avocado oil over medium heat, add the leeks and the onion, stir and sauté for 5 minutes.

Add the rest of the ingredients, toss, simmer over medium heat for 10 minutes, divide into bowls and serve.

Nutrition: calories 238, fat 9, fiber 5.6, carbs 14.4, protein 8.4

Cod With Lentils

Preparation time: 10 minutes

Cooking time: 30 minutes

Servings: 4

Ingredients:

1 red pepper, chopped

1 yellow onion, diced

1 teaspoon ground black pepper

1 teaspoon butter

1 jalapeno pepper, chopped

½ cup lentils

3 cups chicken stock

1 teaspoon salt

1 tablespoon tomato paste

1 teaspoon chili pepper

3 tablespoons fresh cilantro, chopped

8 oz cod, chopped

Directions:

Place butter, red pepper, onion, and ground black pepper in the saucepan.

Roast the vegetables for 5 minutes over the medium heat.

Then add chopped jalapeno pepper, lentils, and chili pepper.

Mix up the mixture well and add chicken stock and tomato paste.

Stir until homogenous. Add cod.

Close the lid and cook chili for 20 minutes over the medium heat.

Nutrition: :calories 187, fat 2.3, fiber 8.8, carbs 21.3, protein 20.6

Honey Garlic Shrimp

Preparation time: 10 minutes

Cooking time: 5 minutes

Servings: 3

Ingredients:

1 lb shrimp, peeled and deveined

1/4 cup honey

1 tbsp garlic, minced

1 tbsp ginger, minced

1 tbsp olive oil

1/4 cup fish stock

Pepper

Salt

Directions:

Add shrimp into the large bowl. Add remaining ingredients over shrimp and toss well.

Transfer shrimp into the instant pot and stir well.

Seal pot with lid and cook on high for 5 minutes.

Once done, release pressure using quick release. Remove lid.

Serve and enjoy.

Nutrition: Calories 240 Fat 5.6 g Carbohydrates 20.9 g Sugar 17.5 g Protein 26.5 g Cholesterol 239 mg

Pepper Salmon Skewers

Preparation time: 10 minutes

Cooking time: 15 minutes

Servings: 5

Ingredients:

1.5-pound salmon fillet

½ cup Plain yogurt

1 teaspoon paprika

1 teaspoon turmeric

1 teaspoon red pepper

1 teaspoon salt

1 teaspoon dried cilantro

1 teaspoon sunflower oil

½ teaspoon ground nutmeg

Directions:

For the marinade: mix up together Plain yogurt, paprika, turmeric red pepper, salt, and ground nutmeg.

Chop the salmon fillet roughly and put it in the yogurt mixture.

Mix up well and marinate for 25 minutes.

Then skew the fish on the skewers.

Sprinkle the skewers with sunflower oil and place in the tray.

Bake the salmon skewers for 15 minutes at 375F.

Nutrition: :calories 217, fat 9.9, fiber 0.6, carbs 4.2, protein 28.1

Orange Salsa

Preparation time: 10 minutes

Cooking time: 30 minutes

Servings: 3

Ingredients

1½ C. fresh mango, cut into chunks

1½ C. fresh pineapple, peeled, pitted and cubed

¼ C. red onion, chopped

2 tbsp. fresh cilantro, chopped

2 tbsp. fresh orange juice

Salt and freshly ground black pepper, to taste

2 tbsp. unsweetened coconut, shredded

Directions

In a large bowl, add all ingredients except coconut and gently toss to coat well.

Serve immediately with the topping of coconut.

Nutrition: 448 Calories 27g fat 41g carbs 15g protein

Raw Broccoli Poppers

Preparation Time: 2 minutes

Cooking Time: 8 minutes

Servings: 4

Ingredients:

1/8 cup water

1/8 tsp. fine sea salt

4 cups broccoli florets, washed and cut into 1-inch pieces

1/4 tsp. turmeric powder

1 cup unsalted cashews, soaked overnight or at least 3-4 hours and drained

1/4 tsp. onion powder

1 red bell pepper, seeded and

2 tbsp. nutritional heaping

2 tbsp. lemon juice

Directions:

Transfer the drained cashews to a high-speed blender and pulse for about 30 seconds. Add in the chopped pepper and pulse again for 30 seconds.

Add 2 tbsp. of lemon juice, 1/8 cup of water, 2 tbsp. of nutritional yeast/ heaping, ¼ tsp. of onion powder, 1/8 of tsp. fine sea salt, and 1/4 tsp. of turmeric powder. Pulse for about 45 seconds until smooth.

Handover the broccoli into a bowl and add in the chopped cheesy cashew mixture. Toss well until coated.

Transfer the pieces of broccoli to the trays of a yeast dehydrator.

Follow the dehydrator's instructions and dehydrate for about 8 minutes at 125°F or until crunchy.

Nutrition:

Calories: 408

Fats: 32 g

Carbs: 22 g

Protein: 15 g

Candied Ginger

Preparation Time: 10 minutes

Cooking Time: 40 minutes

Servings: 3-5

Ingredients:

2 1/2 cups salted pistachios, shelled

1 1/4 tsp. powdered ginger

3 tbsp. pure maple syrup

Directions:

Add 1 1/4 tsp. of powdered ginger to a bowl with pistachios. Stir well until combined. There

Should be no lumps.

Drizzle with 3 tbsp. of maple syrup and stir well.

Transfer to a baking sheet lined with parchment paper and spread evenly.

Cook into a preheated oven at 275°F for about 20 minutes.

Take it out from the oven, stir, and cook again for 10-15 minutes.

Let it cool for about a few minutes until crispy. Enjoy!

Nutrition:

Calories: 378

Fats: 27.6 g

Carbs: 26 g

Protein: 13 g

Chia Crackers

Preparation Time: 20 minutes

Cooking Time: 1 hour

Servings: 24-26

Ingredients:

1/2 cup pecans, chopped

1/2 cup chia seeds

1/2 tsp. cayenne pepper

1 cup water

1/4 cup nutritional yeast

1/2 cup pumpkin seeds

1/4 cup ground flax

Salt and pepper, to taste

Directions:

Mix around 1/2 cup of chia seeds and 1 cup of water. Keep it aside.

Take another bowl and combine all the remaining ingredients. Combine well and stir in the chia water mixture until you obtained dough.

Transfer the dough onto a baking sheet and roll it out into a ¼"-thick dough.

Transfer into a preheated oven at 325ºF and bake for about ½ hour.

Take out from the oven, flip over the dough, and cut it into desired cracker shaped-squares.

Spread and back again for a further half an hour, or until crispy and browned.

Once done, take them out from the oven and let them cool at room temperature. Enjoy!

Nutrition:

Calories: 41

Fats: 3.1 g

Carbs: 2 g

Protein: 2 g

Orange-Spiced Pumpkin Hummus

Preparation Time: 2 minutes

Cooking Time: 5 minutes

Servings: 4

Ingredients:

1 tbsp. maple syrup

1/2 tsp. salt

1 can (16 oz.) garbanzo beans

1/8 tsp. ginger or nutmeg

1 cup canned pumpkin Blend,

1/8 tsp. cinnamon

1/4 cup tahini

1 tbsp. fresh orange juice

Pinch of orange zest, for garnish

1 tbsp. apple cider vinegar

Directions:

Mix all the ingredients in a food processor or blender until slightly chunky.

Serve right away, and enjoy!

Nutrition:

Calories: 291

Fats: 22.9 g

Carbs: 15 g

Protein: 12 g

Superfood Spiced Apricot-Sesame Bliss Balls

Preparation time: 10 minutes

Cooking time: 30 minutes

Servings: 3

Ingredients:

2 tablespoons sesame seeds

1 cup apricots

1 cup natural gluten-free muesli

1 cup almonds

2 tablespoons raw honey

1 teaspoon ground cinnamon

Directions:

In a food processor, process almonds until finely chopped; add in raw honey, muesli, apricots, and cinnamon and process until very smooth.

Add sesame seeds in a shallow dish. Roll two tablespoons of the almond mixture into bite-sized balls and then roll them into the sesame seeds until well coated.

Arrange them on a tray and refrigerate until set. Serve and store the rest in an airtight container.

Nutrition: 448 Calories 27g fat 41g carbs 15g protein

Crunchy Veggie Chips

Preparation time: 10 minutes

Cooking time: 17 minutes

Servings: 3

Ingredients:

1 cup thinly sliced portobello mushrooms

1 cup thinly sliced zucchini

1 cup thinly sliced sweet potatoes

1 tablespoon extra-virgin olive oil

Pinch of sea salt

Pinch of pepper

Directions:

Place veggies in a baking dish and drizzle with olive oil; sprinkle with salt and pepper and toss to coat well; bake at 325°F for about 12 minutes or until crunchy. Enjoy!

Nutrition: 448 Calories 27g fat 41g carbs 15g protein

Superfood Raw Bars

Preparation time: 10 minutes

Cooking time: 5 minutes

Servings: 6

Ingredients:

1/2 cup toasted pistachios

1/4 cup goji berries + 2 tablespoons more

1/2 cup roasted almonds

1/4 cup chia seeds

3/4 cup blackcurrants

3/4 cup coconut flakes, toasted

1/3 cup ginger

1 tablespoon raw cacao nibs

1 tablespoon coconut oil

500g chopped dark chocolate

Pinch of sea salt

Directions:

Preparation are a baking pan by greasing and lining with baking paper.

In a large bowl, combine 1/3 cup of pistachios, blackcurrants, ½ cup of coconut flakes, goji berries, almond, chia pieces, and ginger until well mixed.

In another bowl, stir together cacao nibs, the remaining pistachios and coconut flakes, and more goji berries.

In a saucepan, stir together oil, chocolate and salt until chocolate is melted. Pour the chocolate mixture into the pistachio mixture and stir until well coated; transfer to the pan and sprinkle with the cacao mixture.

Refrigerate for at least 4 hours or until firm. Cut into 24 squares and serve, storing the rest in the refrigerator for up two weeks.

Nutrition: 448 Calories 27g fat 41g carbs 15g protein

Trail Mix

Preparation time: 10 minutes

Cooking time: 0 minutes

Servings: 3

Ingredients:

¼ cup unsalted roasted peanuts

¼ cup whole shelled almonds

¼ cup chopped pitted dates

¼ cup dried cranberries

2 ounces dried apricots

Directions:

In a medium bowl, mix together all the ingredients until well combined. Enjoy!

Nutrition: 448 Calories 27g fat 41g carbs 15g protein

Avocado & Pea Dip with Carrots

Preparation time: 10 minutes

Cooking time: 0 minutes

Servings: 3

Ingredients:

1 avocado, peeled and seed removed

1 1/2 cups steamed snow peas

1/4 teaspoon cayenne pepper

2 tablespoons lime juice

I clove of garlic, diced

Carrots to serve

Directions:

Combine together all ingredients in a blender and blend until very smooth. Serve with fresh carrots.

Nutrition: 448 Calories 27g fat 41g carbs 15g protein

Carrot Chips

Preparation time: 10 minutes

Cooking time: 10 minutes

Servings: 3

Ingredients:

6 large carrots

2 tablespoons extra virgin olive oil

½ teaspoon black pepper

Directions:

Chop the carrots into 2-inch sections and then cut each section into thin sticks.

Toss together the carrots sticks with extra virgin olive oil and pepper in a bowl and spread into a baking sheet lined with parchment paper.

Bake the carrot sticks at 425° for about 20 minutes or until browned.

Nutrition: 448 Calories 27g fat 41g carbs 15g protein

Spiced Spinach Bites

Preparation time: 10 minutes

Cooking time: 20 minutes

Servings: 3

Ingredients:

12 baby spinach leaves

2 chopped limes

½ chopped chilli

1 sliced shallot

1 teaspoon chopped ginger

2 tablespoons peanuts

A pinch of sea salt

1 tablespoon coriander

Directions:

In a bowl, combine peanuts, chilli, shallot, ginger, limes, and coriander; season with a sprinkle of sea salt. Lay spinach leaves on a plate and add a spoonful of the mixture on each; roll them up to make round wraps.

Nutrition: 448 Calories 27g fat 41g carbs 15g protein

Ginger Tahini Dip with Veggies

Preparation time: 10 minutes

Cooking time: 0 minutes

Servings: 3

Ingredients:

½ cup tahini

1 teaspoon grated garlic

2 teaspoons ground turmeric

1 tablespoon grated fresh ginger

¼ cup apple cider vinegar

¼ cup water

½ teaspoon salt

Directions:

In a bowl, whisk together tahini, turmeric, ginger, water, vinegar, garlic, and salt until well blended. Serve with assorted veggies.

Nutrition: 448 Calories 27g fat 41g carbs 15g protein

Spiced Toasted Almonds & Seed Mix

Preparation time: 10 minutes

Cooking time: 10 minutes

Servings: 4

Ingredients:

2 tablespoons olive oil

1/2 cup sunflower seeds

1/2 cup pumpkin seeds

1 cup almonds

1 tablespoon chili paste

1 tablespoon crushed fennel seeds

1 tablespoon ground cumin

½ teaspoon sea salt

Directions:

Heat oil in a skillet set over medium heat; stir in chili paste and fennel seeds and then add in seeds and almonds; sauté for about 5 minutes and then stir in cumin and salt. Remove from heat and let cool before serving.

Nutrition: 448 Calories 27g fat 41g carbs 15g protein

Lime Pea Guacamole

Preparation time: 10 minutes

Cooking time: 0 minutes

Servings: 3

Ingredients:

2 cups thawed frozen green peas

¼ cup fresh lime juice

1 teaspoon crushed garlic

½ teaspoon cumin

1/8 teaspoon hot sauce

½ cup chopped cilantro

4 green onions, chopped

1 tomato, chopped

Black pepper

Directions:

In a food processor, blend together peas, lime juice, garlic, and cumin until very smooth; transfer to a large bowl and stir in hot sauce, cilantro, green onion, tomato and pepper. Refrigerate, covered, for about 30 minutes for flavors to blend. Enjoy!

Nutrition: 324 Calories 24g fat 20g protein 7g carbs

Chili-lime Cucumber, Jicama, & Apple Sticks

Preparation time: 10 minutes

Cooking time: 0 minutes

Servings: 3

Ingredients:

6 spears cucumber

6 spears very ripe apple

6 spears jicama (you can use mango instead)

1 teaspoon chili lime seasoning

2 lime wedges

Directions:

In a bowl, mix together cucumber, apple, jicama, lime juice, chili lime seasoning until well combined. Serve garnished with lime wedges. Enjoy!

Nutrition: 324 Calories 24g fat 20g protein 7g carbs

Savory Trail Mix

Preparation time: 10 minutes

Cooking time: 0 minutes

Servings: 3

Ingredient

¼ cup chopped almonds

1/4 cup pumpkin seeds

1/4 cup sunflower seeds

1/2 teaspoon garlic powder

1/2 teaspoon onion powder

1/4 teaspoon cayenne pepper

Directions:

Mix everything and enjoy!

Nutrition: 324 Calories 24g fat 20g protein 7g carbs

Raw Turmeric Cashew Nut & Coconut Balls

Preparation time: 10 minutes

Cooking time: 0 minutes

Servings: 3

Ingredients:

1 cup raw cashews

1 1/2 cup shredded coconut

1 tablespoon raw honey

3 teaspoons ground turmeric

1 teaspoon cinnamon

1 teaspoon ground ginger

1 teaspoon black pepper

1/2 teaspoon sea salt

Directions:

In a food processor, process coconut until almost oily; add in the rest of the ingredients and process until cashews are finely chopped.

Press the mixture into bite-sized balls and arrange them on a baking tray. Refrigerate until firm before serving

Nutrition: 324 Calories 24g fat 20g protein 7g carbs

Homemade Nutella

Preparation time: 10 minutes

Cooking time: 0 minutes

Servings: 3

Ingredients:

3/4 cup toasted hazelnuts

3 tablespoons peanut oil

2 tablespoons cocoa powder

3 scoops protein powder

1/2 teaspoon vanilla extract

2 tablespoons raw honey

Pinch salt

Directions:

Add hazelnuts to your food processor and grind until finely ground; add in peanut oil and process the mixture into butter; add in the remaining ingredients and process until creamy and smooth. Serve with celery or carrot sticks.

Nutrition: 324 Calories 24g fat 20g protein 7g carbs

Wheat Crackers

Preparation Time: 10 minutes

Cooking Time: 20 minutes

Servings: 4

Ingredients:

1 3/4 cups almond flour

1 1/2 cups coconut flour

3/4 teaspoon sea salt

1/3 cup vegetable oil

1 cup alkaline water

Sea salt for sprinkling

Directions:

Set your oven to 350 degrees F.

Mix coconut flour, almond flour and salt in a bowl.

Stir in vegetable oil and water. Mix well until smooth.

Spread this dough on a floured surface into a thin sheet.

Cut small squares out of this sheet.

Arrange the dough squares on a baking sheet lined with parchment paper.

Bake for 20 minutes until light golden in color.

Serve.

Nutrition:

Calories 64

Total Fat 9.2 g

Saturated Fat 2.4 g

Cholesterol 110 mg

Sodium 276 mg

Total Carbs 9.2 g

Fiber 0.9 g

Sugar 1.4 g

Protein 1.5 g

Potato Chips

Preparation Time: 10 minutes

Cooking Time: 5 minutes

Servings: 4

Ingredients:

1 tablespoon vegetable oil

1 potato, sliced paper thin

Sea salt, to taste

Directions:

Toss potato with oil and sea salt.

Spread the slices in a baking dish in a single layer.

Cook in a microwave for 5 minutes until golden brown.

Serve.

Nutrition:

Calories 80

Total Fat 3.5 g

Saturated Fat 0.1 g

Cholesterol 320 mg

Sodium 350 mg

Total Carbs 11.6 g

Fiber 0.7 g

Sugar 0.7 g

Protein 1.2 g

Rosemary & Garlic Kale Chips

Preparation Time: 10 minutes

Cooking Time: 30 minutes

Servings: 1

Ingredients:

9oz kale chips, chopped into 2inch

2 sprigs of rosemary

2 cloves of garlic

2 tablespoons olive oil

Sea salt

Freshly ground black pepper

Directions:

Gently warm the olive oil, rosemary and garlic over a low heat for 10 minutes. Remove it from the heat and set aside to cool.

Take the rosemary and garlic out of the oil and discard them.

Toss the kale leaves in the oil, making sure they are well coated.

Season with salt and pepper.

Spread the kale leaves onto 2 baking sheets and bake them in the oven at 170C/325F for 15 minutes, until crispy.

Nutrition:

Calories: 249

Sodium: 36 mg

Dietary Fiber: 1.7 g

Total Fat: 4.3 g

Total Carbs: 15.3 g

Protein: 1.4 g

Collard Greens and Tomatoes

Preparation Time: 10 minutes

Cooking Time: 12 minutes

Servings: 5

Ingredients:

1-pound collard greens

3 bacon strips, chopped

¼ cup cherry tomatoes, halved

1 tbsp. apple cider vinegar

2 tbsp. chicken stock

Salt and ground black pepper to taste

Directions:

Heat a pan over medium heat, add the bacon, stir, and cook until it browns. Add the tomatoes, collard greens, vinegar, stock, salt, and pepper, stir, and cook for 8 minutes.

Add more salt, and pepper, stir again gently, divide onto plates, and serve.

Nutrition

Calories 120

Fat 8 g

Carbs 3 g

Protein 7 g

Blueberry Cauliflower

Preparation Time: 2 minutes

Cooking Time: 5 minutes

Servings: 1

Ingredients:

¼ cup frozen strawberries

2 tsp. maple syrup

¾ cup unsweetened cashew milk

1 tsp. vanilla extract

½ cup plain cashew yogurt

5 tbsp. powdered peanut butter

¾ cup frozen wild blueberries

½ cup cauliflower florets, coarsely chopped

Directions:

Add all the smoothie ingredients to a high-speed blender.

Quickly combine until smooth.

Pour into a chilled glass and serve.

Nutrition:

Calories: 340

Fats: 11 g

Carbs: 48 g

Protein: 16 g

Roasted Asparagus

Preparation Time: 10 minutes

Cooking Time: 10 minutes

Servings: 3

Ingredients:

1 asparagus bunch, trimmed

3 tsp. avocado oil

A splash of lemon juice

Salt and ground black pepper to taste

1 tbsp. fresh oregano, chopped

Directions:

Spread the asparagus spears on a lined baking sheet, season with salt, and pepper, drizzle with oil and lemon juice, sprinkle with oregano, and toss to coat well.

Put in an oven at 425ºF, and bake for 10 minutes.

Divide onto plates and serve.

Nutrition

Calories 130

Fat 1 g

Carbs 2 g

Protein 3 g

Asparagus Frittata

Preparation Time: 10 minutes

Cooking Time: 15 minutes

Servings: 4

Ingredients:

¼ cup onion, chopped

Drizzle of olive oil

1-pound asparagus spears, cut into 1-inch pieces

Salt and ground black pepper to taste

4 eggs, whisked

1 cup cheddar cheese, grated

Directions:

Heat a pan with the oil over medium-high heat, add the onions, stir, and cook for 3 minutes. Add the asparagus, stir, and cook for 6 minutes. Add the eggs, stir, and cook for 3 minutes.

Add the salt and pepper sprinkle with the cheese, put in an oven, and broil for 3 minutes.

Divide the frittata onto plates and serve.

Nutrition

Calories 200

Fat 12 g

Carbs 5 g

Protein 14 g

Roasted Radishes

Preparation Time: 10 minutes

Cooking Time: 35 minutes

Servings: 2

Ingredients:

2 cups radishes cut in quarters

Salt and ground black pepper to taste

2 tbsp. butter, melted

1 tbsp. fresh chives, chopped

1 tbsp. lemon zest

Directions:

Spread the radishes on a lined baking sheet. Add the salt, pepper, chives, lemon zest, and butter, toss to coat, and bake in the oven at 375ºF for 35 minutes.

Divide onto plates and serve.

Nutrition:

Calories 122

Fat 12 g

Carbs 3 g

Protein 14 g

Radish Hash Browns

Preparation Time: 10 minutes.

Cooking Time: 10 minutes

Servings: 4

Ingredients:

½ tsp. onion powder

1-pound radishes, shredded

½ tsp. garlic powder

Salt and ground black pepper to taste

4 eggs

⅓ Cup Parmesan cheese, grated

Directions:

In a bowl, mix the radishes with salt, pepper, onion, and garlic powder, eggs, and Parmesan cheese, and stir well.

Spread on a lined baking sheet, put in an oven at 375ºF, and bake for 10 minutes.

Divide the hash browns onto plates and serve.

Nutrition:

Calories 80

Fat 5 g

Carbs 5 g

Protein 7 g

Strawberry Frozen Yogurt

Preparation Time: 10 minutes

Cooking Time: 15 minutes

Servings: 4

Ingredients:

15 ounces of plain yogurt

6 ounces of strawberries

Juice of 1 orange

1 tablespoon honey

Directions:

Place the strawberries and orange juice into a food processor or blender and blitz until smooth.

Press the mixture through a sieve into a large bowl to remove seeds.

Stir in the honey and yogurt. Transfer the mixture to an ice-cream maker and follow the manufacturer's instructions.

Alternatively, pour the mixture into a container and place in the fridge for 1 hour. Use a fork to whisk it and break up the ice crystals and freeze for 2 hours.

Nutrition:

Calories: 238

Sodium: 33 mg

Dietary Fiber: 1.4 g

Total Fat: 1.8 g

Total Carbs: 12.3 g

Protein: 1.3 g

Walnut & Spiced Apple Tonic

Preparation Time: 10 minutes

Cooking Time: 15 minutes

Servings: 1

Ingredients:

6 walnuts halves

1 apple, cored

1 banana

½ teaspoon matcha powder

½ teaspoon cinnamon

Pinch of ground nutmeg

Directions:

Place ingredients into a blender and add sufficient water to cover them. Blitz until smooth and creamy.

Nutrition:

Calories: 124

Sodium: 22 mg

Dietary Fiber: 1.4 g

Total Fat: 2.1 g

Total Carbs: 12.3 g

Protein: 1.2 g

Basil & Walnut Pesto

Preparation Time: 10 minutes

Cooking Time: 30 minutes

Servings: 1

Ingredients:

2oz fresh basil

2oz walnuts

1oz pine nuts

3 cloves of garlic, crushed

2 tablespoons Parmesan, grated

4 tablespoons olive oil

Direction

Place the pesto ingredients into a food processor and process until it becomes a smooth paste.

Serve with meat, fish, salad and pasta dishes.

Nutrition

Calories: 136

Sodium: 23 mg,

Dietary Fiber: 1.2 g,

Total Fat: 3.1 g,

Total Carbs: 14.3 g

Protein: 1.4 g

Honey Chili Nuts

Preparation Time: 10 minutes

Cooking Time: 30 minutes

Servings: 1

Ingredients:

5oz walnuts

5oz pecan nuts

2oz softened butter

1 tablespoon honey

½ bird's-eye chili, very finely chopped and de-seeded

Directions

Preheat the oven to 180C/360F.

Combine the butter, honey and chili in a bowl, then add the nuts and stir them well.

Spread the nuts onto a lined baking sheet and roast them in the oven for 10 minutes, stirring once halfway through.

Remove from the oven and allow them to cool before eating.

Nutrition:

Calories: 295

Sodium: 28 mg

Dietary Fiber: 1.6 g

Total Fat: 4.7 g

Total Carbs: 14.6 g

Protein: 1.3 g

Mozzarella Cauliflower Bars

Preparation Time: 10 minutes

Cooking Time: 40 minutes

Servings: 12

Ingredients:

1 big cauliflower head, riced

½ cup low-fat mozzarella cheese, shredded

¼ cup egg whites

1 teaspoon Italian seasoning

Black pepper to the taste

Directions:

Spread the cauliflower rice on a lined baking sheet, cook in the oven at 375 degrees F for 20 minutes, transfer to a bowl, add black pepper, cheese, seasoning, and egg whites, stir well, spread into a rectangle pan and press on the bottom.

Introduce in the oven at 375 degrees F, bake for 20 minutes, cut into 12 bars, and serve as a snack.

Nutrition:

Calories 140

Fat 1 g

Carbohydrate 6 g

Protein 6 g

Grape, Celery & Parsley Reviver

Preparation Time: 10 minutes

Cooking Time: 0 minutes

Servings: 2

Ingredients:

75g 3ozred grapes

3 sticks of celery

1 avocado, de-stoned and peeled

1 tablespoon fresh parsley

½ teaspoon matcha powder

Directions:

Place all of the ingredients into a blender with enough water to cover them and blitz until smooth and creamy. Add crushed ice to make it even more refreshing.

Nutrition:

Calories 334

Fat 1.5 g

Carbohydrate 42.9 g

Protein 6 g

Roasted Red Endive With Caper Butter

Preparation Time: 10 minutes

Cooking Time: 25 minutes

Servings: 4

Ingredients:

10 – 12 red endives

2 teaspoons extra virgin olive oil

2–5 anchovy fillets, packed in oil

1 small lemon, juiced

3 tablespoons capers, drained

5 tablespoons cold butter, cut into cubes

1 tablespoon fresh parsley, chopped

Salt and pepper as needed

Directions:

Preheat the oven to 425 degrees F.

Toss endives with olive oil, salt, and pepper, and spread out on to a baking sheet cut side down. Bake for about 20-25 minutes or until caramelized.

While they're roasting, add the anchovies to a large pan over medium heat and use a fork to mash them until broken up.

Add lemon juice and mix well, then add capers.

Lower the heat and slowly stir in the butter and parsley.

Drizzle butter over roasted endives, season as necessary and garnish with more fresh parsley.

Nutrition:

Calories 109

Fat 8.6g

Protein1.5 g,

Carbohydrates 4.9 g,

Fiber 4 g

Zucchini Pepper Chips

Preparation Time: 10 minutes

Cooking Time: 15 minutes

Servings: 04

Ingredients:

1 2/3 cups vegetable oil

1 teaspoon garlic powder

1 teaspoon onion powder

1/2 teaspoon black pepper

3 tablespoons crushed red pepper flakes

2 zucchinis, thinly sliced

Directions:

Mix oil with all the spices in a bowl.

Add zucchini slices and mix well.

Transfer the mixture to a Ziplock bag and seal it.

Refrigerate for 10 minutes.

Spread the zucchini slices on a greased baking sheet.

Bake for 15 minutes

Serve.

Nutrition:

Calories 172

Total Fat 11.1 g

Saturated Fat 5.8 g

Cholesterol 610 mg

Sodium 749 mg

Total Carbs 19.9 g

Fiber 0.2 g

Sugar 0.2 g

Protein 13.5 g

Apple Chips

Preparation Time: 5 minutes

Cooking Time: 45 minutes

Servings: 4

Ingredients:

2 Golden Delicious apples, cored and thinly sliced

1 1/2 teaspoons white sugar

1/2 teaspoon ground cinnamon

Directions:

Set your oven to 225 degrees F.

Place apple slices on a baking sheet.

Sprinkle sugar an

d cinnamon over apple slices.

Bake for 45 minutes.

Serve

Nutrition:

Calories 127

Total Fat 3.5 g

Saturated Fat 0.5 g

Cholesterol 162 mg

Sodium 142 mg

Total Carbs 33.6g

Fiber 0.4 g

Sugar 0.5 g

Protein 4.5 g

Carrot Chips

Preparation Time: 5 minutes

Cooking Time: 12 minutes

Servings: 4

Ingredients:

4 carrots, washed, peeled and sliced

2 teaspoons extra-virgin olive oil

1/4 teaspoon sea salt

Directions:

Set your oven to 350 degrees F.

Toss carrots with salt and olive oil.

Spread the slices on two baking sheets in a single layer.

Bake for 6 minutes on upper and lower rack of the oven.

Switch the baking racks and bake for another 6 minutes.

Serve.

Nutrition:

Calories 153

Total Fat 7.5 g

Saturated Fat 1.1 g

Cholesterol 20 mg

Sodium 97 mg

Total Carbs 20.4 g

Fiber 0 g

Sugar 0 g

Protein 3.1g

Chapter 6: Lunch Recipes

Tilapia with Avocado & Red Onion

Preparation Time: 5 minutes

Cooking Time: 15 minutes

Servings: 4

Ingredients:

Olive oil (1 tbsp.)

Sea salt (.25 tsp.)

Fresh orange juice (1 tbsp.)

Tilapia fillets (four 4 oz. - more rectangular than square)

Red onion (.25 cup)

Sliced avocado (1)

Also Needed: 9-inch pie plate

Directions:

Combine the salt, juice, and oil to add into the pie dish. Work with one fillet at a time. Place it in the dish and turn to coat all sides.

Arrange the fillets in a wagon wheel-shaped formation. (Each of the fillets should be in the center of the dish with the other end draped over the edge.)

Place a tablespoon of the onion on top of each of the fillets and fold the end into the center. Cover the dish with plastic wrap, leaving one corner open to vent the steam.

Place in the microwave using the high heat setting for three minutes. It's done when the center can be easily flaked.

Top the fillets off with avocado and serve.

Nutrition:

Calories: 200

Protein: 22 grams

Fat: 11 grams

Berries and Grilled Calamari

Preparation Time: 5 minutes

Cooking Time: 5 minutes

Servings: 4

Ingredients:

¼ cup dried cranberries

¼ cup extra virgin olive oil

¼ cup olive oil

¼ cup sliced almonds

½ lemon, juiced

¾ cup blueberries

1 ½ pounds calamari tube, cleaned

1 granny smith apple, sliced thinly

1 tablespoon fresh lemon juice

2 tablespoons apple cider vinegar

6 cups fresh spinach

Freshly grated pepper to taste

Sea salt to taste

Directions for Cooking:

In a small bowl, make the vinaigrette by mixing well the tablespoon of lemon juice, apple cider vinegar, and extra virgin olive oil. Season with pepper and salt to taste. Set aside.

Turn on the grill to medium fire and let the grates heat up for a minute or two.

In a large bowl, add olive oil and the calamari tube. Season calamari generously with pepper and salt.

Place seasoned and oiled calamari onto heated grate and grill until cooked or opaque. This is around two minutes per side.

As you wait for the calamari to cook, you can combine almonds, cranberries, blueberries, spinach, and the thinly sliced apple in a large salad bowl. Toss to mix.

Remove cooked calamari from grill and transfer on a chopping board. Cut into ¼-inch thick rings and throw into the salad bowl.

Drizzle with vinaigrette and toss well to coat salad.

Serve and enjoy!

Nutrition:

Calories: 567

Fat: 24.5g

Protein: 54.8g

Carbs: 30.6g

Cajun Garlic Shrimp Noodle Bowl

Preparation Time: 7 minutes

Cooking Time: 15 minutes

Servings: 2

Ingredients:

½ teaspoon salt

1 onion, sliced

1 red pepper, sliced

1 tablespoon butter

1 teaspoon garlic granules

1 teaspoon onion powder

1 teaspoon paprika

2 large zucchinis, cut into noodle strips

20 jumbo shrimps, shells removed and deveined

3 cloves garlic, minced

3 tablespoon ghee

A dash of cayenne pepper

A dash of red pepper flakes

Directions for Cooking:

Preparation are the Cajun seasoning by mixing the onion powder, garlic granules, pepper flakes, cayenne pepper, paprika and salt. Toss in the shrimp to coat in the seasoning.

In a skillet, heat the ghee and sauté the garlic. Add in the red pepper and onions and continue sautéing for 4 minutes.

Add the Cajun shrimp and cook until opaque. Set aside.

In another pan, heat the butter and sauté the zucchini noodles for three minutes.

Assemble by the placing the Cajun shrimps on top of the zucchini noodles.

Nutrition:

Calories: 712

Fat: 30.0g

Protein: 97.8g

Carbs: 20.2g

Tarragon Cod Fillets

Preparation Time: 10 minutes

Cooking Time: 12 minutes

Servings: 4

Ingredients:

4 cod fillets, boneless

¼ cup capers, drained

1 tablespoon tarragon, chopped

Sea salt and black pepper to the taste

2 tablespoons olive oil

2 tablespoons parsley, chopped

1 tablespoon olive oil

1 tablespoon lemon juice

Directions:

Heat up a pan with the oil over medium-high heat, add the fish and cook for 3 minutes on each side.

Add the rest of the ingredients, cook everything for 7 minutes more, divide between plates and serve.

Nutrition:

Calories 162

Fat 9.6 g

Fiber 4.3 g

Carbs 12.4 g

Protein 16.5 g

Chicken And White Bean

Preparation time: 10 minutes

Cooking time: 60 minutes

Servings: 3

Ingredients:

2 tbsp fresh cilantro, chopped

2 cups grated Monterey Jack cheese

3 cups water

1/8 tsp cayenne pepper

2 tsp pure chile powder

2 tsp ground cumin

1 4-oz can chopped green chiles

1 cup corn kernels

2 15-oz cans shite beans, drained and rinsed

2 garlic cloves

1 medium onion, diced

2 tbsp extra virgin olive oil

1 lb. chicken breasts, boneless and skinless

Directions:

Slice chicken breasts into ½-inch cubes and with pepper and salt, season it.

On high fire, place a large nonstick fry pan and heat oil.

Sauté chicken pieces for three to four minutes or until lightly browned.

Reduce fire to medium and add garlic and onion.

Cook for 5 to 6 minutes or until onions are translucent.

Add water, spices, chilies, corn and beans. Bring to a boil.

Once boiling, slow fire to a simmer and continue simmering for an hour, uncovered.

To serve, garnish with a sprinkling of cilantro and a tablespoon of cheese.

Nutrition: Calories per serving: 433; Protein: 30.6g; Carbs: 29.5g; Fat: 21.8g

Quinoa & Black Bean Stuffed Sweet Potatoes

Preparation time: 10 minutes

Cooking time: 60 minutes

Servings: 8

Ingredients:

4 sweet potatoes

½ onion, diced

1 garlic glove, crushed and diced

½ large bell pepper diced (about 2/3 cups)

Handful of diced cilantro

½ cup cooked quinoa

½ cup black beans

1 tbsp olive oil

1 tbsp chili powder

½ tbsp cumin

½ tbsp paprika

½ tbsp oregano

2 tbsp lime juice

2 tbsp honey

Sprinkle salt

1 cup shredded cheddar cheese

Chopped spring onions, for garnish (optional)

Directions:

Preheat oven to 400oF.

Wash and scrub outside of potatoes. Poke with fork a few times and then place on parchment paper on cookie sheet. Bake for 40-45 minutes or until it is cooked.

While potatoes are baking, sauté onions, garlic, olive oil and spices in a pan on the stove until onions are translucent and soft.

In the last 10 minutes while the potatoes are cooking, in a large bowl combine the onion mixture with the beans, quinoa, honey, lime juice, cilantro and ½ cup cheese. Mix well.

When potatoes are cooked, remove from oven and let cool slightly. When cool to touch, cut in half (hot dog style) and scoop out most of the insides. Leave a thin ring of potato so that it will hold its shape. You can save the sweet potato guts for another recipe, such as my veggie burgers (recipe posted below).

Fill with bean and quinoa mixture. Top with remaining cheddar cheese.

(If making this a freezer meal, stop here. Individually wrap potato skins in plastic wrap and place on flat surface to freeze. Once frozen, place all potatoes in large zip lock container or Tupperware.)

Return to oven for an additional 10 minutes or until cheese is melted.

Nutrition: Calories per serving: 243; Carbs: 37.6g; Protein: 8.5g; Fat: 7.3g

Feta, Eggplant And Sausage Penne

Preparation time: 10 minutes

Cooking time: 30 minutes

Servings: 6

Ingredients:

¼ cup chopped fresh parsley

½ cup crumbled feta cheese

6 cups hot cooked penne

1 14.5oz can diced tomatoes

¼ tsp ground black pepper

1 tsp dried oregano

2 tbsp tomato paste

4 garlic cloves, minced

½ lb. bulk pork breakfast sausage

4 ½ cups cubed peeled eggplant

Directions:

On medium high fire, place a nonstick, big fry pan and cook for seven minutes garlic, sausage and eggplant or until eggplants are soft and sausage are lightly browned.

Stir in diced tomatoes, black pepper, oregano and tomato paste. Cover and simmer for five minutes while occasionally stirring.

Remove pan from fire, stir in pasta and mix well.

Transfer to a serving dish, garnish with parsley and cheese before serving.

Nutrition: Calories per Serving: 376; Carbs: 50.8g; Protein: 17.8g; Fat: 11.6g

Bell Peppers 'n Tomato-chickpea Rice

Preparation time: 10 minutes

Cooking time: 35 minutes

Servings: 4

Ingredients:

2 tablespoons olive oil

1/2 chopped red bell pepper

1/2 chopped green bell pepper

1/2 chopped yellow pepper

1/2 chopped red pepper

1 medium onion, chopped

1 clove garlic, minced

2 cups cooked jasmine rice

1 teaspoon tomato paste

1 cup chickpeas

salt to taste

1/2 teaspoon paprika

1 small tomato, chopped

Parsley for garnish

Directions:

In a large mixing bowl, whisk well olive oil, garlic, tomato paste, and paprika. Season with salt generously.

Mix in rice and toss well to coat in the dressing.

Add remaining ingredients and toss well to mix.

Let salad rest to allow flavors to mix for 15 minutes.

Toss one more time and adjust salt to taste if needed.

Garnish with parsley and serve.

Nutrition: Calories per serving: 490; Carbs: 93.0g; Protein: 10.0g; Fat: 8.0g

Lipsmacking Chicken Tetrazzini

Preparation time: 10 minutes

Cooking time: 3Hours

Servings: 3

Ingredients:

Toasted French bread slices

¾ cup thinly sliced green onion

2/3 cup grated parmesan cheese

10 oz dried spaghetti or linguine, cooked and drained

¼ tsp ground nutmeg

¼ tsp ground black pepper

2 tbsp dry sherry

¼ cup chicken broth or water

1 16oz jar of Alfredo pasta sauce

2 4.5oz jars of sliced mushrooms, drained

2.5 lbs. skinless chicken breasts cut into ½ inch slices

Directions:

In a slow cooker, mix mushrooms and chicken.

In a bowl, mix well nutmeg, pepper, sherry, broth and alfredo sauce before pouring over chicken and mushrooms.

Set on high heat, cover and cook for two to three hours.

Once chicken is cooked, pour over pasta, garnish with green onion and serve with French bread on the side.

Nutrition: Calories per Serving: 505; Carbs: 24.7g; Protein: 35.1g; Fat: 30.2g

Spaghetti In Lemon Avocado White Sauce

Preparation time: 10 minutes

Cooking time: 30 minutes

Servings: 3

Ingredients:

Freshly ground black pepper

Zest and juice of 1 lemon

1 avocado, pitted and peeled

1-pound spaghetti

Salt

1 tbsp Olive oil

8 oz small shrimp, shelled and deveined

¼ cup dry white wine

1 large onion, finely sliced

Directions:

Let a big pot of water boil. Once boiling add the spaghetti or pasta and cook following manufacturer's instructions until al dente. Drain and set aside.

In a large fry pan, over medium fire sauté wine and onions for ten minutes or until onions are translucent and soft.

Add the shrimps into the fry pan and increase fire to high while constantly sautéing until shrimps are cooked around five minutes. Turn the fire off. Season with salt and add the oil right away. Then quickly toss in the cooked pasta, mix well.

In a blender, until smooth, puree the lemon juice and avocado. Pour into the fry pan of pasta, combine well. Garnish with pepper and lemon zest then serve.

Nutrition: Calories per Serving: 206; Carbs: 26.3g; Protein: 10.2g; Fat: 8.0g

Kidney Beans And Beet Salad

Preparation time: 10 minutes

Cooking time: 15 minutes

Servings: 3

Servings: 4

Cooking Time: 15 Minutes

Ingredients:

1 14.5-ounce can kidney beans, drained and rinsed

1 tablespoon pomegranate syrup or juice

2 tablespoons olive oil

4 beets, scrubbed and stems removed

4 green onions, chopped

Juice of 1 lemon

Salt and pepper to taste

Directions:

Bring a pot of water to boil and add beets. Simmer for 10 minutes or until tender. Drain beets and place in ice bath for 5 minutes.

Peel bets and slice in halves.

Toss to mix the pomegranate syrup, olive oil, lemon juice, green onions, and kidney beans in a salad bowl.

Stir in beets. Season with pepper and salt to taste.

Serve and enjoy.

Nutrition: Calories per serving: 175; Protein: 6.0g; Carbs: 22.0g; Fat: 7.0g

Filling Macaroni Soup

Preparation time: 10 minutes

Cooking time: 45 minutes

Servings: 6

Ingredients:

1 cup of minced beef or chicken or a combination of both

1 cup carrots, diced

1 cup milk

½ medium onion, sliced thinly

3 garlic cloves, minced

Salt and pepper to taste

2 cups broth (chicken, vegetable or beef)

½ tbsp olive oil

1 cup uncooked whole wheat pasta like macaroni, shells, even angel hair broken to pieces

1 cup water

Directions:

In a heavy bottomed pot on medium high fire heat oil.

Add garlic and sauté for a minute or two until fragrant but not browned.

Add onions and sauté for 3 minutes or until soft and translucent.

Add a cup of minced meat. You can also use whatever leftover frozen meat you have.

Sauté the meat well until cooked around 8 minutes. While sautéing, season meat with pepper and salt.

Add water and broth and bring to a boil.

Once boiling, add pasta. I use any leftover pasta that I have in the pantry. If all you have left is spaghetti, lasagna, angel hair or fettuccine, just break them into pieces—around 1-inch in length before adding to the pot.

Slow fire to a simmer and cook while covered until pasta is soft.

Halfway through cooking the pasta, around 8 minutes I add the carrots.

Once the pasta is soft, turn off fire and add milk.

Mix well and season to taste again if needed.

Serve and enjoy.

Nutrition: Calories per Serving: 125; Carbs: 11.4g; Protein: 10.1g; Fat: 4.3g

Simple Penne Anti-pasto

Preparation time: 10 minutes

Cooking time: 15 minutes

Servings: 5

Ingredients:

¼ cup pine nuts, toasted

½ cup grated Parmigiano-Reggiano cheese, divided

8oz penne pasta, cooked and drained

1 6oz jar drained, sliced, marinated and quartered artichoke hearts

1 7 oz jar drained and chopped sun-dried tomato halves packed in oil

3 oz chopped prosciutto

1/3 cup pesto

½ cup pitted and chopped Kalamata olives

1 medium red bell pepper

Directions:

Slice bell pepper, discard membranes, seeds and stem. On a foiled lined baking sheet, place bell pepper halves, press down by hand and broil in oven for eight minutes. Remove from oven, put in a sealed bag for 5 minutes before peeling and chopping.

Place chopped bell pepper in a bowl and mix in artichokes, tomatoes, prosciutto, pesto and olives.

Toss in ¼ cup cheese and pasta. Transfer to a serving dish and garnish with ¼ cup cheese and pine nuts. Serve and enjoy!

Nutrition: Calories per Serving: 606; Carbs: 70.3g; Protein: 27.2g; Fat: 27.6g

Squash And Eggplant Casserole

Preparation time: 10 minutes

Cooking time: 45 minutes

Servings: 2

Ingredients:

½ cup dry white wine

1 eggplant, halved and cut to 1-inch slices

1 large onion, cut into wedges

1 red bell pepper, seeded and cut to julienned strips

1 small butternut squash, cut into 1-inch slices

1 tbsp olive oil

12 baby corn

2 cups low sodium vegetable broth

Salt and pepper to taste

¼ cup parmesan cheese, grated

1 cup instant polenta

2 tbsp fresh oregano, chopped

1 garlic clove, chopped

2 tbsp slivered almonds

5 tbsp parsley, chopped

Grated zest of 1 lemon

Directions:

Preheat the oven to 350 degrees Fahrenheit.

In a casserole, heat the oil and add the onion wedges and baby corn. Sauté over medium high heat for five minutes. Stir occasionally to prevent the onions and baby corn from sticking at the bottom of the pan.

Add the butternut squash to the casserole and toss the vegetables. Add the eggplants and the red pepper.

Cover the vegetables and cook over low to medium heat.

Cook for about ten minutes before adding the wine. Let the wine sizzle before stirring in the broth. Bring to a boil and cook in the oven for 30 minutes.

While the casserole is cooking inside the oven, make the topping by spreading the slivered almonds on a baking tray and toasting under the grill until they are lightly browned.

Place the toasted almonds in a small bowl and mix the remaining ingredients for the toppings.

Preparation are the polenta. In a large saucepan, bring 3 cups of water to boil over high heat.

Add the polenta and continue whisking until it absorbs all the water.

Reduce the heat to medium until the polenta is thick. Add the parmesan cheese and oregano.

Serve the polenta on plates and add the casserole on top. Sprinkle the toppings on top.

Nutrition: Calories per Serving: 579.3; Carbs: 79.2g; Protein: 22.2g; Fat: 19.3g

Blue Cheese And Grains Salad

Preparation time: 10 minutes

Cooking time: 40 minutes

Servings: 4

Ingredients:

¼ cup thinly sliced scallions

½ cup millet, rinsed

½ cup quinoa, rinsed

1 ½ tsp olive oil

1 Bartlett pear, cored and diced

1/8 tsp ground black pepper

2 cloves garlic, minced

2 oz blue cheese

2 tbsp fresh lemon juice

2 tsp dried rosemary

4 4-oz boneless, skinless chicken breasts

6 oz baby spinach

olive oil cooking spray

¼ cup fresh raspberries

1 tbsp pure maple syrup

1 tsp fresh thyme leaf

2 tbsp grainy mustard

6 tbsp balsamic vinegar

Directions:

Bring millet, quinoa, and 2 ¼ cups water on a small saucepan to a boil. Once boiling, slow fire to a simmer and stir once. Cover and cook until water is fully absorbed and grains are soft around 15 minutes. Turn off fire, fluff grains with a fork and set aside to cool a bit.

Arrange one oven rack to highest position and preheat broiler. Line a baking sheet with foil, and grease with cooking spray.

Whisk well pepper, oil, rosemary, lemon juice and garlic. Rub onto chicken.

Place chicken on preparation ared pan, pop into the broiler and broil until juices run clear and no longer pin inside around 12 minutes.

Meanwhile, make the dressing by combining all ingredients in a blender. Blend until smooth.

Remove chicken from oven, cool slightly before cutting into strips, against the grain.

To assemble, place grains in a large salad bowl. Add in dressing and spinach, toss to mix well.

Add scallions and pear, mix gently and evenly divide into four plates. Top each salad with cheese and chicken.

Serve and enjoy.

Nutrition: Calories per Serving: 530.4; Carbs: 77g; Protein: 21.4g; Fat: 15.2g

Creamy Artichoke Lasagna

Preparation time: 10 minutes

Cooking time: 70 minutes

Servings: 3

Ingredients:

1 cup shredded mozzarella cheese

2 cups light cream

¼ cup all-purpose flour

1 cup vegetable broth

¾ tsp salt

1 egg

1 cup snipped fresh basil

1 cup finely shredded Parmesan cheese

1 15-oz carton ricotta cheese

4 cloves garlic, minced

½ cup pine nuts

3 tbsp olive oil

9 dried lasagna noodles, cooked, rinsed in cold water and drained

15 fresh baby artichokes

¼ cup lemon juice

3 cups water

Directions:

Preparation are in a medium bowl lemon juice and water. Put aside. Slice off artichoke base and remove yellowed outer leaves and cut into quarters. Immediately soak sliced artichokes in preparation ared liquid and drain after a minute.

Over medium fire, place a big saucepan with 2 tbsp oil and fry half of garlic, pine nuts and artichokes. Stir frequently and cook until artichokes are soft around ten minutes. Turn off fire and transfer mixture to a big bowl and quickly stir in salt, egg, ½ cup of basil, ½ cup of parmesan cheese and ricotta cheese. Mix thoroughly.

In a small bowl mix flour and broth. In same pan, add 1 tbsp oil and fry remaining garlic for half a minute. Add light cream and flour mixture. Stir constantly and cook until thickened. Remove from fire and stir in ½ cup of basil.

In a separate bowl mix ½ cup parmesan and mozzarella cheese.

Assemble the lasagna by layering the following in a greased rectangular glass dish: lasagna, 1/3 of artichoke mixture, 1/3 of sauce, sprinkle with the dried cheeses and repeat layering procedure until all ingredients are used up.

For forty minutes, bake lasagna in a preheated oven of 350oF. Remove lasagna from oven and before serving, let it stand for fifteen minutes.

Nutrition: Calories per Serving: 425; Carbs: 41.4g; Protein: 21.3g; Fat: 19.8g

Brown Rice Pilaf With Butternut Squash

Preparation time: 10 minutes

Cooking time: 50 minutes

Servings: 3

Ingredients:

Pepper to taste

A pinch of cinnamon

1 tsp salt

2 tbsp chopped fresh oregano

½ cup chopped fennel fronds

½ cup white wine

1 ¾ cups water + 2 tbsp, divided

1 cup instant or parboiled brown rice

1 tbsp tomato paste

1 garlic clove, minced

1 large onion, finely chopped

3 tbsp extra virgin olive oil

2 lbs. butternut squash, peeled, halved and seeded

Directions:

In a large hole grater, grate squash.

On medium low fire, place a large nonstick skillet and heat oil for 2 minutes.

Add garlic and onions. Sauté for 8 minutes or until lightly colored and soft.

Add 2 tbsp water and tomato paste. Stir well to combine and cook for 3 minutes.

Add rice, mix well to coat in mixture and cook for 5 minutes while stirring frequently.

If needed, add squash in batches until it has wilted so that you can cover pan.

Add remaining water and increase fire to medium high.

Add wine, cover and boil. Once boiling, lower fire to a simmer and cook for 20 to 25 minutes or until liquid is fully absorbed.

Stir in pepper, cinnamon, salt, oregano, and fennel fronds.

Turn off fire, cover and let it stand for 5 minutes before serving.

Nutrition: Calories per Serving: 147; Carbs: 22.1g; Protein: 2.3g; Fat: 5.5g

Cranberry And Roasted Squash Delight

Preparation time: 10 minutes

Cooking time: 60 minutes

Servings: 8

Ingredients:

¼ cup chopped walnuts

¼ tsp thyme

½ tbsp chopped Italian parsley

1 cup diced onion

1 cup fresh cranberries

1 small orange, peeled and segmented

2 tsp canola oil, divided

4 cups cooked wild rice

4 cups diced winter squash, peeled and cut into ½-inch cubes

Pepper to taste

Directions:

Grease roasting pan with cooking spray and preheat oven to 400oF.

In preparation ped roasting pan place squash cubes, add a teaspoon of oil and toss to coat. Place in oven and roast until lightly browned, around 40 minutes.

On medium high fire, place a nonstick fry pan and heat remaining oil. Once hot, add onions and sauté until lightly browned and tender, around 5 minutes.

Add cranberries and continue stir frying for a minute.

Add remaining ingredients into pan and cook until heated through around four to five minutes.

Best served warm.

Nutrition: Calories per Serving: 166.2; Protein: 4.8g; Carbs: 29.1g; Fat: 3.4g

Spanish Rice Casserole With Cheesy Beef

Preparation time: 10 minutes

Cooking time: 32 minutes

Servings: 2

Ingredients:

2 tablespoons chopped green bell pepper

1/4 teaspoon Worcestershire sauce

1/4 teaspoon ground cumin

1/4 cup shredded Cheddar cheese

1/4 cup finely chopped onion

1/4 cup chile sauce

1/3 cup uncooked long grain rice

1/2-pound lean ground beef

1/2 teaspoon salt

1/2 teaspoon brown sugar

1/2 pinch ground black pepper

1/2 cup water

1/2 (14.5 ounce) can canned tomatoes

1 tablespoon chopped fresh cilantro

Directions:

Place a nonstick saucepan on medium fire and brown beef for 10 minutes while crumbling beef. Discard fat.

Stir in pepper, Worcestershire sauce, cumin, brown sugar, salt, chile sauce, rice, water, tomatoes, green bell pepper, and onion. Mix well and cook for 10 minutes until blended and a bit tender.

Transfer to an ovenproof casserole and press down firmly. Sprinkle cheese on top and cook for 7 minutes at 400oF preheated oven. Broil for 3 minutes until top is lightly browned.

Serve and enjoy with chopped cilantro.

Nutrition: Calories per serving: 460; Carbohydrates: 35.8g; Protein: 37.8g; Fat: 17.9g

Kidney Bean And Parsley-lemon Salad

Preparation time: 10 minutes

Cooking time: 0 minutes

Servings: 6

Ingredients:

¼ cup lemon juice (about 1 ½ lemons)

¼ cup olive oil

¾ cup chopped fresh parsley

¾ teaspoon salt

1 can (15 ounces) chickpeas, rinsed and drained, or 1 ½ cups cooked chickpeas

1 medium cucumber, peeled, seeded and diced

1 small red onion, diced

2 cans (15 ounces each) red kidney beans, rinsed and drained, or 3 cups cooked kidney beans

2 stalks celery, sliced in half or thirds lengthwise and chopped

2 tablespoons chopped fresh dill or mint

3 cloves garlic, pressed or minced

Small pinch red pepper flakes

Directions:

Whisk well in a small bowl the pepper flakes, salt, garlic, and lemon juice until emulsified.

In a serving bowl, combine the preparation ared kidney beans, chickpeas, onion, celery, cucumber, parsley and dill (or mint).

Drizzle salad with the dressing and toss well to coat.

Serve and enjoy.

Nutrition: Calories per serving: 228; Protein: 8.5g; Carbs: 26.2g; Fat: 11.0g

Italian White Bean Soup

Preparation time: 10 minutes

Cooking time: 50 minutes

Servings: 4

Ingredients:

1 (14 ounce) can chicken broth

1 bunch fresh spinach, rinsed and thinly sliced

1 clove garlic, minced

1 stalk celery, chopped

1 tablespoon lemon juice

1 tablespoon vegetable oil

1 onion, chopped

1/4 teaspoon ground black pepper

1/8 teaspoon dried thyme

2 (16 ounce) cans white kidney beans, rinsed and drained

2 cups water

Directions:

Place a pot on medium high fire and heat pot for a minute. Add oil and heat for another minute.

Stir in celery and onion. Sauté for 7 minutes.

Stir in garlic and cook for another minute.

Add water, thyme, pepper, chicken broth, and beans. Cover and simmer for 15 minutes.

Remove 2 cups of the bean and celery mixture with a slotted spoon and set aside.

With an immersion blender, puree remaining soup in pot until smooth and creamy.

Return the 2 cups of bean mixture. Stir in spinach and lemon juice. Cook for 2 minutes until heated through and spinach is wilted.

Serve and enjoy.

Nutrition: Calories per serving: 245; Protein: 12.0g; Carbs: 38.1g; Fat: 4.9g

Mexican Quinoa Bake

Preparation time: 10 minutes

Cooking time: 40 minutes

Servings: 4

Ingredients:

3 cups sweet potato, peeled, diced very small (about 1 large sweet potato)

2 cups cooked quinoa

1 cup shredded sharp cheddar cheese

2 Tbs chili powder

T Tbs paprika

1 1/4 cup salsa of your choice

1 red bell pepper, diced

1 large carrot, diced

3 Tbs canned green chiles

1 small onion, diced

3 garlic cloves, minced

2 cups cooked black beans

Directions:

Preheat oven to 400oF.

Dice, chop, measure and preparation all ingredients.

Combine all ingredients in one big bowl and toss ingredients well.

Spray a 9 X 13-inch pan with cooking spray and pour all ingredients in.

Bake for 35-40 minutes or until sweet potato pieces are slightly mushy, cheese is melted and items are heated all the way through.

Let sit for about 5 minutes, scoop into bowls and enjoy!

Nutrition: Calories per serving: 414; Carbs: 56.6g; Protein: 22.0g; Fat: 13.0g

Citrus Quinoa & Chickpea Salad

Preparation time: 10 minutes

Cooking time: 0 minutes

Servings: 4

Ingredients:

2 cups cooked quinoa

1 can chickpeas, drained & rinsed

1 ripe avocado, diced

1 red bell pepper, diced

1/2 red onion, diced

1/4 cup lime juice

1/2 tbsp garlic powder

1/2 tbsp paprika

1/4-1/2 cup chopped cilantro

1 tbsp chopped jalapenos

Sea salt to taste

Directions:

Add all ingredients in a large bowl and mix well.

Enjoy right away or refrigerate for later.

Nutrition: Calories per serving: 300; Carbs: 43.5g; Protein: 10.3g; Fat: 10.9g

Chickpea Salad Moroccan Style

Preparation time: 10 minutes

Cooking time: 0 minutes

Servings: 6

Ingredients:

1/3 cup crumbled low-fat feta cheese

¼ cup fresh mint, chopped

¼ cup fresh cilantro, chopped

1 red bell pepper, diced

2 plum tomatoes, diced

3 green onions, sliced thinly

1 large carrot, peeled and julienned

3 cups BPA free canned chickpeas or garbanzo beans

Pinch of cayenne pepper

¼ tsp salt

¼ tsp pepper

2 tsp ground cumin

3 tbsp fresh lemon juice

3 tbsp olive oil

Directions:

Make the dressing by whisking cayenne, black pepper, salt, cumin, lemon juice and oil in a small bowl and set aside.

Mix together feta, mint, cilantro, red pepper, tomatoes, onions, carrots and chickpeas in a large salad bowl.

Pour dressing over salad and toss to coat well.

Serve and enjoy.

Nutrition: Calories per serving: 300; Protein: 13.2g; Carbs: 35.4g; Fat: 12.8g

Garlicky Peas And Clams On Veggie Spiral

Preparation time: 10 minutes

Cooking time: 15 minutes

Servings: 4

Ingredients:

2 tbsp chopped fresh basil

½ cup pre-shredded Parmesan cheese

1 cup frozen green peas

¼ tsp crushed red pepper

¼ cup dry white wine

1 cup organic vegetable broth

3 cans chopped clams, clams and juice separated

1 ½ tsp bottled minced garlic

2 tbsp olive oil

6 cups zucchini, spiral

Directions:

Bring a pot of water to a rolling boil and blanch zucchini for 4 minutes on high fire. Drain and let stand for a couple of minutes to continue cooking.

On medium high fire, add a large nonstick saucepan and heat oil. Add and sauté for a minute the garlic. Pour in wine, broth and clam juice.

Once liquid is boiling, low fire to a simmer and add pepper. Continue cooking and stirring for 5 minutes.

Add peas and clams, cook until heated through or around two minutes.

Toss in zucchini, mix well. Cook until heated through.

Add basil and cheese, toss to mix well then remove from fire.

Transfer equally to four serving bowls and enjoy.

Nutrition: Calories per Serving: 210; Carbs: 24.0g; Protein: 8.5g; Fat: 9.2g

Leek, Bacon And Pea Risotto

Preparation time: 10 minutes

Cooking time: 60 minutes

Servings: 4

Ingredients:

Salt and pepper to taste

2 tbsp fresh lemon juice

½ cup grated parmesan cheese

¾ cup frozen peas

1 cup dry white wine

2 ½ cups Arborio rice

4 slices bacon (cut into strips)

12 cups low sodium chicken broth

2 leeks cut lengthwise

Directions:

In a saucepan, bring the broth to a simmer over medium flame.

On another skillet, cook bacon and stir continuously to avoid the bacon from burning. Cook more for five minutes and add the leeks and cook for two more minutes.

Increase the heat to medium high and add the rice until the grains become translucent.

Add the wine and stir until it evaporates.

Add 1 cup of broth to the mixture and reduce the heat to medium low. Stir constantly for two minutes.

Gradually add the remaining broth until the rice becomes al dente and it becomes creamy.

Add the peas and the rest of the broth.

Remove the skillet or turn off the heat and add the Parmesan cheese.

Cover the skillet and let the cheese melt. Season the risotto with lemon juice, salt and pepper.

Serve the risotto with more parmesan cheese.

Nutrition: Calories per Serving: 742; Carbs: 57.6g; Protein: 38.67g; Fat: 39.6g

Chickpea Fried Eggplant Salad

Preparation time: 10 minutes

Cooking time: 10 minutes

Servings: 3

Ingredients:

1 cup chopped dill

1 cup chopped parsley

1 cup cooked or canned chickpeas, drained

1 large eggplant, thinly sliced (no more than 1/4 inch in thickness)

1 small red onion, sliced in 1/2 moons

1/2 English cucumber, diced

3 Roma tomatoes, diced

3 tbsp Za'atar spice, divided

oil for frying, preferably extra virgin olive oil

Salt

1 large lime, juice of

1/3 cup extra virgin olive oil

1-2 garlic cloves, minced

Salt & Pepper to taste

Directions:

On a baking sheet, spread out sliced eggplant and season with salt generously. Let it sit for 30 minutes. Then pat dry with paper towel.

Place a small pot on medium high fire and fill halfway with oil. Heat oil for 5 minutes. Fry eggplant in batches until golden brown, around 3 minutes per side. Place cooked eggplants on a paper towel lined plate.

Once eggplants have cooled, assemble the eggplant on a serving dish. Sprinkle with 1 tbsp of Za'atar.

Mix dill, parsley, red onions, chickpeas, cucumbers, and tomatoes in a large salad bowl. Sprinkle remaining Za'atar and gently toss to mix.

Whisk well the vinaigrette ingredients in a small bowl. Drizzle 2 tbsp of the dressing over the fried eggplant. Add remaining dressing over the chickpea salad and mix.

Add the chickpea salad to the serving dish with the fried eggplant.

Serve and enjoy.

Nutrition: Calories per serving: 642; Protein: 16.6g; Carbs: 25.9g; Fat: 44.0g

Turkey And Quinoa Stuffed Peppers

Preparation time: 10 minutes

Cooking time: 55 minutes

Servings: 6

Ingredients:

3 large red bell peppers

2 tsp chopped fresh rosemary

2 tbsp chopped fresh parsley

3 tbsp chopped pecans, toasted

¼ cup extra virgin olive oil

½ cup chicken stock

½ lb. fully cooked smoked turkey sausage, diced

½ tsp salt

2 cups water

1 cup uncooked quinoa

Directions:

On high fire, place a large saucepan and add salt, water and quinoa. Bring to a boil.

Once boiling, reduce fire to a simmer, cover and cook until all water is absorbed around 15 minutes.

Uncover quinoa, turn off fire and let it stand for another 5 minutes.

Add rosemary, parsley, pecans, olive oil, chicken stock and turkey sausage into pan of quinoa. Mix well.

Slice peppers lengthwise in half and discard membranes and seeds. In another boiling pot of water, add peppers, boil for 5 minutes, drain and discard water.

Grease a 13 x 9 baking dish and preheat oven to 350oF.

Place boiled bell pepper onto preparation ared baking dish, evenly fill with the quinoa mixture and pop into oven.

Bake for 15 minutes.

Nutrition: Calories per Serving: 255.6; Carbs: 21.6g; Protein: 14.4g; Fat: 12.4g

Pastitsio An Italian Dish

Preparation time: 10 minutes

Cooking time: 30 minutes

Servings: 8

Ingredients:

2 tbsp chopped fresh flat leaf parsley

¾ cup shredded mozzarella cheese

1 3oz package of fat free cream cheese

½ cup 1/3 less fat cream cheese

1 can 14.5-oz of diced tomatoes, drained

2 cups fat free milk

1 tbsp all-purpose flour

¾ tsp kosher salt

5 garlic cloves, minced

1 ½ cups chopped onion

1 tbsp olive oil

1 lb. ground sirloin

Cooking spray

8 oz penne, cooked and drained

Directions:

On medium high fire, place a big nonstick saucepan and for five minutes sauté beef. Keep on stirring to break up the pieces of ground meat. Once cooked, remove from pan and drain fat.

Using same pan, heat oil and fry onions until soft around four minutes while occasionally stirring.

Add garlic and continue cooking for another minute while constantly stirring.

Stir in beef and flour, cook for another minute. Mix constantly.

Add the fat free cream cheese, less fat cream cheese, tomatoes and milk. Cook until mixture is smooth and heated. Toss in pasta and mix well.

Transfer pasta into a greased rectangular glass dish and top with mozzarella. Cook in a preheated broiler for four minutes. Remove from broiler and garnish with parsley before serving.

Nutrition: Calories per Serving: 263; Carbs: 17.8g; Protein: 24.1g; Fat: 10.6g

Spiced Eggplant Stew

Preparation time: 10 minutes

Cooking time: 45 minutes

Servings: 4

Ingredients:

4 eggplants, cubed

Salt and black pepper to the taste

2 yellow onions, chopped

2 red bell peppers, chopped

30 ounces canned tomatoes, chopped

1 cup black olives, pitted and chopped

¼ teaspoon allspice, ground

½ teaspoon cinnamon powder

1 teaspoon oregano, dried

A drizzle of olive oil

A pinch of red chili flakes

3 tablespoons Greek yogurt

Directions:

Heat up a pot with the oil over medium high heat, add the onions, bell pepper, oregano, cinnamon and the allspice and sauté fro 5 minutes.

Add the rest of the ingredients except the flakes and the yogurt, bring to a simmer and cook over medium heat for 40 minutes.

Divide the stew into bowls, top each serving with the flakes and the yogurt and serve.

Nutrition: calories 256, fat 3.5, fiber 25.4, carbs 53.3, protein 8.8

Shrimp Soup

Preparation time: 10 minutes

Cooking time: 5 minutes

Servings: 3

Ingredients:

1 cucumber, chopped

3 cups tomato juice

3 roasted red peppers, chopped

3 tablespoons olive oil

2 tablespoons balsamic vinegar

1 garlic clove, minced

Salt and black pepper to the taste

½ teaspoon cumin, ground

1 pounds shrimp, peeled and deveined

1 teaspoon thyme, chopped

Directions:

In your blender, mix cucumber with tomato juice, red peppers, 2 tablespoons oil, the vinegar, cumin, salt, pepper and the garlic, pulse well, transfer to a bowl and keep in the fridge for 10 minutes.

Heat up a pot with the rest of the oil over medium heat, add the shrimp, salt, pepper and the thyme and cook for 2 minutes on each side.

Divide cold soup into bowls, top with the shrimp and serve.

Nutrition: calories 263, fat 11.1, fiber 2.4, carbs 12.5, protein 6.32

Halloumi, Grape Tomato And Zucchini Skewers With Spinach-basil Oil

Preparation time: 10 minutes

Cooking time: 10 minutes

Ingredients:

1 large zucchini, halved lengthways, cut into 8 pieces

16 grape tomatoes

180 g halloumi cheese, cut into 16 pieces

Olive oil spray

For the spinach-basil oil:

2 cups baby spinach leaves

2 cups fresh basil leaves

185 ml (3/4 cup) extra-virgin olive oil

125 ml (1/2 cup) light olive oil

Directions:

In a saucepan of boiling water, cook the spinach and the basil for about 30 seconds or until just wilted. Drain and cool under running cold water.

Place the cooked spinach and basil into a food processor. Add the light olive oil and the extra-virgin olive oil; process until the mixture is smooth. Transfer into an airtight container, refrigerate for 8 hours to develop the flavors.

Preheat the barbecue grill to medium-high.

Thread a piece of zucchini, halloumi cheese, and tomato into each skewer. Lightly spray with the olive oil spray.

Grill for about4 minutes per side or until cooked through and golden brown.

Arrange the grilled skewers on to serving platter; serve immediately with the preparation ared spinach-basil oil.

Nutrition: :192.2Cal, 20 g total fat (4 g sat. fat), 1 g carb., 1 g fiber, 1 g sugar, 3 g protein, and 328.8 mg sodium.

Beef Bourguignon

Preparation time: 10 minutes

Cooking time: 2 Hours

Servings: 3

Ingredients:

3 tablespoons olive oil

2 pounds beef roast, cubed

1 tablespoon all-purpose flour

3 sweet onions, chopped

2 carrots, sliced

4 garlic cloves, minced

1 chili pepper, sliced

1 pound button mushrooms

1 ½ cups beef stock

½ cup dark beer

2 bay leaves

1 thyme sprig

1 rosemary sprig

Salt and pepper to taste

Directions:

Sprinkle the beef with flour.

Heat the oil in a deep heavy pot and add the beef roast.

Cook on all sides for 5 minutes or until browned.

Add the onions, carrots and chili and cook for 5 more minutes.

Add the mushrooms, stock, beer, bay leaves, thyme, rosemary, salt and pepper.

Cover the pot and cook on low heat for 1 ½ hours.

Serve the stew warm and fresh.

Nutrition: Per Serving:Calories:306 Fat:12.6g Protein:37.6g Carbohydrates:9.0g

Flank Steak

Preparation time: 10 minutes

Cooking time: 40 minutes

Servings: 3

Ingredients:

4 flank steaks

1 lemon, juiced

1 orange, juiced

4 garlic cloves, chopped

1 teaspoon Dijon mustard

1 teaspoon chopped thyme

1 teaspoon dried sage

2 tablespoons olive oil

Salt and pepper to taste

Directions:

Combine the flank steaks and the rest of the ingredients in a zip lock bag.

Refrigerate for 30 minutes.

Heat a grill pan over medium flame and place the steaks on the grill.

Cook on each side for 6-7 minutes.

Serve the steaks warm and fresh.

Nutrition: Per Serving:Calories:234 Fat:13.4g Protein:21.6g Carbohydrates:6.7g

Spiced Grilled Flank Steak

Preparation time: 10 minutes

Cooking time: 40 minutes

Servings: 3

Ingredients:

4 flank steaks

1 teaspoon chili powder

1 teaspoon ground coriander

1 teaspoon ground cumin

1 teaspoon mustard powder

Salt and pepper to taste

Directions:

Season the steaks with salt and pepper then sprinkle with chili, coriander, cumin and mustard powder.

Allow to rest for 20 minutes then heat a grill pan over medium flame and place the steaks on the grill.

Cook on each side for 5-7 minutes and serve the steaks warm and fresh.

Nutrition: Per Serving:Calories:202 Fat:8.8g Protein:28.2g Carbohydrates:0.9g

Pan Roasted Chicken With Olives And Lemon

Preparation time: 10 minutes

Cooking time: 50 minutes

Servings: 4

Ingredients:

4 chicken legs

Salt and pepper to taste

3 tablespoons olive oil

1 lemon, juiced

1 orange, juiced

1 jalapeno, sliced

2 garlic cloves, chopped

½ cup green olives, sliced

¼ cup black olives, pitted and sliced

1 thyme sprig

1 rosemary sprig

Directions:

Season the chicken with salt and pepper.

Heat the oil in a skillet and add the chicken.

Cook on each side for 5 minutes until golden brown then add the rest of the ingredients and continue cooking on medium heat for 15 minutes.

Serve the chicken and the sauce warm.

Nutrition: Per Serving:Calories:319 Fat:18.9g Protein:29.7g Carbohydrates:8.0g

Creamy Salmon Soup

Preparation time: 10 minutes

Cooking time: 30 minutes

Servings: 6

Ingredients:

2 tablespoon olive oil

1 red onion, chopped

Salt and white pepper to the taste

3 gold potatoes, peeled and cubed

2 carrots, chopped

4 cups fish stock

4 ounces salmon fillets, boneless and cubed

½ cup heavy cream

1 tablespoon dill, chopped

Directions:

Heat up a pan with the oil over medium heat, add the onion, and sauté for 5 minutes.

Add the rest of the ingredients expect the cream, salmon and the dill, bring to a simmer and cook for 5-6 minutes more.

Add the salmon, cream and the dill, simmer for 5 minutes more, divide into bowls and serve.

Nutrition: calories 214, fat 16.3, fiber 1.5, carbs 6.4, protein 11.8

Grilled Salmon With Cucumber Dill Sauce

Preparation time: 10 minutes

Cooking time: 30 minutes

Servings: 4

Ingredients:

4 salmon fillets

1 teaspoon smoked paprika

1 teaspoon dried sage

Salt and pepper to taste

4 cucumbers, sliced

2 tablespoons chopped dill

½ cup Greek yogurt

1 tablespoon lemon juice

1 tablespoon olive oil

Directions:

Season the salmon with salt, pepper, paprika and sage.

Heat a grill pan over medium flame and place the salmon on the grill.

Cook on each side for 4 minutes.

For the sauce, mix the cucumbers, dill, yogurt, lemon juice and oil in a bowl. Add salt and pepper and mix well.

Serve the salmon with the cucumber sauce.

Nutrition: Per Serving:Calories:224 Fat:10.3g Protein:26.3g Carbohydrates:8.9g

Grilled Basil-lemon Tofu Burgers

Preparation time: 10 minutes

Cooking time: 6 minutes

Servings: 5

Ingredients:

6 slices (1/4-inch thick each) tomato

6 pieces (1 1/2-ounce) whole-wheat hamburger buns

1 pound tofu, firm or extra-firm, drained

1 cup watercress, trimmed

Cooking spray

1/3 cup fresh basil, finely chopped

2 tablespoons Dijon mustard

2 tablespoons honey

1/4 cup freshly squeezed lemon juice

2 teaspoons grated lemon rind

1 tablespoon olive oil, extra-virgin,

1/2 teaspoon salt

1/4 teaspoon black pepper (freshly ground)

3 garlic cloves, minced

1 garlic cloves, minced

1/3 cup Kalamata olives, finely, chopped pitted

3 tablespoons sour cream, reduced-fat

3 tablespoons light mayonnaise

Directions:

Combine the marinade ingredients in a small-sized bowl. In a crosswise direction, cut the tofu into 6 slices. Pat each piece dry using paper towels. Place them in a jelly roll pan and brush both sides of the slices with the marinade mixture; reserve any leftover marinade. Marinate for 1 hour.

Preheat the grill and coated the grill rack with cooking spray. Place the tofu slices; grill for about 3 minutes per side, brushing the tofu with the reserved marinade mixture.

In a small-sized bowl, combine the garlic-olive mayonnaise ingredients. Spread about 1 1/2 tablespoons of the mixture over the bottom half of the hamburger buns. Top each with 1 slice tofu, 1 slice tomato, about 2 tablespoons of watercress, and top with the top buns.

Nutrition: :276 Cal, 11.3 g total fat (1.9 g sat. fat, 5.7 g mono fat, 2.2 g poly fat), 10.5 g protein, 34.5 g carb., 1.5 g fiber, 5 mg chol., 2.4 mg iron, 743 mg sodium, and 101 mg calcium.

Creamy Green Pea Pasta

Preparation time: 10 minutes

Cooking time: 25 minutes

Servings: 4

Ingredients:

8 oz. whole wheat spaghetti

1 cup green peas

1 avocado, peeled and cubed

2 tablespoons olive oil

2 garlic cloves, chopped

2 mint leaves

1 tablespoon lemon juice

¼ cup heavy cream

2 tablespoons vegetable stock

Salt and pepper to taste

Directions:

Pour a few cups of water in a deep pot and bring to a boil with a pinch of salt.

Add the spaghetti and cook for 8 minutes then drain well.

For the sauce, combine the remaining ingredients in a blender and pulse until smooth.

Mix the cooked the spaghetti with the sauce and serve the pasta fresh.

Nutrition: Per Serving:Calories:294 Fat:20.1g Protein:6.4g Carbohydrates:25.9g

Meat Cakes

Preparation time: 10 minutes

Cooking time: 10 minutes

Servings: 4

Ingredients:

1 cup broccoli, shredded

½ cup ground pork

2 eggs, beaten

1 teaspoon salt

1 tablespoon Italian seasonings

1 teaspoon olive oil

3 tablespoons wheat flour, whole grain

1 tablespoon dried dill

Directions:

In the mixing bowl combine together shredded broccoli and ground pork,

Add salt, Italian seasoning, flour, and dried dill.

Mix up the mixture until homogenous.

Then add eggs and stir until smooth.

Heat up olive oil in the skillet.

With the help of the spoon make latkes and place them in the hot oil.

Roast the latkes for 4 minutes from each side over the medium heat.

The cooked latkes should have a light brown crust.

Dry the latkes with the paper towels if needed.

Nutrition: :calories 143, fat 6, fiber 0.9, carbs 7, protein 15.1

Herbed Roasted Cod

Preparation time: 10 minutes

Cooking time: 45 minutes

Servings: 3

Ingredients:

4 cod fillets

4 parsley sprigs

2 cilantro sprigs

2 basil sprigs

1 lemon, sliced

Salt and pepper to taste

2 tablespoons olive oil

Directions:

Season the cod with salt and pepper.

Place the parsley, cilantro, basil and lemon slices at the bottom of a deep dish baking pan.

Place the cod over the herbs and cook in the preheated oven at 350F for 15 minutes.

Serve the cod warm and fresh with your favorite side dish.

Nutrition: Per Serving:Calories:192 Fat:8.1g Protein:28.6g Carbohydrates:0.1g

Mushroom Soup

Preparation time: 10 minutes

Cooking time: 20 minutes

Servings: 2

Ingredients:

1 cup cremini mushrooms, chopped

1 cup Cheddar cheese, shredded

2 cups of water

½ teaspoon salt

1 teaspoon dried thyme

½ teaspoon dried oregano

1 tablespoon fresh parsley, chopped

1 tablespoon olive oil

1 bell pepper, chopped

Directions:

Pour olive oil in the pan.

Add mushrooms and bell pepper. Roast the vegetables for 5 minutes over the medium heat.

Then sprinkle them with salt, thyme, and dried oregano.

Add parsley and water. Stir the soup well.

Cook the soup for 10 minutes.

After this, blend the soup until it is smooth and simmer it for 5 minutes more.

Add cheese and stir until cheese is melted.

Ladle the cooked soup into the bowls. It is recommended to serve soup hot.

Nutrition: :calories 320, fat 26, fiber 1.4, carbs 7.4, protein 15.7

Salmon Parmesan Gratin

Preparation time: 10 minutes

Cooking time: 45 minutes

Servings: 3

Ingredients:

4 salmon fillets, cubed

2 garlic cloves, chopped

1 fennel bulb, sliced

½ teaspoon ground coriander

½ teaspoon Dijon mustard

½ cup vegetable stock

1 cup heavy cream

2 eggs

Salt and pepper to taste

1 cup grated Parmesan cheese

Directions:

Combine the salmon, garlic, fennel, coriander and mustard in a small deep dish baking pan.

Mix the eggs with cream and stock and pour the mixture over the fish.

Top with Parmesan cheese and bake in the preheated oven at 350F for 25 minutes.

Serve the gratin right away.

Nutrition: Per Serving:Calories:414 Fat:25.9g Protein:41.0g Carbohydrates:6.1g

Chicken Souvlaki 2

Preparation time: 10 minutes

Cooking time: 30 minutes

Servings: 3

Ingredients:

4-6 chicken breasts, boneless, skinless

For the marinade:

1 tablespoon dried oregano (use Greek or Turkish oregano)

1 tablespoon garlic, finely minced (or garlic puree from a jar)

1 tablespoon red wine vinegar

1 teaspoon dried thyme

1/2 cup lemon juice, freshly squeezed

1/2 cup olive oil

Directions:

If there are any visible fat on the chicken, trim them off. Cut each breasts into 5-6 pieces 1-inch thick crosswise strips. Put them in a Ziploc bag or a container with tight lid.

Whisk the marinade ingredients together until combined. Pour into the bag or container with the chicken, seal, and shake the bag or the container to coat the chicken. Marinade for 6 to 8 hours or more in the refrigerator.

When marinated, remove the chicken from the fridge, let thaw to room temperature, and drain; discard the marinade. Thread the chicken strips into skewers, about 6 pieces on each skewer, the meat folded over to it would not spin around on the skewers.

Mist the grill with olive oil. Preheat the charcoal or gas grill to medium high.

Grill the skewers for about 12-15 minutes, turning once as soon as you see grill marks. Souvlaki is done when the chicken is slightly browned and firm, but not hard to the touch.

Nutrition: :360 cal., 26 g total fat (4.5 g sat fat), 90 mg chol., 170 mg sodium, 570 mg potassium, 3 g carb., 0 g fiber, <1 g sugar, and 30 g protein.

Rosemary Roasted New Potatoes

Preparation time: 10 minutes

Cooking time: 1 Hour 30 minutes

Servings: 3

Ingredients:

2 pounds new potatoes, washed

3 tablespoons olive oil

2 rosemary sprigs

4 garlic cloves, crushed

Salt and pepper to taste

Directions:

Place the new potatoes in a large pot and cover them with water. Cook for 15 minutes then drain well.

Heat the oil in a skillet and add the rosemary and garlic.

Stir in the potatoes and continue cooking on medium flame for 20 minutes or until evenly golden brown.

Serve the potatoes warm.

Nutrition: Per Serving:Calories:168 Fat:7.2g Protein:2.7g Carbohydrates:24.6g

Artichoke Feta Penne

Preparation time: 10 minutes

Cooking time: 30 minutes

Servings: 4

Ingredients:

8 oz. penne pasta

2 tablespoons olive oil

1 shallot, chopped

4 garlic cloves, chopped

1 jar artichoke hearts, drained and chopped

1 cup diced tomatoes

¼ cup white wine

½ cup vegetable stock

Salt and pepper to taste

4 oz. feta cheese, crumbled

Directions:

Heat the oil in a skillet and stir in the shallot and garlic. Cook for 2 minutes until softened.

Add the artichoke hearts, tomatoes, wine and stock, as well as salt and pepper to taste.

Cook on low heat for 15 minutes.

In the meantime, cook the penne in a large pot of water until al dente, not more than 8 minutes.

Drain the pasta well and mix it with the artichoke sauce.

Serve the penne with crumbled feta cheese.

Nutrition: Per Serving:Calories:325 Fat:14.4g Protein:11.1g Carbohydrates:35.8g

Grilled Chicken And Rustic Mustard Cream

Preparation time: 10 minutes

Cooking time: 12 minutes

Servings: 3

Ingredients:

1 tablespoon plus 1 teaspoon whole-grain Dijon mustard, divided

1 tablespoon water

1 teaspoon fresh rosemary, chopped

1/4 teaspoon black pepper

1/4 teaspoon of salt

1 tablespoon olive oil

3 tablespoons light mayonnaise

4 pieces (6-ounces each) chicken breast halves, skinless, boneless

Rosemary sprigs (optional)

Cooking spray

Directions:

Preheat the grill.

In a small-sized bowl, combine the olive oil, 1-teaspoon of mustard; brush evenly over each chicken breast.

Coat the grill rack with the cooking spray, place and chicken, and grill for 6 minutes per side or until cooked.

While the chicken is grilling, combine the mayonnaise, the 1 tablespoon of mustard, and the water in a bowl.

Serve the grilled chicken with the mustard cream. If desired garnish with some rosemary sprigs.

Nutrition: :262 Cal, 10 g total fat (1 g sat. fat, 4 g mono fat, 3 g poly fat), 39.6 g protein, 1.7 g carb., 0.2 g fiber, 102 mg chol., 1.4 mg iron, 448 mg sodium, and 25 mg calcium.

Balsamic Steak With Feta, Tomato, And Basil

Preparation time: 10 minutes

Cooking time: 20 minutes

Servings: 4

Ingredients:

1 tablespoon balsamic vinegar

1/4 cup basil leaves

175 g Greek fetta, crumbled

2 tablespoons olive oil

2 teaspoons baby capers

4 sirloin steaks, trimmed

4 whole garlic cloves, skin on

6 roma tomatoes, halved

Olive oil spray

Salt and cracked black pepper

Directions:

Preheat the oven to 200C.

Line a baking tray with baking paper. Place the tomatoes and then scatter with the capers, crumbled feta, and the garlic cloves. Drizzle with 1 tablespoon of the olive oil and season with salt and pepper; cook for about 15 minutes or until the tomatoes are soft. Remove from the oven, set aside.

In a large non-metallic bowl, toss the steak with the remaining 1 tablespoon of olive oil, vinegar, salt and pepper; cover and refrigerate for 5 minutes.

Preheat the grill pan to high heat; grill the steaks for about 4 minutes per side or until cooked to your preference.

Serve with the preparation ared tomato mixture and sprinkle with basil.

Nutrition: :520.3 Cal, 30 g total fat (12 g sat. fat), 3 g carb., 2 g fiber, 2 g sugar, 59 g protein, and 622.82 mg sodium.

Fried Chicken With Tzatziki Sauce

Preparation time: 10 minutes

Cooking time: 30 minutes

Servings: 4

Ingredients:

4 chicken breasts, cubed

4 tablespoons olive oil

1 teaspoon dried basil

1 teaspoon dried oregano

½ teaspoon chili flakes

Salt and pepper to taste

1 cup Greek yogurt

1 cucumber, grated

4 garlic cloves, minced

1 teaspoon lemon juice

1 teaspoon chopped mint

2 tablespoons chopped parsley

Directions:

Season the chicken with salt, pepper, basil, oregano and chili.

Heat the oil in a skillet and add the chicken. Cook on each side for 5 minutes on high heat just until golden brown.

Cover the chicken with a lid and continue cooking for 15-20 more minutes.

For the sauce, mix the yogurt, cucumber, garlic, lemon juice, mint and parsley, as well as salt and pepper.

Serve the chicken and the sauce fresh.

Nutrition: Per Serving:Calories:366 Fat:22.6g Protein:34.8g Carbohydrates:6.2g

Green smoothie bowl

Preparation time: 10 minutes

Cooking time: 15 inutes

Servings: 3

Ingredients:

200 g natural yogurt (1.5% fat)

1 medium apple

4 apricots

2 tbsp oatmeal

50 g fresh baby spinach

1 tbsp ground flaxseed

Directions:

Wash the spinach, remove the dead leaves and pat dry with a piece of kitchen paper. Wash apricots, remove stones and cut into small pieces. Wash, quarter and core the apple. Then cut into small pieces.

Put the spinach and fruit in a bowl and puree with a hand blender.

Divide the yoghurt into two bowls and pour the green mixture over them. Sprinkle with the oatmeal and flaxseed and serve.

Nutrition:Calories: 300 Total Fat: 17g Saturated Fat: 4g Cholesterol: 16mg Sodium: 59mg Total Carbohydrates: 34g Fiber: 2g Protein: 7g

Sweet cream cheese breakfast

Preparation time: 10 minutes

Cooking time: 30 minutes

Servings: 3

Ingredients:

400 g of grainy cream cheese

120 g strawberries

100 g blueberries

1 tbsp lemon juice

Fresh mint

Directions:

Wash and clean the strawberries and cut into small pieces. Wash blueberries.

Pour the cream cheese into a bowl and mix with the berries and lemon juice.

Wash the mint, shake dry and pluck some leaves.

Fill the cream cheese into two bowls, garnish with a few mint leaves and serve.

Note: Grainy cream cheese is recommendedparticularly for fatty liver because the fat content is low and the protein content is high. An ideal alternative is not only for breakfast, but also as a spread or instead of high-fat cheeses for warm meals.

Nutrition:Calories: 300 Total Fat: 17g Saturated Fat: 4g Cholesterol: 16mg Sodium: 59mg Total Carbohydrates: 34g Fiber: 2g Protein: 7g

Avocado boat with salsa

Preparation time: 10 minutes

Cooking time: 30 minutes

2 servings

Ingredients:

1 medium avocado

2 medium-sized eggs

1 large tomato

1 teaspoon lemon juice

½ red onion

1 teaspoon olive oil

1 tsp white wine vinegar

Salt and pepper

Directions:

Preheat the oven to 175 degrees top and bottom heat.

Halve the avocado lengthways, remove the stone and brush the flesh with the lemon juice.

Line a baking sheet with a piece of parchment paper and spread the avocado halves on top. Slide an egg into the hollow of the core and sprinkle with a little salt.

Bake on the middle rack for 15-20 minutes.

In the meantime, preparation are the salsa. To do this, peel and finely chop the onion and wash the tomato and cut into fine cubes. Mix both together with the olive oil and vinegar in a bowl. Season to taste with salt and pepper.

Take the avocado out of the oven and serve with the salsa on two plates.

Nutrition:Calories: 300 Total Fat: 17g Saturated Fat: 4g Cholesterol: 16mg Sodium: 59mg Total Carbohydrates: 34g Fiber: 2g Protein: 7g

Vegetable ribbon noodles with chicken breast fillet

Preparation time: 10 minutes

Cooking time: 30 minutes

2 servings

Ingredients:

250 g chicken breast fillet

1 medium-sized carrot

2 small zucchini

2 medium-sized tomatoes

1 tbsp tomato paste

50 ml vegetable broth

1 tbsp olive oil

½ teaspoon paprika powder

Salt and pepper

Directions:

Cut the chicken breast fillet into bite-sized pieces. Heat the olive oil in a pan and add the paprika powder. Now sear the meat until it is completely cooked through. Season with a little salt and pepper.

In the meantime, wash and peel the carrots and cut lengthways into thin strips. Wash the zucchini and cut lengthways into thin strips.

Take the chicken out of the pan and sear the vegetable noodles in the remaining gravy for 3-4 minutes.

Wash tomatoes and cut into small pieces. Then add to the vegetable noodles together with the tomato paste. Simmer for 3-4 minutes over medium heat. Season to taste with salt and pepper.

Add the chicken pieces and sear everything for 2-3 minutes.

Arrange on two plates and serve.

Nutrition:Calories: 300 Total Fat: 17g Saturated Fat: 4g Cholesterol: 16mg Sodium: 59mg Total Carbohydrates: 34g Fiber: 2g Protein: 7g

Zucchini and mozzarella casserole

Preparation time: 10 minutes

Cooking time: 30 minutes

2 servings

Ingredients:

400 g ground poultry

125 g mozzarella

2 medium zucchini

1 medium onion

1 clove of garlic

1 tbsp tomato paste

100 ml vegetable broth

2 teaspoons of olive oil

½ teaspoon dried thyme

½ teaspoon dried oregano

½ teaspoon dried basil

Salt and pepper

Directions:

Preheat the oven to 150 degrees top and bottom heat.

Wash the zucchini and cut into thin slices.

Grease a baking dish with 1 teaspoon of olive oil and arrange some of the zucchini slices evenly in the dish.

Peel onions and cut them into fine pieces. Heat the remaining olive oil in a pan and fry the onion, garlic and minced meat in it until the minced meat has a crumbly consistency. Then stir in the tomato paste and season with a little salt and pepper and season with thyme, oregano and basil.

Spread part of the minced meat mixture over the zucchini slices. Put another zucchini slices on top and distribute the remaining minced meat mixture on top.

Drain the mozzarella, cut into slices and spread on the casserole.

Bake on the middle rack for 20-25 minutes.

Take out of the oven, let cool down a little and serve.

Nutrition:Calories: 300 Total Fat: 17g Saturated Fat: 4g Cholesterol: 16mg Sodium: 59mg Total Carbohydrates: 34g Fiber: 2g Protein: 7g

Oven vegetables with salmon fillet

Preparation time: 10 minutes

Cooking time: 30 minutes

2 servings

Ingredients:

250 g salmon fillet

1 medium zucchini

1 red pepper

300 g cherry tomatoes

150 g mushrooms

100 g of low-fat feta

1 tbsp olive oil

Salt and pepper

Directions:

Preheat the oven to 180 degrees top and bottom heat.

Rub the salmon fillet with salt and pepper.

Wash the zucchini and cut into large pieces. Wash the peppers, remove the core and cut into strips. Wash the cherry tomatoes and cut in half. Clean the mushrooms then cut off the hard stem ends and quarter. Put the vegetables and mushrooms in a bowl, drizzle with the olive oil, season with salt and pepper and mix well.

Drain the feta and cut into cubes.

Spread the vegetables in a baking dish, sprinkle with the feta cubes and serve the salmon fillet on top.

Cook on the middle rack for 30-35 minutes.

Take out of the oven, let cool down a little and serve.

Nutrition:Calories: 300 Total Fat: 17g Saturated Fat: 4g Cholesterol: 16mg Sodium: 59mg Total Carbohydrates: 34g Fiber: 2g Protein: 7g

Smoked Salmon and Watercress Salad

Preparation Time: 5 minutes

Cooking Time: 0 minutes

Servings: 4

Ingredients:

2 bunches watercress

1 pound smoked salmon, skinless, boneless and flaked

2 teaspoons mustard

¼ cup lemon juice

½ cup Greek yogurt

Salt and black pepper to the taste

1 big cucumber, sliced

2 tablespoons chives, chopped

Directions:

In a salad bowl, combine the salmon with the watercress and the rest of the ingredients toss and serve right away.

Nutrition:

Calories 244

Fat 16.7 g

Fiber 4.5 g

Carbs 22.5 g

Protein 15.6 g

Salmon and Corn Salad

Preparation Time: 5 minutes

Cooking Time: 0 minutes

Servings: 4

Ingredients:

½ cup pecans, chopped

2 cups baby arugula

1 cup corn

¼ pound smoked salmon, skinless, boneless and cut into small chunks

2 tablespoons olive oil

2 tablespoon lemon juice

Sea salt and black pepper to the taste

Directions:

In a salad bowl, combine the salmon with the corn and the rest of the ingredients, toss and serve right away.

Nutrition:

Calories 284

Fat 18.4 g

Fiber 5.4 g

Carbs 22.6 g

Protein 17.4 g

Stuffed Eggplants

Preparation time: 10 minutes

Cooking time: 35 minutes

Servings: 3

Ingredients:

2 eggplants, halved lengthwise and 2/3 of the flesh scooped out

3 tablespoons olive oil

1 red onion, chopped

2 garlic cloves, minced

1 pint white mushrooms, sliced

2 cups kale, torn

2 cups quinoa, cooked

1 tablespoon thyme, chopped

Zest and juice of 1 lemon

Salt and black pepper to the taste

½ cup Greek yogurt

3 tablespoons parsley, chopped

Directions:

Rub the inside of each eggplant half with half of the oil and arrange them on a baking sheet lined with parchment paper.

Heat up a pan with the rest of the oil over medium heat, add the onion and the garlic and sauté for 5 minutes.

Add the mushrooms and cook for 5 minutes more.

Add the kale, salt, pepper, thyme, lemon zest and juice, stir, cook for 5 minutes more and take off the heat.

Stuff the eggplant halves with the mushroom mix, introduce them in the oven and bake 400 degrees F for 20 minutes.

Divide the eggplants between plates, sprinkle the parsley and the yogurt on top and serve for lunch.

Nutrition: calories 512, fat 16.4, fiber 17.5, carbs 78, protein 17.2

Mushroom Pilaf

Preparation time: 10 minutes

Cooking time: 50 minutes

Servings: 3

Ingredients:

2 tablespoons olive oil

1 shallot, chopped

2 garlic cloves, minced

1 pound button mushrooms

1 cup brown rice

2 cups chicken stock

1 bay leaf

1 thyme sprig

Salt and pepper to taste

Directions:

Heat the oil in a skillet and stir in the shallot and garlic. Cook for 2 minutes until softened and fragrant.

Add the mushrooms and rice and cook for 5 minutes.

Add the stock, bay leaf and thyme, as well as salt and pepper and continue cooking for 20 more minutes on low heat.

Serve the pilaf warm and fresh.

Nutrition: Per Serving:Calories:265 Fat:8.9g Protein:7.6g Carbohydrates:41.2g

Cream Cheese Artichoke Mix

Preparation time: 10 minutes

Cooking time: 45 minutes

Servings: 6

Ingredients:

4 sheets matzo

½ cup artichoke hearts, canned

1 cup cream cheese

1 cup spinach, chopped

½ teaspoon salt

1 teaspoon ground black pepper

3 tablespoons fresh dill, chopped

3 eggs, beaten

1 teaspoon canola oil

½ cup cottage cheese

Directions:

In the bowl combine together cream cheese, spinach, salt, ground black pepper, dill, and cottage cheese.

Pour canola oil in the skillet, add artichoke hearts and roast them for 2-3 minutes over the medium heat. Stir them from time to time.

Then add roasted artichoke hearts in the cheese mixture.

Add eggs and stir until homogenous.

Place one sheet of matzo in the casserole mold.

Then spread it with cheese mixture generously.

Cover the cheese layer with the second sheet of matzo.

Repeat the steps till you use all ingredients.

Then preheat oven to 360F.

Bake matzo mina for 40 minutes.

Cut the cooked meal into the servings.

Nutrition: :calories 272, fat 17.3, fiber 4.3, carbs 20.2, protein 11.8

Caramelized Shallot Steaks

Preparation time: 10 minutes

Cooking time: 45 minutes

Servings: 7

Ingredients:

6 flank steaks

Salt and pepper to taste

1 teaspoon dried oregano

1 teaspoon dried basil

6 shallots, sliced

4 tablespoons olive oil

¼ cup dry white wine

Directions:

Season the steaks with salt, pepper, oregano and basil.

Heat a grill pan over medium flame and place the steaks on the grill.

Cook on each side for 6-7 minutes.

Heat the oil in a skillet and stir in the shallots. Cook for 15 minutes, stirring often, until the shallots are caramelized.

Add the wine and cook for another 5 minutes.

Serve the steaks with shallots.

Nutrition: Per Serving:Calories:258 Fat:16.3g Protein:23.5g Carbohydrates:2.1g

Carrot And Potato Soup

Preparation time: 10 minutes

Cooking time: 35 minutes

Servings: 6

Ingredients:

5 cups beef broth

4 carrots, peeled

1 teaspoon dried thyme

½ teaspoon ground cumin

1 teaspoon salt

1 ½ cup potatoes, chopped

1 tablespoon olive oil

½ teaspoon ground black pepper

1 tablespoon lemon juice

1/3 cup fresh parsley, chopped

1 chili pepper, chopped

1 tablespoon tomato paste

1 tablespoon sour cream

Directions:

Line the baking tray with baking paper.

Put sweet potatoes and carrot on the tray and sprinkle with olive oil and salt.

Bake the vegetables for 25 minutes at 365F.

Meanwhile, pour the beef broth in the pan and bring it to boil.

Add dried thyme, ground cumin, chopped chili pepper, and tomato paste.

When the vegetables are cooked, add them in the pan.

Boil the vegetables until they are soft.

Then blend the mixture with the help of the blender until smooth.

Simmer it for 2 minutes and add lemon juice. Stir well.

Then add sour cream and chopped parsley. Stir well.

Simmer the soup for 3 minutes more.

Nutrition: :calories 123, fat 4.1, fiber 2.9, carbs 16.4, protein 5.3

Macedonian Greens And Cheese Pie

Preparation time: 10 minutes

Cooking time: 50 minutes

Servings: 3

Ingredients:

1 bunch chicory

1 bunch rocket or arugula

1 bunch mint

1 bunch dill

10 sheets whole-wheat filo pastry

150 g halloumi, finely diced

150 g ricotta

200 g baby spinach

250 g Greek feta, crumbled

4 eggs

50 g dried whole-wheat breadcrumbs

6 green onions, trimmed

Olive oil, to brush

Directions:

Trim the rocket stalks and the chicory. Finely chop the green onions and the dill (include the dill stems). Strip the mint leaves.

Pour water into a large-sized pan; bring to boil. Ready a bowl with iced water beside the stove. Add the chicory into the boiling water; blanch for 3 minutes and using a slotted spoon, transfer to the bowl with iced water. Repeat the process with the spinach and the rocket, blanching each for 1 minute; drain well.

A handful at a time, tightly wring the greens to squeeze out the excess liquid, then pat dry with paper towel. Finely chop the blanched greens. Combine them with the eggs, herbs, feta, 30 g of the breadcrumbs, ricotta, and 3/4 of the halloumi; season.

Preheat the oven to 180C.

Grease a 5-cm deep 25cmx pie tin.

Brush a filo sheet with the olive oil, place it in the pie tin, extending the edge of the filo outside the edge of the tin. Brush the remaining sheets of filo and add them to the pie tin, arranging them like wheel spokes.

Sprinkle the remaining breadcrumbs over the base of the layered filo sheets. Top with the filling mixture. Loosely fold the filo sheets over to cover the filling, brush with oil, sprinkle with water, and scatter the halloumi over.

Bake for 45 minutes. After 45 minutes, cover, and bake for additional 15 minutes, or until heated through.

Nutrition: :374.8 Cal, 20 g total fat (12 g sat. fat), 22 g carb., 2 g fiber, 3 g sugar, 25g protein, and 1506.7 mg sodium.

Chicken Stuffed Peppers

Preparation time: 10 minutes

Cooking time: 0 minutes

Servings: 6

Ingredients:

1 cup Greek yogurt

2 tablespoons mustard

Salt and black pepper to the taste

1 pound rotisserie chicken meat, cubed

4 celery stalks, chopped

2 tablespoons balsamic vinegar

1 bunch scallions, sliced

¼ cup parsley, chopped

1 cucumber, sliced

3 red bell peppers, halved and deseeded

1 pint cherry tomatoes, quartered

Directions:

In a bowl, mix the chicken with the celery and the rest of the ingredients except the bell peppers and toss well.

Stuff the peppers halves with the chicken mix and serve for lunch.

Nutrition: calories 266, fat 12.2, fiber 4.5, carbs 15.7, protein 3.7

Turkey Fritters And Sauce

Preparation time: 10 minutes

Cooking time: 30 minutes

Servings: 3

Ingredients:

2 garlic cloves, minced

1 egg

1 red onion, chopped

1 tablespoon olive oil

¼ teaspoon red pepper flakes

1 pound turkey meat, ground

½ teaspoon oregano, dried

Cooking spray

For the sauce:

1 cup Greek yogurt

1 cucumber, chopped

1 tablespoon olive oil

¼ teaspoon garlic powder

2 tablespoons lemon juice

¼ cup parsley, chopped

Directions:

Heat up a pan with 1 tablespoon oil over medium heat, add the onion and the garlic, sauté for 5 minutes, cool down and transfer to a bowl.

Add the meat, turkey, oregano and pepper flakes, stir and shape medium fritters out of this mix.

Heat up another pan greased with cooking spray over medium-high heat, add the turkey fritters and brown for 5 minutes on each side.

Introduce the pan in the oven and bake the fritters at 375 degrees F for 15 minutes more.

Meanwhile, in a bowl, mix the yogurt with the cucumber, oil, garlic powder, lemon juice and parsley and whisk really well.

Divide the fritters between plates, spread the sauce all over and serve for lunch.

Nutrition: calories 364, fat 16.8, fiber 5.5, carbs 26.8, protein 23.4

Garlic Clove Roasted Chicken

Preparation time: 10 minutes

Cooking time: 40 minutes

Servings: 5

Ingredients:

8 chicken legs

40 garlic cloves, crushed

1 shallot, sliced

½ cup white wine

1 bay leaf

1 thyme sprig

Salt and pepper to taste

Directions:

Season the chicken with salt and pepper.

Combine it with the rest of the ingredients in a deep dish baking pan.

Cover the pan with aluminum foil and cook in the preheated oven at 350F for 1 hour.

Serve the chicken warm and fresh.

Nutrition: Per Serving:Calories:225 Fat:7.5g Protein:29.9g Carbohydrates:5.6g

Chickpeas, Spinach And Arugula Bowl

Preparation time: 10 minutes

Cooking time: 25 minutes

Servings: 5

Ingredients:

1 cup chickpeas, canned, drained

½ teaspoon butter

½ teaspoon salt

½ teaspoon ground paprika

¾ teaspoon onion powder

6 oz quinoa, dried

12 oz chicken stock

2 tomatoes, chopped

1 cucumber, chopped

½ cup fresh spinach, chopped

½ cup arugula, chopped

½ cup lettuce chopped

1 tablespoon olive oil

4 teaspoons hummus

Directions:

Place chickpeas in the skillet. Add butter and salt.

Roast the chickpeas for 5 minutes over the high heat. Stir them from time to time.

After this, place quinoa and chicken stock in the pan.

Cook the quinoa for 15 minutes over the medium heat.

Then make the salad: mix up together tomatoes, cucumber, spinach, arugula, lettuce, and olive oil. Shake the salad gently.

Arrange roasted chickpeas in every serving bowl.

Add salad and hummus.

Then add quinoa. Buddha bowl is cooked.

Nutrition: :calories 330, fat 8.4, fiber 10.9, carbs 51.6, protein 14.1

Tuna Sandwiches

Preparation time: 10 minutes

Cooking time: 10 minutes

Servings: 3

Ingredients:

1/3 cup sun-dried tomato packed in oil, drained

1/4 cup red bell pepper, finely chopped (optional)

1/4 cup red onions or 1/4 cup sweet Spanish onion, finely chopped

1/4 cup ripe green olives or 1/4 cup ripe olives, sliced

1/4 teaspoon black pepper, fresh ground

2 cans (6 ounce) tuna in water, drained, flaked

2 teaspoons capers (more to taste)

4 romaine lettuce or curly green lettuce leaves

4 teaspoons balsamic vinegar

4 teaspoons roasted red pepper

8 slices whole-grain bread (or 8 slices whole-wheat pita bread)

Olive oil

Optional:

3 tablespoons mayonnaise (or low-fat mayonnaise)

Directions:

Toast the bread, if desired.

In a small mixing bowl, mix the vinegar and the olive oil. Brush the oil mixture over 1 side of each bread slices or on the inside of the pita pockets.

Except for the lettuce, combine the remaining of the ingredients in a mixing bowl.

Place 1 lettuce leaf on the oiled side of 4 bread slices.

Top the leaves with the tuna mix; top with the remaining bread slices with the oiled side in.

If using pita, place 1 lettuce leave inside each pita slices, then fill with the tuna mixture; serve immediately.

Nutrition: :338.1 Cal, 11.7 g total fat (2.1 g sat. fat), 28.5 g carb., 4.7 g sugar, 5.5 g fiber, 29.4 g protein, and 801.9 mg sodium.

Cream Cheese Tart

Preparation time: 10 minutes

Cooking time: 20 minutes

Servings: 6

Ingredients:

1 cup wheat flour, whole grain

½ teaspoon salt

1/3 cup butter, softened

1 cup Mozzarella, shredded

3 tablespoons chives, chopped

1 tablespoon cream cheese

½ teaspoon ground paprika

4 eggs, beaten

1 teaspoon dried oregano

Directions:

In the mixer bowl combine together flour and salt. Add butter and blend the mixture until you get non-sticky dough or knead it with the help of the fingertips.

Roll up the dough and arrange it in the round tart mold.

Flatten it gently and bake for 10 minutes at 365F.

Meanwhile, mix up together eggs with Mozzarella cheese, cream cheese, and chives.

Remove the tart crust from the oven and chill for 5-10 minutes.

Then place the cheese mixture in the tart crust and flatten it well with the help of a spatula.

Bake the tart for 10 minutes.

Use the kitchen torch to make the grilled tart surface.

Chill the cooked tart well and only after this slice it onto the servings.

Nutrition: :calories 229, fat 14.8, fiber 0.8, carbs 16.7, protein 7.5

Cherry Tomato Caper Chicken

Preparation time: 10 minutes

Cooking time: 30 minutes

Servings: 4

Ingredients:

4 chicken breasts

3 tablespoons olive oil

4 garlic cloves, chopped

2 cups cherry tomatoes, halved

1 teaspoon capers, chopped

½ cup black olives, pitted and sliced

1 thyme sprig

Directions:

Heat the oil in a skillet and add the chicken. Cook on high heat for 5 minutes on each side.

Add the rest of the ingredients and season with salt and pepper.

Cook in the preheated oven at 350F for 35 minutes.

Serve the chicken and the sauce warm and fresh.

Nutrition: Per Serving:Calories:320 Fat:19.9g Protein:30.1g Carbohydrates:5.6g

Shrimp Pancakes

Preparation time: 10 minutes

Cooking time: 10 minutes

Servings: 4

Ingredients:

4 eggs, beaten

4 teaspoons sour cream

1 cup shrimps, peeled, boiled

1 teaspoon butter

1 teaspoon olive oil

1/3 cup Mozzarella, shredded

½ teaspoon salt

1 teaspoon dried oregano

Directions:

In the mixing bowl, combine together sour cream, eggs, salt, and dried oregano.

Place butter and olive oil in the crepe skillet and heat the ingredients up.

Separate the egg liquid into 4 parts.

Ladle the first part of the egg liquid in the skillet and flatten it in the shape of crepe.

Sprinkle the egg crepe with ¼ part of shrimps and a small amount of Mozzarella.

Roast the crepe for 2 minutes from one side and then flip it onto another.

Cook the crepe for 30 seconds more.

Repeat the same steps with all remaining ingredients.

Nutrition: :calories 148, fat 8.5, fiber 0.2, carbs 1.5, protein 16.1

Herbed Chicken Stew

Preparation time: 10 minutes

Cooking time: 1 hour 30 minutes

Ingredients:

3 tablespoons olive oil

6 chicken legs

2 shallots, chopped

4 garlic cloves, minced

2 tablespoons pesto sauce

½ cup chopped cilantro

½ cup chopped parsley

2 tablespoons lemon juice

4 tablespoons vegetable stock

Salt and pepper to taste

Directions:

Heat the oil in a skillet and place the chicken in the hot oil.

Cook on each side until golden brown then add the shallots, garlic and pesto sauce.

Cook for 2 more minutes then add the rest of the ingredients.

Season with salt and pepper and continue cooking on low heat, covered with a lid, for 30 minutes.

Serve the stew warm and fresh.

Nutrition: Per Serving:Calories:357 Fat:19.6g Protein:41.4g Carbohydrates:2.0g

Spiced Seared Scallops With Lemon Relish

Preparation time: 10 minutes

Cooking time: 40 minutes

Servings: 3

Ingredients:

2 pounds scallops, cleaned

½ teaspoon cumin powder

¼ teaspoon ground ginger

½ teaspoon ground coriander

½ teaspoon smoked paprika

½ teaspoon salt

3 tablespoons olive oil

Directions:

Pat the scallops dry with a paper towel.

Sprinkle them with spices and salt.

Heat the oil in a skillet and place half of the scallops in the hot oil. Cook for 1-2 minutes per side, just until the scallops look golden brown on the sides.

Remove the scallops and place the remaining ones in the hot oil.

Serve the scallops warm and fresh with your favorite side dish.

Nutrition: Per Serving:Calories:292 Fat:12.3g Protein:38.2g Carbohydrates:5.7g

White Bean Soup

Preparation time: 10 minutes

Cooking time: 8 hours 30 minutes

Servings: 6

Ingredients:

1 cup celery, chopped

1 cup carrots, chopped

1 yellow onion, chopped

6 cups veggie stock

4 garlic cloves, minced

2 cup navy beans, dried

½ teaspoon basil, dried

½ teaspoon sage, dried

1 teaspoon thyme, dried

A pinch of salt and black pepper

Directions:

In your slow cooker, combine the beans with the stock and the rest of the ingredients, put the lid on and cook on Low for 8 hours.

Divide the soup into bowls and serve right away.

Nutrition: calories 264, fat 17.5, fiber 4.5, carbs 23.7, protein 11.5

Coriander Pork And Chickpeas Stew

Preparation time: 10 minutes

Cooking time: 8 hours 30 minutes

Servings: 3

Ingredients:

½ cup beef stock

1 tablespoon ginger, grated

1 teaspoon coriander, ground

2 teaspoons cumin, ground

Salt and black pepper to the taste

2 and ½ pounds pork stew meat, cubed

28 ounces canned tomatoes, drained and chopped

1 red onion, chopped

4 garlic cloves, minced

½ cup apricots, cut into quarters

15 ounces canned chickpeas, drained

1 tablespoon cilantro, chopped

Directions:

In your slow cooker, combine the meat with the stock, ginger and the rest of the ingredients except the cilantro and the chickpeas, put the lid on and cook on Low for 7 hours and 40 minutes.

Add the cilantro and the chickpeas, cook the stew on Low for 20 minutes more, divide into bowls and serve.

Nutrition: calories 283, fat 11.9, fiber 4.5, carbs 28.8, protein 25.4

Crispy Pollock And Gazpacho

Preparation time: 10 minutes

Cooking time: 15 minutes

Servings: 3

Ingredients:

85 g whole-wheat bread, torn into chunks

4 tablespoons olive oil

4 pieces Pollock fillets, skinless

4 large tomatoes, cut into chunks

3/4 cucumber, cut into chunks

2 tablespoons sherry vinegar

2 garlic cloves, crushed

1/2 red onion, thinly sliced

1 yellow pepper, deseeded, cut into chunks

Directions:

Preheat the oven to 200C, gas to 6, or fan to 180C.

Over a baking tray, scatter the chunks of bread. Toss with 1 tablespoon of the olive oil and bake for about 10 minutes, or until golden and crispy.

Meanwhile, mix the cucumber, tomatoes, onion, pepper, crushed garlic, sherry vinegar, and 2 tablespoons of the olive oil; season well.

Heat a non-stick large frying pan. Add the remaining 1 tablespoon of the olive oil and heat. When the oil is hot, add the fish; cook for about 4 minutes or until golden. Flip the fillet; cook for additional 1 to 2 minutes or until the fish cooked through.

In a mixing bowl, quickly toss the salad and the croutons; divide among 4 plates and then serve with the fish.

Nutrition: :296 Cal, 13 g total fat (2 g sat. fat), 19 g carb., 9 g sugar, 3 g fiber, 27 g protein, and 0.67 g sodium.

Falafel

Preparation time: 10 minutes

Cooking time: 40 minutes

Servings: 3

Ingredients:

1 pound (about 2 cups) dry chickpeas or garbanzo beans (use dry, DO NOT use canned)

1 1/2 tablespoons flour

1 3/4 teaspoons salt

1 small onion, roughly chopped

1 teaspoon ground coriander

1/4 cup fresh parsley, chopped

1/4 teaspoon black pepper

1/4 teaspoon cayenne pepper

2 teaspoons cumin

3-5 cloves garlic, roasted, if desired

Pinch ground cardamom

Canola, grapeseed, peanut oil, or oil with high smoking point, for frying

Directions:

Pour the chickpeas into a large-sized bowl, cover with about 3-inch cold water, and soak overnight. The chickpeas will double to about 4-5 cups after soaking.

Drain and then rinse well, pour into a food processor. Except for the oil for frying, add the remaining of the ingredients into the processor; pulse until the texture resembles a coarse meal. Periodically scrape the sides of the processor, pushing the mixture down the sides, process until the mixture resembles a texture that is between couscous and paste, making sure not to over process or they will turn into hummus.

Transfer into a bowl. With a fork, stir the mixture, removing any large chickpeas that remained unprocessed. Cover the bowl with a plastic wrap; refrigerate for about 1 to 2 hours.

Fill a skillet with 1 1/2-inch worth of oil. Slowly heat the oil over medium flame or heat.

Meanwhile, scoop out 2 tablespoons worth of the falafel mixture; with wet hands form it into round ball or slider-shaped. You can make them smaller or larger if you want. They may stick together loosely, but when they start to fry, they will bind nicely. If the balls won't hold, add flour by the 1 tablespoon-worth until they hold. If they still don't hold, add 1-2 eggs.

Test the hotness of your oil with 1 piece falafel in the center of the pan. If the oil is at the right temperature the falafel will brown 5-6 minutes total or 2-3 minutes each side. If it browns faster, the oil is too hot. Slightly cool the oil down and then test again. When you reach the right temperature, cook the falafel in 5-6 pieces batches until both sides are golden brown. With a slotted spoon, remove from the skillet, and drain on paper towels.

Serve fresh and hot with hummus and then topped with tahini sauce.

Nutrition: :60 cal., 1.5 g total fat (0 g sat fat), 0 mg chol., 135 mg sodium, 140 mg potassium, 10 g carb., 3 g fiber, 2 g sugar, and 3 g protein.

Prosciutto Balls

Preparation time: 10 minutes

Cooking time: 10 minutes

Servings: 4

Ingredients:

8 Mozzarella balls, cherry size

4 oz bacon, sliced

¼ teaspoon ground black pepper

¾ teaspoon dried rosemary

1 teaspoon butter

Directions:

Sprinkle the sliced bacon with ground black pepper and dried rosemary.

Wrap every Mozzarella ball in the sliced bacon and secure them with toothpicks.

Melt butter.

Brush wrapped Mozzarella balls with butter.

Line the tray with the baking paper and arrange Mozzarella balls in it.

Bake the meal for 10 minutes at 365F.

Nutrition: :calories 323, fat 26.8, fiber 0.1, carbs 0.6, protein 20.6

Chicken Skillet

Preparation time: 10 minutes

Cooking time: 35 minutes

Servings: 3

Ingredients:

6 chicken thighs, bone-in and skin-on

Juice of 2 lemons

1 teaspoon oregano, dried

1 red onion, chopped

Salt and black pepper to the taste

1 teaspoon garlic powder

2 garlic cloves, minced

2 tablespoons olive oil

2 and ½ cups chicken stock

1 cup white rice

1 tablespoon oregano, chopped

1 cup green olives, pitted and sliced

1/3 cup parsley, chopped

½ cup feta cheese, crumbled

Directions:

Heat up a pan with the oil over medium heat, add the chicken thighs skin side down, cook for 4 minutes on each side and transfer to a plate.

Add the garlic and the onion to the pan, stir and sauté for 5 minutes.

Add the rice, salt, pepper, the stock, oregano, and lemon juice, stir, cook for 1-2 minutes more and take off the heat.

Add the chicken to the pan, introduce the pan in the oven and bake at 375 degrees F for 25 minutes.

Add the cheese, olives and the parsley, divide the whole mix between plates and serve for lunch.

Nutrition: calories 435, fat 18.5, fiber 13.6, carbs 27.8, protein 25.6

Salmon Bowls

Preparation time: 10 minutes

Cooking time: 40 minutes

Servings: 3

Ingredients:

2 cups farro

Juice of 2 lemons

1/3 cup olive oil+ 2 tablespoons

Salt and black pepper

1 cucumber, chopped

¼ cup balsamic vinegar

1 garlic cloves, minced

¼ cup parsley, chopped

¼ cup mint, chopped

2 tablespoons mustard

4 salmon fillets, boneless

Directions:

Put water in a large pot, bring to a boil over medium-high heat, add salt and the farro, stir, simmer for 30 minutes, drain, transfer to a bowl, add the lemon juice, mustard, garlic, salt, pepper and 1/3 cup oil, toss and leave aside for now.

In another bowl, mash the cucumber with a fork, add the vinegar, salt, pepper, the parsley, dill and mint and whisk well.

Heat up a pan with the rest of the oil over medium heat, add the salmon fillets skin side down, cook for 5 minutes on each side, cool them down and break into pieces.

Add over the farro, add the cucumber dressing, toss and serve for lunch.

Nutrition: calories 281, fat 12.7, fiber 1.7, carbs 5.8, protein 36.5

Cod and Mushrooms Mix

Preparation Time: 10 minutes

Cooking Time: 25 minutes

Servings: 4

Ingredients:

2 cod fillets, boneless

4 tablespoons olive oil

4 ounces mushrooms, sliced

Sea salt and black pepper to the taste

12 cherry tomatoes, halved

8 ounces lettuce leaves, torn

1 avocado, pitted, peeled and cubed

1 red chili pepper, chopped

1 tablespoon cilantro, chopped

2 tablespoons balsamic vinegar

1 ounce feta cheese, crumbled

Directions:

Put the fish in a roasting pan, brush it with 2 tablespoons oil, sprinkle salt and pepper all over and broil under medium-high heat for 15 minutes. Meanwhile, heat up a pan with the rest of the oil over medium heat, add the mushrooms, stir and sauté for 5 minutes.

Add the rest of the ingredients, toss, cook for 5 minutes more and divide between plates.

Top with the fish and serve right away.

Nutrition:

Calories 257

Fat 10 g

Fiber 3.1 g

Carbs 24.3 g

Protein 19.4 g

Salmon Panatela

Preparation Time: 5 minutes

Cooking Time: 22 minutes

Servings: 4

Ingredients:

1 lb skinned salmon, cut into 4 steaks each

1 cucumber, peeled, seeded, cubed

Salt and black pepper to taste

8 black olives, pitted and chopped

1 tbsp capers, rinsed

2 large tomatoes, diced

3 tbsp red wine vinegar

¼ cup thinly sliced red onion

3 tbsp olive oil

2 slices zero carb bread, cubed

¼ cup thinly sliced basil leaves

Directions:

Preheat a grill to 350ºF and preparation are the salad. In a bowl, mix the cucumbers, olives, pepper, capers, tomatoes, wine vinegar, onion, olive oil, bread, and basil leaves. Let sit for the flavors to incorporate.

Season the salmon steaks with salt and pepper; grill them on both sides for 8 minutes in total. Serve the salmon steaks warm on a bed of the veggies' salad.

Nutrition:

Calories 338,

Fat 27g

Net Carbs 1g

Protein 25g

Blackened Fish Tacos with Slaw

Preparation Time: 5 minutes

Cooking Time: 20 minutes

Servings: 4

Ingredients:

1 tbsp olive oil

1 tsp chili powder

2 tilapia fillets

1 tsp paprika

4 low carb tortillas

Slaw: ½ cup red cabbage, shredded

1 tbsp lemon juice

1 tsp apple cider vinegar

1 tbsp olive oil

Salt and black pepper to taste

Directions:

Season the tilapia with chili powder and paprika. Heat the olive oil in a skillet over medium heat.

Add tilapia and cook until blackened, about 3 minutes per side. Cut into strips. Divide the tilapia between the tortillas. Combine all slaw ingredients in a bowl and top the fish to serve.

Nutrition:

Calories 268,

Fat: 20g

Net Carbs: 5g

Protein: 18g

Red Cabbage Tilapia Taco Bowl

Preparation Time: 5 minutes

Cooking Time: 20 minutes

Servings: 4

Ingredients:

2 cups caulis rice

2 tsp ghee

4 tilapia fillets, cut into cubes

¼ tsp taco seasoning

Salt and chili pepper to taste

¼ head red cabbage, shredded

1 ripe avocado, pitted and chopped

Directions:

Sprinkle caulis rice in a bowl with a little water and microwave for 3 minutes. Fluff after with a fork and set aside. Melt ghee in a skillet over medium heat, rub the tilapia with the taco seasoning, salt, and chili pepper, and fry until brown on all sides, for about 8 minutes in total.

Transfer to a plate and set aside. In 4 serving bowls, share the caulis rice, cabbage, fish, and avocado. Serve with chipotle lime sour cream dressing.

Nutrition:

Calories 269,

Fat 24g

Net Carbs 4g

Protein 15g

Sicilian-Style Zoodle Spaghetti

Preparation Time: 5 minutes

Cooking Time: 10 minutes

Servings: 2

Ingredients:

4 cups zoodles (spiraled zucchini)

2 ounces cubed bacon

4 ounces canned sardines, chopped

½ cup canned chopped tomatoes

1 tbsp capers

1 tbsp parsley

1 tsp minced garlic

Directions:

Pour some of the sardine oil in a pan. Add garlic and cook for 1 minute. Add the bacon and cook for 2 more minutes. Stir in the tomatoes and let simmer for 5 minutes. Add zoodles and sardines and cook for 3 minutes.

Nutrition:

Calories 172,

Fat 4g

Fiber 0.6g

Carbs 3g,

Protein 34g

Sour Cream Salmon with Parmesan

Preparation Time: 5 minutes

Cooking Time: 25 minutes

Servings: 4

Ingredients:

1 cup sour cream

½ tbsp minced dill

½ lemon, zested and juiced

Pink salt and black pepper to season

4 salmon steaks

½ cup grated Parmesan cheese

Directions:

Preheat oven to 400ºF and line a baking sheet with parchment paper; set aside. In a bowl, mix the sour cream, dill, lemon zest, juice, salt and black pepper, and set aside.

Season the fish with salt and black pepper, drizzle lemon juice on both sides of the fish and arrange them in the baking sheet. Spread the sour cream mixture on each fish and sprinkle with Parmesan.

Bake the fish for 15 minutes and after broil the top for 2 minutes with a close watch for a nice a brown color. Plate the fish and serve with buttery green beans.

Nutrition:

Calories 355,

Fat: 31g

Net Carbs: 6g

Protein: 20g

Vegetable Buckwheat Pasta

Preparation time: 10 minutes

Cooking time: 15 minutes

Servings: 4

Ingredients:

4 tablespoons coconut oil

500g buckwheat pasta

2 garlic cloves, diced

1 medium white onion, cut into rings

3 carrots, sliced

1 head broccoli

1 red bell pepper, chopped into strips

3 medium tomatoes, diced

1 teaspoon vegetable broth

1 tablespoon fresh lemon juice

1 teaspoon oregano

A pinch of Sea salt

A pinch of pepper

Directions:

Chop al the veggies read to cook. Cook buckwheat pasta in boiling salt water. In a separate pot, boil broccoli in boiling salt water.

Meanwhile, heat two tablespoons of oil in a pan and sauté garlic and onion until fragrant and translucent. Remove from pan and set aside.

Heat the remaining oil in the same pan and cook veggies for a few minutes until tender. Add broccoli and onions to the pan and stir in broth, lemon juice, oregano, salt and pepper.

Stir to mix well and serve the veggie mix over the buckwheat pasta.

Pan-Seared Salmon Salad with Snow Peas & Grapefruit

Preparation time: 10 minutes

Cooking time: 0 minutes

Servings: 3

Ingredients:

4 (100g) skin-on salmon fillets

1/8 teaspoon sea salt

2 teaspoons extra virgin olive oil

4 cups arugula

8 leaves Boston lettuce, washed and dried

1 cup snow peas, cooked

2 avocados, diced

For Grapefruit-Dill Dressing:

1/4 cup grapefruit juice

1/4 cup extra virgin olive oil

1 teaspoon raw honey

1 tablespoon Dijon mustard

1 tablespoon chopped fresh dill

2 garlic cloves, minced

1/2 teaspoon pepper

Directions:

Sprinkle fish with about 1/8 teaspoon salt and cook in 2 teaspoons of olive oil over medium heat for about 4 minutes per side or until golden.

In a small bowl, whisk together al dressing ingredients and set aside. Divide arugula and lettuce among four serving plates.

Divide lettuce and arugula among 4 plates and add the remaining salad ingredients; top each with seared fish and drizzle with dressing. Enjoy!

Cleansing Vegetable Broth

Preparation time: 10 minutes

Cooking time: 20 minutes

Servings: 6

Ingredients:

1/4 cup water

2 cloves garlic, minced

1/2 cup chopped red onion

1 tablespoon minced fresh ginger

1 cup chopped tomatoes

1 small head of broccoli, chopped into florets

3 medium carrots, diced

3 celery stalks, diced

1/8 teaspoon cayenne pepper

1/4 teaspoon cinnamon

1 teaspoon turmeric

Sea salt and pepper

6 cups vegetable broth

¼ cup fresh lemon juice

1 cup chopped purple cabbage

2 cups chopped kale

Directions:

Boil ¼ cup of water in a large pot; add garlic and onion and sauté for about 2 minutes, stirring.

Stir in ginger, tomatoes, broccoli, carrots and celery and cook for about 3 minutes. Stir in spices.

Add in vegetable broth and bring the mixture to a boil; lower heat and simmer for about 15 minutes or until veggies are tender.

Stir in lemon juice, cabbage and kale and cook for about 2 minutes or until kale is wilted. Adjust the seasoning and serve hot.

Nutrition:Calories: 300 Total Fat: 17g Saturated Fat: 4g Cholesterol: 16mg Sodium: 59mg Total Carbohydrates: 34g Fiber: 2g Protein: 7g

Barbecued Spiced Tuna with Avocado-Mango Salsa

Preparation time: 10 minutes

Cooking time: 10 minutes

Servings: 4

Ingredients:

4 (120g each) skinless tuna fillets

1 teaspoon dried oregano

1 teaspoon onion powder

1 teaspoon ground paprika

1 teaspoon ground coriander

1 teaspoon ground cumin

1 tablespoon olive oil

Thinly shaved fennel

Baby rocket leaves

Avocado-Mango Salsa:

1/2 red onion, chopped

1 cucumber, chopped

1 avocado, diced

1 mango, diced

1 long red chilli, chopped

2 tablespoons lime juice

1/2 cup chopped coriander

Directions:

In a bowl, mix together onion powder, paprika, coriander, cumin, and oil until well combined; add in tuna and turn until well coated; sprinkle with salt and pepper.

Preheat the BBQ grill on medium high and grill the fish for about 3 minutes per side or until cooked to your liking. Wrap in foil and let set for at least 5 minutes.

In the meantime, in a bowl, mix together avocado, mango, red onion, cucumber, chili, coriander, and fresh lime juice until well combined.

Divide fennel and rocket on serving plates and top each with the grilled tuna and mango-avocado salsa. Serve right away.

Nutrition:Calories: 300 Total Fat: 17g Saturated Fat: 4g Cholesterol: 16mg Sodium: 59mg Total Carbohydrates: 34g Fiber: 2g Protein: 7g

Low Carb Berry Salad with Citrus Dressing

Preparation time: 10 minutes

Cooking time: 0 minutes

Servings: 3

Ingredients:

Salad:

¼ cup blueberries

½ cup chopped strawberries

1 cup mixed greens (kale and chard)

2 cups baby spinach

2 chopped green onions

½ cup chopped avocado

1 shredded carrots

Citrus Dressing:

1 tablespoon extra-virgin olive oil

2 tablespoons apple cider vinegar

¼ cup fresh orange juice

5 strawberries chopped

Directions:

In a blender, blend together all dressing ingredients until very smooth; set aside.

Combine all salad ingredients in a large bowl; drizzle with dressing and toss to coat well before serving.

Nutrition:Calories: 300 Total Fat: 17g Saturated Fat: 4g Cholesterol: 16mg Sodium: 59mg Total Carbohydrates: 34g Fiber: 2g Protein: 7g

Tasty Lime Cilantro Cauliflower Rice

Preparation time: 10 minutes

Cooking time: 10 minutes

Servings: 3

Ingredients:

1 head cauliflower, rinsed

1 tablespoon extra-virgin olive oil

2 garlic cloves, minced

2 scallions, chopped

½ teaspoon sea salt

Pinch of pepper

4 tablespoons fresh lime juice

1/4 cup chopped fresh cilantro

Directions:

Chop cauliflower into florets and transfer to a food processor; pulse into rice texture.

Heat a large skillet over medium heat and add olive oil; sauté garlic and scallions for about 4 minutes or until fragrant and tender.

Increase heat to medium high and stir in cauliflower rice; cook, covered, for about 6 minutes or until cauliflower is crispy on outside and soft inside.

Season with salt and pepper and transfer to a bowl. Toss with freshly squeezed lime juice and cilantro and serve right away.

Nutrition:Calories: 300 Total Fat: 17g Saturated Fat: 4g Cholesterol: 16mg Sodium: 59mg Total Carbohydrates: 34g Fiber: 2g Protein: 7g

Citrus Chicken with Delicious Cold Soup

Preparation time: 10 minutes

Cooking time: 30 minutes

Servings: 3

Ingredients:

2 tablespoons extra-virgin olive oil

500g ounces chicken breast

1 teaspoon fresh rosemary

1 lemon, sliced

1 orange, sliced

For the Cold Soup:

2 tablespoons apple cider vinegar

1/4 cup green pepper, chopped

1/4 cup cucumber, chopped

1/2 cup onion, chopped

3 cloves garlic, minced

1 cup stewed tomatoes

Directions:

Generously coat chicken with extra virgin olive oil and cover with rosemary, lemon and orange slices. Bake in the oven at 350°F for about 30 minutes.

In a blender, blend together all the soup ingredients until very smooth and then serve with chicken and cooked brown rice.

Nutrition: Calories: 384, Fat: 19.8g, Total Carbs: 42.9g, Sugars: 3.6g, Protein: 11.7g

Pan-Fried Chicken with Oregano-Orange Chimichurri & Arugula Salad

Preparation time: 10 minutes

Cooking time: 5 minutes

Servings: 3

Ingredients:

1 tablespoon orange juice

1 teaspoon orange zest

1 teaspoon dried oregano

1 small garlic clove, grated

2 teaspoon apple cider vinegar

1/2 cup chopped parsley

1 1/2 pound chicken, cut into 4 pieces

1 tablespoon lemon juice

A pinch of pepper

1/4 cup olive oil

4 cups arugula

2 bulbs fennel, shaved

2 tablespoons whole-grain mustard

Directions:

Make chimichurri: In a medium bowl, combine orange zest, oregano and garlic. Mix in vinegar, orange juice and parsley and then slowly whisk in ¼ cup of olive oil until emulsified. Season with black pepper.

Sprinkle the chicken with lemon juice and pepper; heat the remaining olive oil in a large skillet and cook the chicken over medium high heat for about 6 minutes per side or until browned.

Remove from heat and let rest for at least 10 minutes. Toss chicken, greens, and fennel with mustard in a medium bowl; season with salt and pepper.

Serve steak with chimichurri and salad. Enjoy!

Nutrition: Calories: 384, Fat: 19.8g, Total Carbs: 42.9g, Sugars: 3.6g, Protein: 11.7g

Cauliflower Couscous Salad

Preparation time: 10 minutes

Cooking time: 0 minutes

Servings: 3

Ingredients:

1 large head cauliflower, cut into florets

3-4 green onions, thinly sliced

2 garlic cloves, finely minced

1 jalapeño, seeds and ribs removed, minced

1 cup shredded carrots

1 cup diced celery

1 cup diced cucumber

1 green apple, diced

Juice of 1 lemon

1 tablespoon extra-virgin olive oil

Sea salt

Freshly ground black pepper

Directions:

Using two batches, set your cauliflower to pulse in a food processor until finely chopped.

Transfer to a mixing bowl with the remaining ingredients then gently toss until combined.

Serve and enjoy.

Nutrition: Calories: 384, Fat: 19.8g, Total Carbs: 42.9g, Sugars: 3.6g, Protein: 11.7g

Ultimate Liver Detox Soup

Preparation time: 10 minutes

Cooking time: 20 minutes

Servings: 5

Ingredients:

2 tablespoons extra-virgin olive oil

1 cup chopped shallot

1 tablespoon grated ginger

2 cloves garlic, minced

4 cups homemade chicken broth

1 medium golden beet, diced

1 large carrot, sliced

1 cup shredded red cabbage

1 cup sliced mushrooms

a handful of pea pods, halved

1 hot chili pepper, sliced

1 cup chopped cauliflower

1 cup chopped broccoli

1 bell pepper, diced

A pinch of cayenne pepper

A pinch of sea salt

1 cup baby spinach

1 cup chopped kale

1 cup grape tomatoes, halved

Directions:

In a large skillet, heat olive oil until hot but not smoky; sauté in shallots, ginger and garlic for about 2 minutes or until tender; stir in broth and bring the mixture to a gentle simmer.

Add in beets and carrots and simmer for about 5 minutes. Stir in hot pepper, cauliflower and broccoli and cook for about 3 minutes. stir in bell pepper, red cabbage, mushrooms, and peas and cook for 1 minute.

Remove from heat and stir in salt and pepper. Stir in leafy greens and tomatoes and cover the pot for about 5 minutes. Serve.

Nutrition: Calories: 384, Fat: 19.8g, Total Carbs: 42.9g, Sugars: 3.6g, Protein: 11.7g

Brown Rice and Grilled Chicken Salad

Preparation time: 10 minutes

Cooking time: 15 minutes

Servings: 3

Ingredients:

300g grilled chicken breasts

3/4 cup brown rice

1 1/4 cup coconut water

1 teaspoon minced garlic

2 tablespoons teriyaki sauce

1 tablespoon extra-virgin olive oil

2 tablespoons cider vinegar

1 small red onion, chopped

5 radishes, sliced

1 cup broccoli, chopped

Dash of pepper

Directions:

Cook rice in coconut water following package instructions. Remove from heat and let cool completely, and then fluff with a fork.

Whisk together garlic, teriyaki sauce, extra virgin olive oil, and vinegar. Stir in red onion, radishes, broccoli and rice. Season with pepper and stir until well blended. Serve with grilled chicken breasts.

Nutrition: Calories: 384, Fat: 19.8g, Total Carbs: 42.9g, Sugars: 3.6g, Protein: 11.7g

Superfood Liver Cleansing Soup

Preparation time: 10 minutes

Cooking time: 20 minutes

Servings: 3

Ingredients:

1/4 cup water

2 cloves garlic, minced

1/2 of a red onion, diced

1 tablespoon fresh ginger, peeled and minced

1 cup chopped tomatoes

1 small head of broccoli, florets

3 medium carrots, diced

3 celery stalks, diced

6 cups water

1/4 teaspoon cinnamon

1 teaspoon turmeric

1/8 teaspoon cayenne pepper

Freshly ground black pepper

juice of 1 lemon

1 cup purple cabbage, chopped

2 cups kale, torn in pieces

Directions:

Bring a large pot of water to a gentle boil over medium heat. Add garlic and onion and cook for about 2 minutes, stirring occasionally.

Stir in carrots, broccoli, tomatoes, fresh ginger, celery and cook for another 3 minutes. Stir in cayenne, turmeric, cinnamon, and black pepper.

Add half cup of water to the pot and bring to a gentle boil; lower heat and simmer until the veggies and tender, for about 15 minutes.

Stir in kale, cabbage, and fresh lemon juice during the last 2 minutes of cooking. Serve hot or warm.

Nutrition: Calories: 384, Fat: 19.8g, Total Carbs: 42.9g, Sugars: 3.6g, Protein: 11.7g

Toxin Flush & Detox Salad

Preparation time: 10 minutes

Cooking time: 10 minutes

Servings: 3

Ingredients:

For the salad:

2 cups broccoli florets

2 cups red cabbage, thinly sliced

2 cups chopped kale

1 cup grated carrot

1 red bell pepper, sliced into strips

2 avocados, diced

1/2 cup chopped parsley

1 cup walnuts

1 tablespoon sesame seeds

For the dressing:

2 teaspoons gluten-free mustard

1 tablespoon freshly grated ginger

1/2 cup fresh lemon juice

1/3 cup grapeseed oil

1 teaspoon raw honey

1/4 teaspoon salt

Directions:

In a blender, blend all the dressing ingredients until well blended; set aside.

In a salad bowl, mix broccoli, cabbage, kale, carrots and bell pepper; pour the dressing over the salad and toss until well coated.

Add diced avocado, parsley, walnuts and sesame seed; toss again to coat and serve.

Nutrition: Calories: 384, Fat: 19.8g, Total Carbs: 42.9g, Sugars: 3.6g, Protein: 11.7g

Grilled Chicken Salad

Preparation time: 10 minutes

Cooking time: 15 minutes

Servings: 3

Ingredients:

4 cups chopped broccoli

1/4 cup extra virgin olive oil

1/2 small red onion, thinly sliced

1 carrot, coarsely grated

4 chicken thighs, skinless

1 1/2 tablespoons Cajun seasoning

1/4 cup lemon juice

1 tablespoon drained baby capers

1 lemon, cut into wedges, to serve

Directions:

Drizzle chicken with oil and sprinkle with seasoning; rub to coat well.

Heat your grill to medium heat and grill the chicken for about 8 minutes per side or until cooked through and golden browned on the outside.

In the meantime, place the grated broccoli in a bowl and add in red onion, carrots, capers, lime juice and the remaining oil, salt and pepper; toss to combine well and serve with grilled chicken garnished with lemon wedges.

Nutrition: Calories: 384, Fat: 19.8g, Total Carbs: 42.9g, Sugars: 3.6g, Protein: 11.7g

Chicken Stir Fry with Red Onions & Cabbage

Preparation time: 10 minutes

Cooking time: 10 minutes

Servings: 3

Ingredients:

550g chicken, thinly sliced strips

1 tablespoon apple cider wine

2 teaspoons balsamic vinegar

Pinch of sea salt

pinch of pepper

4 tablespoons extra-virgin olive oil

1 large yellow onion, thinly chopped

1/2 red bell pepper, sliced

1/2 green bell pepper, sliced

1 tablespoon toasted sesame seeds

1 teaspoon crushed red pepper flakes

4 cups cabbage

1 ½ avocados, diced

Directions:

Place meat in a bowl; stir in rice wine and vinegar, sea salt and pepper. Toss to coat well.

Heat a tablespoon of olive oil in a pan set over medium high heat; add meat and cook for about 2 minutes or until meat is browned; stir for another 2 minutes and then remove from heat.

Heat the remaining oil to the pan and sauté onions for about 2 minutes or until caramelized; stir in pepper and cook for 2 minutes more.

Stir in cabbage and cook for 2 minutes; return meat to pan and stir in sesame seeds and red pepper flakes. Serve hot topped with diced avocado!

Nutrition: Calories: 384, Fat: 19.8g, Total Carbs: 42.9g, Sugars: 3.6g, Protein: 11.7g

Green Salad w/ Herbs

Preparation time: 10 minutes

Cooking time: 0 minutes

Servings: 3

Ingredients:

1 bunch rocket

2 baby cos, outer leaves discarded, roughly chopped

1 curly endive, outer leaves removed, roughly chopped

2 tablespoons chopped parsley

2 tablespoons chopped fresh dill

2 tablespoons snipped chives

1/2 cup extra-virgin olive oil

2 tablespoons fresh lemon juice

Directions:

In a large bowl, mix rocket, cos and endive and herbs.

In another small bowl, whisk together olive oil, fresh lemon juice, salt and pepper until well blended; pour over the salad and toss to coat well. Serve.

Nutrition: Calories: 384, Fat: 19.8g, Total Carbs: 42.9g, Sugars: 3.6g, Protein: 11.7g

Chilled Green Goddess Soup

Preparation time: 10 minutes

Cooking time: 0 minutes

Servings: 3

Ingredients:

6 cups cucumber

2 stalks celery chopped

1-2 cups water (depending how thin you want it)

2 tablespoons fresh lime juice

1 cup watercress leaves

1 cup rocket leaves

½ cup mashed avocado (roughly 1 avocado)

1 teaspoon wheatgrass power or a mixed green powder, optional

Sea salt to taste

Directions:

Blend all ingredients except the avocado in a blender until a broth forms. Strain the liquid through a cheesecloth or fine sieve. Then return to blender and add the avocado and blend until smooth.

Garnish with a few watercress leaves and cracked black pepper.

Nutrition: Calories: 384, Fat: 19.8g, Total Carbs: 42.9g, Sugars: 3.6g, Protein: 11.7g

Chicken Avocado Wrap

Preparation time: 10 minutes

Cooking time: 2 minutes

Servings: 3

Ingredients:

3-4 cups chopped cooked chicken (boiled or grilled with minimal oil)

1 large tomato, chopped

2 avocados, chopped

1 cup green onions, chopped, or purple onion

juice of 2-3 fresh limes

1/3 cup fresh cilantro, chopped

3 jalapenos, minced (more or less)

1 tablespoon fajita seasoning

10 whole wheat tortillas

minimal monterey jack cheese, shredded

Directions:

Combine all ingredients except for the tortillas and cheese, mixing well.

Place tortillas on a baking sheet, very lightly coated with oil. Top each tortilla with a light sprinkle of cheese and bake at 400 degrees for about a minute or until cheese melts.

Spoon chicken mixture evenly on tortillas. Roll up and place on plate or serving platter seam side down.

Nutrition: Calories: 384, Fat: 19.8g, Total Carbs: 42.9g, Sugars: 3.6g, Protein: 11.7g

Broccoli and Brown Rice Pasta Shells with Garlic

Preparation time: 10 minutes

Cooking time: 8 minutes

Servings: 3

Ingredients:

1 large head broccoli, cut into chunks and florets (peel the stem and cut into chunks)

1 pound brown rice pasta shells

1/3 cup extra-virgin olive oil

2-3 large garlic cloves, minced

crushed red pepper flakes to taste

low sodium salt and fresh ground pepper to taste

Directions:

Fill a large pasta pot 3/4 full with low sodium salted water and bring to a boil. Add pasta shells and bring back to boiling.

Add broccoli stem chunks and let cook for about 1 minute, then add florets. Continue boiling until pasta is cooked. Strain and return to pot.

Meanwhile, in a large frying pan over medium heat, combine olive oil, garlic, red pepper, salt and pepper and heat until almost sizzling, but don't let the garlic brown.

Pour the garlic mixture over the broccoli/pasta mixture and toss until a moist sauce starts to form.

You can sprinkle a little bit of parmesan on top of it while serving.

Nutrition: Calories: 384, Fat: 19.8g, Total Carbs: 42.9g, Sugars: 3.6g, Protein: 11.7g

Chicken with Potatoes Olives & Sprouts

Preparation Time: 15 minutes

Cooking Time: 35 minutes

Servings: 4

Ingredients:

1 lb. chicken breasts, skinless, boneless, and cut into pieces

¼ cup olives, quartered

1 tsp oregano

1 ½ tsp Dijon mustard

1 lemon juice

1/3 cup vinaigrette dressing

1 medium onion, diced

3 cups potatoes cut into pieces

4 cups Brussels sprouts, trimmed and quartered

¼ tsp pepper

¼ tsp salt

Directions:

Warm-up oven to 400 F. Place chicken in the center of the baking tray, then place potatoes, sprouts, and onions around the chicken.

In a small bowl, mix vinaigrette, oregano, mustard, lemon juice, and salt and pour over chicken and veggies. Sprinkle olives and season with pepper.

Bake in preheated oven for 20 minutes. Transfer chicken to a plate. Stir the vegetables and roast for 15 minutes more. Serve and enjoy.

Nutrition:

Calories: 397

Fat: 13g

Protein: 38.3g

Carbs: 31.4g

Sodium 175 mg

Garlic Mushroom Chicken

Preparation Time: 15 minutes

Cooking Time: 15 minutes

Servings: 4

Ingredients:

4 chicken breasts, boneless and skinless

3 garlic cloves, minced

1 onion, chopped

2 cups mushrooms, sliced

1 tbsp olive oil

½ cup chicken stock

¼ tsp pepper

½ tsp salt

Directions:

Season chicken with pepper and salt. Warm oil in a pan on medium heat, then put season chicken in the pan and cook for 5-6 minutes on each side. Remove and place on a plate.

Add onion and mushrooms to the pan and sauté until tender, about 2-3 minutes. Add garlic and sauté for a minute. Add stock and bring to boil. Stir well and cook for 1-2 minutes. Pour over chicken and serve.

Nutrition:

Calories: 331

Fat: 14.5g

Protein: 43.9g

Carbs: 4.6g

Sodium 420 mg

Grilled Chicken

Preparation Time: 15 minutes

Cooking Time: 15 minutes

Servings: 4

Ingredients:

4 chicken breasts, skinless and boneless

1 ½ tsp dried oregano

1 tsp paprika

5 garlic cloves, minced

½ cup fresh parsley, minced

½ cup olive oil

½ cup fresh lemon juice

Pepper

Salt

Directions:

Add lemon juice, oregano, paprika, garlic, parsley, and olive oil to a large zip-lock bag. Season chicken with pepper and salt and add to bag. Seal bag and shake well to coat chicken with marinade. Let sit chicken in the marinade for 20 minutes.

Remove chicken from marinade and grill over medium-high heat for 5-6 minutes on each side. Serve and enjoy.

Nutrition:

Calories: 512

Fat: 36.5g

Protein: 43.1g

Carbs: 3g

Sodium 110mg

Roasted Tomato And Chicken Pasta

Preparation Time: 20 min

Cooking Time: 30 min

Servings: 4

Ingredients:

1 pound boneless, skinless chicken thighs, cut into bite-size pieces

⅛ Teaspoon kosher salt (optional)

¼ teaspoon freshly ground black pepper (optional)

4 cups cherry tomatoes, halved 4 garlic cloves, minced

1 tablespoon canola or sunflower oil

1 teaspoon dried basil

8 ounces uncooked whole-wheat rotini

10 kalamata olives, pitted and sliced

¼ teaspoon red pepper flakes (optional)

¼ cup grated Parmesan cheese (optional)

Directions:

Preheat the oven to 450°F.

Season the chicken with salt and pepper, if desired. Toss the chicken in a large bowl with the tomatoes, garlic, oil, and basil. Transfer to a rimmed baking sheet, and spread out evenly.

Roast until the chicken is cooked through, 15 to 20 minutes, tossing halfway though. A meat thermometer should read 165°F.

Meanwhile, cook the pasta to al dente according to the package directions. Drain.

In a large serving bowl, toss the chicken and tomatoes with the pasta, olives, and pepper flakes (if using). Top with Parmesan, if desired.

Nutrition:

Calories: 458

Total Fat: 14g

Saturated Fat: 3g

Cholesterol: 110mg

Sodium: 441mg

Carbohydrates: 52g

Fiber: 8g

Protein: 34g

Oat Risotto With Mushrooms, Kale, And Chicken

Preparation Time: 30 minutes

Cooking Time: 30 minutes

Servings: 4

Ingredients:

4 cups reduced-sodium chicken broth

1 tablespoon extra-virgin olive oil

1 small onion, finely chopped

1 pound sliced mushrooms

1 pound boneless, skinless chicken thighs, cut into bite-size pieces

1¼ cups quick-cooking steel-cut oats

1 (10-ounce) package frozen chopped kale (about 4 cups)

½ cup grated Parmesan cheese (optional)

Freshly ground black pepper (optional)

Directions:

In a medium saucepan, bring the broth to a simmer over medium-low heat.

Warm the olive oil in a large, nonstick skillet over medium-high heat. Sauté the onion and mushrooms until the onion is translucent, about 5 minutes. Push the vegetables to the side, and add the chicken. Let it sit untouched until it browns, about 2 minutes.

Add the oats. Cook for 1 minute, stirring constantly. Add ½ cup of the hot broth, and stir until it is completely absorbed. Continue stirring in broth, ½ cup at a time, until it is absorbed and the oats and chicken are cooked, about 10 minutes. If you run out of broth, switch to hot water.

Stir in the frozen kale, and cook until it's warm. Top with Parmesan and black pepper, if you like.

FLAVOR BOOST: Garnish with minced parsley and red pepper flakes. You can also substitute ½ cup dry white wine for ½ cup of the chicken broth.

INGREDIENT TIP: All varieties of oats have similar amounts of fiber, vitamins, and minerals. The main difference is in how quickly they're digested, with the steel-cut and old-fashioned/rolled oats breaking down more slowly, which is helpful for blood sugar control. The quick-cooking steel-cut oats used in this risotto are simply cut into smaller pieces, enabling you to make this dish in under 30 minutes.

Nutrition:

Calories: 470

Total Fat: 16g

Saturated Fat: 4g

Cholesterol: 118mg

Sodium: 389mg

Carbohydrates: 44g

Fiber: 9g

Protein: 40g

Turkey with Leeks and Radishes

Preparation Time: 10 minutes

Cooking Time: 6 hours

Servings: 2

Ingredients:

1-pound turkey breast, skinless, boneless and cubed

1 leek, sliced

1 cup radishes, sliced

1 red onion, chopped

1 tablespoon olive oil

A pinch of salt and black pepper

1 cup chicken stock

½ teaspoon sweet paprika

½ teaspoon coriander, ground

1 tablespoon cilantro, chopped

Directions:

In your slow cooker, combine the turkey with the leek, radishes, onion and the other ingredients toss, put the lid on and cook on High for 6 hours.

Divide everything between plates and serve.

Nutrition:

Calories 226,

Fat 9g

Fiber 1g

Carbs 6g,

Protein 12g

Easy Mozzarella & Pesto Chicken Casserole

Preparation Time: 5 minutes

Cooking Time: 30 minutes

Servings: 4

Ingredients:

¼ - cup pesto

8 - Oz cream cheese softened

¼ - ½ - cup heavy cream

8 - Oz mozzarella cubed

2 - Lb cooked cubed chicken breasts

8 - Oz mozzarella shredded

Directions:

Preheat stove to 400. Splash a vast meal dish with cooking shower.

Consolidate the initial three fixings and blend until smooth in an extensive bowl. Include the chicken and cubed mozzarella. Exchange to the goulash dish. Sprinkle the destroyed mozzarella to finish everything.

Preparation are for 25-30 minutes. Present with zoodles, spinach, or squashed cauliflower.

Nutrition:

Calories: 404

Fat 23g

Net carbs: 8g

Protein: 31g

Chapter 7: Dinner Recipes

Chicken And Butter Sauce

Preparation time: 10 minutes

Cooking time: 30 minutes

Servings: 5

Ingredients:

1-pound chicken fillet

1/3 cup butter, softened

1 tablespoon rosemary

½ teaspoon thyme

1 teaspoon salt

½ lemon

Directions:

Churn together thyme, salt, and rosemary.

Chop the chicken fillet roughly and mix up with churned butter mixture.

Place the preparation ared chicken in the baking dish.

Squeeze the lemon over the chicken.

Chop the squeezed lemon and add in the baking dish.

Cover the chicken with foil and bake it for 20 minutes at 365F.

Then discard the foil and bake the chicken for 10 minutes more.

Nutrition: :calories 285, fat 19.1, fiber 0.5, carbs 1, protein 26.5

Turkey And Cranberry Sauce

Preparation time: 10 minutes

Cooking time: 50 minutes

Servings: 3

Ingredients:

1 cup chicken stock

2 tablespoons avocado oil

½ cup cranberry sauce

1 big turkey breast, skinless, boneless and sliced

1 yellow onion, roughly chopped

Salt and black pepper to the taste

Directions:

Heat up a pan with the avocado oil over medium-high heat, add the onion and sauté for 5 minutes.

Add the turkey and brown for 5 minutes more.

Add the rest of the ingredients, toss, introduce in the oven at 350 degrees F and cook for 40 minutes

Nutrition: calories 382, fat 12.6, fiber 9.6, carbs 26.6, protein 17.6

Coriander And Coconut Chicken

Preparation time: 10 minutes

Cooking time: 30 minutes

Servings: 4

Ingredients:

2 pounds chicken thighs, skinless, boneless and cubed

2 tablespoons olive oil

Salt and black pepper to the taste

3 tablespoons coconut flesh, shredded

1 and ½ teaspoons orange extract

1 tablespoon ginger, grated

¼ cup orange juice

2 tablespoons coriander, chopped

1 cup chicken stock

¼ teaspoon red pepper flakes

Directions:

Heat up a pan with the oil over medium-high heat, add the chicken and brown for 4 minutes on each side.

Add salt, pepper and the rest of the ingredients, bring to a simmer and cook over medium heat for 20 minutes.

Divide the mix between plates and serve hot.

Nutrition: calories 297, fat 14.4, fiber 9.6, carbs 22, protein 25

Chicken Pilaf

Preparation time: 10 minutes

Cooking time: 30 minutes

Servings: 4

Ingredients:

4 tablespoons avocado oil

2 pounds chicken breasts, skinless, boneless and cubed

½ cup yellow onion, chopped

4 garlic cloves, minced

8 ounces brown rice

4 cups chicken stock

½ cup kalamata olives, pitted

½ cup tomatoes, cubed

6 ounces baby spinach

½ cup feta cheese, crumbled

A pinch of salt and black pepper

1 tablespoon marjoram, chopped

1 tablespoon basil, chopped

Juice of ½ lemon

¼ cup pine nuts, toasted

Directions:

Heat up a pot with 1 tablespoon avocado oil over medium-high heat, add the chicken, some salt and pepper, brown for 5 minutes on each side and transfer to a bowl.

Heat up the pot again with the rest of the avocado oil over medium heat, add the onion and garlic and sauté for 3 minutes.

Add the rice, the rest of the ingredients except the pine nuts, also return the chicken, toss, bring to a simmer and cook over medium heat for 20 minutes.

Divide the mix between plates, top each serving with some pine nuts and serve.

Nutrition: calories 283, fat 12.5, fiber 8.2, carbs 21.5, protein 13.4

Chicken And Black Beans

Preparation time: 10 minutes

Cooking time: 20 minutes

Servings: 3

Ingredients:

12 oz chicken breast, skinless, boneless, chopped

1 tablespoon taco seasoning

1 tablespoon nut oil

½ teaspoon cayenne pepper

½ teaspoon salt

½ teaspoon garlic, chopped

½ red onion, sliced

1/3 cup black beans, canned, rinsed

½ cup Mozzarella, shredded

Directions:

Rub the chopped chicken breast with taco seasoning, salt, and cayenne pepper.

Place the chicken in the skillet, add nut oil and roast it for 10 minutes over the medium heat. Mix up the chicken pieces from time to time to avoid burning.

After this, transfer the chicken in the plate.

Add sliced onion and garlic in the skillet. Roast the vegetables for 5 minutes. Stir them constantly. Then add black beans and stir well. Cook the ingredients for 2 minute more.

Add the chopped chicken and mix up well. Top the meal with Mozzarella cheese.

Close the lid and cook the meal for 3 minutes.

Nutrition: :calories 209, fat 6.4, fiber 2.8, carbs 13.7, 22.7

Coconut Chicken

Preparation time: 10 minutes

Cooking time: 5 minutes

Servings: 3

Ingredients:

6 oz chicken fillet

¼ cup of sparkling water

1 egg

3 tablespoons coconut flakes

1 tablespoon coconut oil

1 teaspoon Greek Seasoning

Directions:

Cut the chicken fillet on small pieces (nuggets).

Then crack the egg in the bowl and whisk it.

Mix up together egg and sparkling water.

Add Greek seasoning and stir gently.

Dip the chicken nuggets in the egg mixture and then coat in the coconut flakes.

Melt the coconut oil in the skillet and heat it up until it is shimmering.

Then add preparation ared chicken nuggets.

Roast them for 1 minute from each or until they are light brown.

Dry the cooked chicken nuggets with the help of the paper towel and transfer in the serving plates.

Nutrition:calories 141, fat 8.9, fiber 0.3, carbs 1, protein 13.9

Ginger Chicken Drumsticks

Preparation time: 10 minutes

Cooking time: 30 minutes

Servings: 4

Ingredients:

4 chicken drumsticks

1 apple, grated

1 tablespoon curry paste

4 tablespoons milk

1 teaspoon coconut oil

1 teaspoon chili flakes

½ teaspoon minced ginger

Directions:

Mix up together grated apple, curry paste, milk, chili flakes, and minced garlic.

Put coconut oil in the skillet and melt it.

Add apple mixture and stir well.

Then add chicken drumsticks and mix up well.

Roast the chicken for 2 minutes from each side.

Then preheat oven to 360F.

Place the skillet with chicken drumsticks in the oven and bake for 25 minutes.

Nutrition: :calories 150, fat 6.4, fiber 1.4, carbs 9.7, protein 13.5

Parmesan Chicken

Preparation time: 10 minutes

Cooking time: 30 minutes

Servings: 3

Ingredients:

1-pound chicken breast, skinless, boneless

2 oz Parmesan, grated

1 teaspoon dried oregano

½ teaspoon dried cilantro

1 tablespoon Panko bread crumbs

1 egg, beaten

1 teaspoon turmeric

Directions:

Cut the chicken breast on 3 servings.

Then combine together Parmesan, oregano, cilantro, bread crumbs, and turmeric.

Dip the chicken servings in the beaten egg carefully.

Then coat every chicken piece in the cheese-bread crumbs mixture.

Line the baking tray with the baking paper.

Arrange the chicken pieces in the tray.

Bake the chicken for 30 minutes at 365F.

Nutrition: :calories 267, fat 9.5, fiber 0.5, carbs 3.2, protein 40.4

Pomegranate Chicken

Preparation time: 10 minutes

Cooking time: 30 minutes

Servings: 6

Ingredients:

1-pound chicken breast, skinless, boneless

1 tablespoon za'atar

½ teaspoon salt

1 tablespoon pomegranate juice

1 tablespoon olive oil

Directions:

Rub the chicken breast with za'atar seasoning, salt, olive oil, and pomegranate juice.

Marinate the chicken or 15 minutes and transfer in the skillet.

Roast the chicken for 15 minutes over the medium heat.

Then flip the chicken on another side and cook for 10 minutes more.

Slice the chicken and place in the serving plates.

Nutrition: :calories 107, fat 4.2, fiber 0, carbs 0.2, protein 16.1

Chicken With Artichokes And Beans

Preparation time: 10 minutes

Cooking time: 30 minutes

Servings: 3

Ingredients:

2 tablespoons olive oil

2 chicken breasts, skinless, boneless and halved

Zest of 1 lemon, grated

3 garlic cloves, crushed

Juice of 1 lemon

Salt and black pepper to the taste

1 tablespoon thyme, chopped

6 ounces canned artichokes hearts, drained

1 cup canned fava beans, drained and rinsed

1 cup chicken stock

A pinch of cayenne pepper

Salt and black pepper to the taste

Directions:

Heat up a pan with the oil over medium-high heat, add chicken and brown for 5 minutes.

Add lemon juice, lemon zest, salt, pepper and the rest of the ingredients, bring to a simmer and cook over medium heat for 35 minutes.

Divide the mix between plates and serve right away.

Nutrition: calories 291, fat 14.9, fiber 10.5, carbs 23.8, protein 24.2

Chicken Pie

Preparation time: 10 minutes

Cooking time: 50 minutes

Servings: 3

Ingredients:

¼ cup green peas, frozen

1 carrot, chopped

1 cup ground chicken

5 oz puff pastry

1 tablespoon butter, melted

¼ cup cream

1 teaspoon ground black pepper

1 oz Parmesan, grated

Directions:

Roll up the puff pastry and cut it on 2 parts.

Place one puff pastry part in the non-sticky springform pan and flatten.

Then mix up together green peas, chopped carrot, ground chicken, and ground black pepper.

Place the chicken mixture in the puff pastry.

Pour cream over mixture and sprinkle with Parmesan.

Cover the mixture with second puff pastry half and secure the edges of it with the help of the fork.

Brush the surface of the pie with melted butter and bake it for 50 minutes at 365F.

Nutrition: :calories 223, fat 14.3, fiber 1, carbs 13.2, protein 10.5

Chicken And Semolina Meatballs

Preparation time: 10 minutes

Cooking time: 10 minutes

Servings: 3

Ingredients:

1/3 cup carrot, grated

1 onion, diced

2 cups ground chicken

1 tablespoon semolina

1 egg, beaten

½ teaspoon salt

1 teaspoon dried oregano

1 teaspoon dried cilantro

1 teaspoon chili flakes

1 tablespoon coconut oil

Directions:

In the mixing bowl combine together grated carrot, diced onion, ground chicken, semolina, egg, salt, dried oregano, cilantro, and chili flakes.

With the help of scooper make the meatballs.

Heat up the coconut oil in the skillet.

When it starts to shimmer, put meatballs in it.

Cook the meatballs for 5 minutes from each side over the medium-low heat.

Nutrition: :calories 102, fat 4.9, fiber 0.5, carbs 2.9, protein 11.2

Lemon Chicken Mix

Preparation time: 10 minutes

Cooking time: 10 minutes

Servings: 3

Ingredients:

8 oz chicken breast, skinless, boneless

1 teaspoon Cajun seasoning

1 teaspoon balsamic vinegar

1 teaspoon olive oil

1 teaspoon lemon juice

Directions:

Cut the chicken breast on the halves and sprinkle with Cajun seasoning.

Then sprinkle the poultry with olive oil and lemon juice.

Then sprinkle the chicken breast with the balsamic vinegar.

Preheat the grill to 385F.

Grill the chicken breast halves for 5 minutes from each side.

Slice Cajun chicken and place in the serving plate.

Nutrition: :calories 150, fat 5.2, fiber 0, carbs 0.1, protein 24.1

Turkey And Chickpeas

Preparation time: 10 minutes

Cooking time: 5 hours

Servings: 3

Ingredients:

2 tablespoons avocado oil

1 big turkey breast, skinless, boneless and roughly cubed

Salt and black pepper to the taste

1 red onion, chopped

15 ounces canned chickpeas, drained and rinsed

15 ounces canned tomatoes, chopped

1 cup kalamata olives, pitted and halved

2 tablespoons lime juice

1 teaspoon oregano, dried

Directions:

Heat up a pan with the oil over medium-high heat, add the meat and the onion, brown for 5 minutes and transfer to a slow cooker.

Add the rest of the ingredients, put the lid on and cook on High for 5 hours.

Divide between plates and serve right away!

Nutrition: calories 352, fat 14.4, fiber 11.8, carbs 25.1, protein 26.4

Cardamom Chicken And Apricot Sauce

Preparation time: 10 minutes

Cooking time: 7 Hours minutes

Servings: 3

Ingredients:

Juice of ½ lemon

Zest of ½ lemon, grated

2 teaspoons cardamom, ground

Salt and black pepper to the taste

2 chicken breasts, skinless, boneless and halved

2 tablespoons olive oil

2 spring onions, chopped

2 tablespoons tomato paste

2 garlic cloves, minced

1 cup apricot juice

½ cup chicken stock

¼ cup cilantro, chopped

Directions:

In your slow cooker, combine the chicken with the lemon juice, lemon zest and the other ingredients except the cilantro, toss, put the lid on and cook on Low for 7 hours.

Divide the mix between plates, sprinkle the cilantro on top and serve.

Nutrition: calories 323, fat 12, fiber 11, carbs 23.8, protein 16.4

Chicken And Artichokes

Preparation time: 10 minutes

Cooking time: 20 minutes

Servings: 3

Ingredients:

2 pounds chicken breast, skinless, boneless and sliced

A pinch of salt and black pepper

4 tablespoons olive oil

8 ounces canned roasted artichoke hearts, drained

6 ounces sun-dried tomatoes, chopped

3 tablespoons capers, drained

2 tablespoons lemon juice

Directions:

Heat up a pan with half of the oil over medium-high heat, add the artichokes and the other ingredients except the chicken, stir and sauté for 10 minutes.

Transfer the mix to a bowl, heat up the pan again with the rest of the oil over medium-high heat, add the meat and cook for 4 minutes on each side.

Return the veggie mix to the pan, toss, cook everything for 2-3 minutes more, divide between plates and serve.

Nutrition: calories 552, fat 28, fiber 6, carbs 33, protein 43

Buttery Chicken Spread

Preparation time: 10 minutes

Cooking time: 20 minutes

Servings: 5

Ingredients:

8 oz chicken liver

3 tablespoon butter

1 white onion, chopped

1 bay leaf

1 teaspoon salt

½ teaspoon ground black pepper

½ cup of water

Directions:

Place the chicken liver in the saucepan.

Add onion, bay leaf, salt, ground black pepper, and water.

Mix up the mixture and close the lid.

Cook the liver mixture for 20 minutes over the medium heat.

Then transfer it in the blender and blend until smooth.

Add butter and mix up until it is melted.

Pour the pate mixture in the pate ramekin and refrigerate for 2 hours.

Nutrition: :calories 122, fat 8.3, fiber 0.5, carbs 2.3, protein 9.5

Chicken And Spinach Cakes

Preparation time: 10 minutes

Cooking time: 15 minutes

Servings: 3

Ingredients:

8 oz ground chicken

1 cup fresh spinach, blended

1 teaspoon minced onion

½ teaspoon salt

1 red bell pepper, grinded

1 egg, beaten

1 teaspoon ground black pepper

4 tablespoons Panko breadcrumbs

Directions:

In the mixing bowl mix up together ground chicken, blended spinach, minced garlic, salt, grinded bell pepper, egg, and ground black pepper.

When the chicken mixture is smooth, make 4 burgers from it and coat them in Panko breadcrumbs.

Place the burgers in the non-sticky baking dish or line the baking tray with baking paper.

Bake the burgers for 15 minutes at 365F.

Flip the chicken burgers on another side after 7 minutes of cooking.

Nutrition: :calories 171, fat 5.7, fiber 1.7, carbs 10.5, protein 19.4

Cream Cheese Chicken

Preparation time: 10 minutes

Cooking time: 30 minutes

Servings: 3

Ingredients:

1 onion, chopped

1 sweet red pepper, roasted, chopped

1 cup spinach, chopped

½ cup cream

1 teaspoon cream cheese

1 tablespoon olive oil

½ teaspoon ground black pepper

8 oz chicken breast, skinless, boneless, sliced

Directions:

Mix up together sliced chicken breast with ground black pepper and put in the saucepan.

Add olive oil and mix up.

Roast the chicken for 5 minutes over the medium-high heat. Stir it from time to time.

After this, add chopped sweet pepper, onion, and cream cheese.

Mix up well and bring to boil.

Add spinach and cream. Mix up well.

Close the lid and cook chicken Alfredo for 10 minutes more over the medium heat.

Nutrition: :calories 279, fat 14, fiber 2.5, carbs 12.4, protein 26.4

Chicken And Lemongrass Sauce

Preparation time: 10 minutes

Cooking time: 20 minutes

Servings: 3

Ingredients:

1 tablespoon dried dill

1 teaspoon butter, melted

½ teaspoon lemongrass

½ teaspoon cayenne pepper

1 teaspoon tomato sauce

3 tablespoons sour cream

1 teaspoon salt

10 oz chicken fillet, cubed

Directions:

Make the sauce: in the saucepan whisk together lemongrass, tomato sauce, sour cream, salt, and dried dill.

Bring the sauce to boil.

Meanwhile, pour melted butter in the skillet.

Add cubed chicken fillet and roast it for 5 minutes. Stir it from time to time.

Then place the chicken cubes in the hot sauce.

Close the lid and cook the meal for 10 minutes over the low heat.

Nutrition: :calories 166, fat 8.2, fiber 0.2, carbs 1.1, protein 21

Spiced Chicken Meatballs

Preparation time: 10 minutes

Cooking time: 20 minutes

Servings: 3

Ingredients:

1 pound chicken meat, ground

1 tablespoon pine nuts, toasted and chopped

1 egg, whisked

2 teaspoons turmeric powder

2 garlic cloves, minced

Salt and black pepper to the taste

1 and ¼ cups heavy cream

2 tablespoons olive oil

¼ cup parsley, chopped

1 tablespoon chives, chopped

Directions:

In a bowl, combine the chicken with the pine nuts and the rest of the ingredients except the oil and the cream, stir well and shape medium meatballs out of this mix.

Heat up a pan with the oil over medium-high heat, add the meatballs and cook them for 4 minutes on each side.

Add the cream, toss gently, cook everything over medium heat for 10 minutes more, divide between plates and serve.

Nutrition: calories 283, fat 9.2, fiber 12.8, carbs 24.4, protein 34.5

Paprika Chicken Wings

Preparation time: 10 minutes

Cooking time: 8 minutes

Servings: 3

Ingredients:

4 chicken wings, boneless

1 tablespoon honey

½ teaspoon paprika

¼ teaspoon cayenne pepper

¾ teaspoon ground black pepper

1 tablespoon lemon juice

½ teaspoon sunflower oil

Directions:

Make the honey marinade: whisk together honey, paprika, cayenne pepper, ground black pepper, lemon juice, and sunflower oil.

Then brush the chicken wings with marinade carefully.

Preheat the grill to 385F.

Place the chicken wings in the grill and cook them for 4 minutes from each side.

Nutrition: :calories 26, fat 0.8, fiber 0.3, carbs 5.1, protein 0.3

Chicken And Parsley Sauce

Preparation time: 10 minutes

Cooking time: 25 minutes

Servings: 3

Ingredients:

1 cup ground chicken

2 oz Parmesan, grated

1 tablespoon olive oil

2 tablespoons fresh parsley, chopped

1 teaspoon chili pepper

1 teaspoon paprika

½ teaspoon dried oregano

¼ teaspoon garlic, minced

½ teaspoon dried thyme

1/3 cup crushed tomatoes

Directions:

Heat up olive oil in the skillet.

Add ground chicken and sprinkle it with chili pepper, paprika, dried oregano, dried thyme, and parsley. Mix up well.

Cook the chicken for 5 minutes and add crushed tomatoes. Mix up well.

Close the lid and simmer the chicken mixture for 10 minutes over the low heat.

Then add grated Parmesan and mix up.

Cook chicken bolognese for 5 minutes more over the medium heat.

Nutrition: :calories 154, fat 9.3, fiber 1.1, carbs 3, protein 15.4

Sage Turkey Mix

Preparation time: 10 minutes

Cooking time: 40 minutes

Servings: 3

Ingredients:

1 big turkey breast, skinless, boneless and roughly cubed

Juice of 1 lemon

2 tablespoons avocado oil

1 red onion, chopped

2 tablespoons sage, chopped

1 garlic clove, minced

1 cup chicken stock

Directions:

Heat up a pan with the avocado oil over medium-high heat, add the turkey and brown for 3 minutes on each side.

Add the rest of the ingredients, bring to a simmer and cook over medium heat for 35 minutes.

Divide the mix between plates and serve with a side dish.

Nutrition: calories 382, fat 12.6, fiber 9.6, carbs 16.6, protein 33.2

Chipotle Turkey And Tomatoes

Preparation time: 10 minutes

Cooking time: 1 Hour

Servings: 3

Ingredients:

2 pounds cherry tomatoes, halved

3 tablespoons olive oil

1 red onion, roughly chopped

1 big turkey breast, skinless, boneless and sliced

3 garlic cloves, chopped

3 red chili peppers, chopped

4 tablespoons chipotle paste

Zest of ½ lemon, grated

Juice of 1 lemon

Salt and black pepper to the taste

A handful coriander, chopped

Directions:

Heat up a pan with the oil over medium-high heat, add the turkey slices, cook for 4 minutes on each side and transfer to a roasting pan.

Heat up the pan again over medium-high heat, add the onion, garlic and chili peppers and sauté for 2 minutes.

Add chipotle paste, sauté for 3 minutes more and pour over the turkey slices.

Toss the turkey slices with the chipotle mix, also add the rest of the ingredients except the coriander, introduce in the oven and bake at 400 degrees F for 45 minutes.

Divide everything between plates, sprinkle the coriander on top and serve.

Nutrition: calories 264, fat 13.2, fiber 8.7, carbs 23.9, protein 33.2

Curry Chicken, Artichokes And Olives

Preparation time: 10 minutes

Cooking time: 7 Hours

Servings: 3

Ingredients:

2 pounds chicken breasts, boneless, skinless and cubed

12 ounces canned artichoke hearts, drained

1 cup chicken stock

1 red onion, chopped

1 tablespoon white wine vinegar

1 cup kalamata olives, pitted and chopped

1 tablespoon curry powder

2 teaspoons basil, dried

Salt and black pepper to the taste

¼ cup rosemary, chopped

Directions:

In your slow cooker, combine the chicken with the artichokes, olives and the rest of the ingredients, put the lid on and cook on Low for 7 hours.

Divide the mix between plates and serve hot.

Nutrition: calories 275, fat 11.9, fiber 7.6, carbs 19.7, protein 18.7

Roasted Chicken

Preparation time: 10 minutes

Cooking time: 1 Hour 30 minutes

Servings: 3

Ingredients:

1 (5-lb.) whole chicken

1 TB. extra-virgin olive oil

2 TB. minced garlic

1 tsp. salt

1 tsp. paprika

1 tsp. black pepper

1 tsp. ground coriander

1 tsp. seven spices

1/2 tsp. ground cinnamon

1/2 large lemon, cut in 1/2

1/2 large yellow onion, cut in 1/2

2 sprigs fresh rosemary

2 sprigs fresh thyme

2 sprigs fresh sage

2 large carrots, cut into 1-in. pieces

6 small red potatoes, washed and cut in 1/2

4 cloves garlic

Directions:

Preheat the oven to 450ºF. Wash chicken and pat dry with paper towels. Place chicken in a roasting pan, and drizzle and then rub chicken with extra-virgin olive oil.

In a small bowl, combine garlic, salt, paprika, black pepper, coriander, seven spices, and cinnamon. Sprinkle and then rub entire chicken with spice mixture to coat.

Place 1/4 lemon, 1/4 yellow onion, 1 sprig rosemary, 1 sprig thyme, and 1 sprig sage in chicken cavity.

Place remaining rosemary, thyme, sage, lemon, and onion around chicken in the roasting pan. Add carrots, red potatoes, and garlic cloves to the roasting pan.

Roast for 15 minutes. Reduce temperature to 375ºF, and roast for 1 more hour, basting chicken every 20 minutes.

Let chicken rest for 15 minutes before serving.

Nutrition: Calories: 200, Fat: 6.0g, Total Carbs: 32.4g, Sugars: 15.3g, Protein: 11.7g

Rosemary Cauliflower Rolls

Preparation Time: 10 minutes

Cooking Time: 30 minutes

Servings: 3

Ingredients:

1/3 cup of almond flour

4 cups of riced cauliflower

1/3 cup of reduced-fat, shredded mozzarella or cheddar cheese

2 eggs

2 tablespoon of fresh rosemary, finely chopped

½ teaspoon of salt

Directions:

Preheat your oven to 4000F

Combine all the listed ingredients in a medium-sized bowl

Scoop cauliflower mixture into 12 evenly-sized rolls/biscuits onto a lightly-greased and foil-lined baking sheet.

Bake until it turns golden brown, which should be achieved in about 30 minutes.

Note: if you want to have the outside of the rolls/biscuits crisp, then broil for some minutes before serving.

Nutrition:

Calories: 254

Protein: 24g

Carbohydrate: 7g

Fat: 8 g

Delicious Lemon Chicken Salad

Preparation Time: 15 minutes

Cooking Time: 5 minutes

Servings: 4

Ingredients:

1 lb. chicken breast, cooked and diced

1 tbsp fresh dill, chopped

2 tsp olive oil

1/4 cup low-fat yogurt

1 tsp lemon zest, grated

2 tbsp onion, minced

¼ tsp pepper

¼ tsp salt

Directions:

Put all your fixing into the large mixing bowl and toss well. Season with pepper and salt. Cover and place in the refrigerator. Serve chilled and enjoy.

Nutrition:

Calories: 165

Fat: 5.4g

Protein: 25.2g

Carbs: 2.2g

Sodium 153mg

Healthy Chicken Orzo

Preparation Time: 15 minutes

Cooking Time: 15 minutes

Servings: 4

Ingredients:

1 cup whole wheat orzo

1 lb. chicken breasts, sliced

½ tsp red pepper flakes

½ cup feta cheese, crumbled

½ tsp oregano

1 tbsp fresh parsley, chopped

1 tbsp fresh basil, chopped

¼ cup pine nuts

1 cup spinach, chopped

¼ cup white wine

½ cup olives, sliced

1 cup grape tomatoes, cut in half

½ tbsp garlic, minced

2 tbsp olive oil

½ tsp pepper

½ tsp salt

Directions:

Add water in a small saucepan and bring to boil. Heat 1 tablespoon of olive oil in a pan over medium heat. Season chicken with pepper and salt and cook in the pan for 5-7 minutes on each side. Remove from pan and set aside.

Add orzo in boiling water and cook according to the packet directions. Heat remaining olive oil in a pan on medium heat, then put garlic in the pan and sauté for a minute. Stir in white wine and cherry tomatoes and cook on high for 3 minutes.

Add cooked orzo, spices, spinach, pine nuts, and olives and stir until well combined. Add chicken on top of orzo and sprinkle with feta cheese. Serve and enjoy.

Nutrition:

Calories: 518

Fat: 27.7g

Protein: 40.6g

Carbs: 26.2g

Sodium 121mg

Lemon Garlic Chicken

Preparation Time: 15 minutes

Cooking Time: 12 minutes

Servings: 3

Ingredients:

3 chicken breasts, cut into thin slices

2 lemon zest, grated

¼ cup olive oil

4 garlic cloves, minced

Pepper

Salt

Directions:

Warm-up olive oil in a pan over medium heat. Add garlic to the pan and sauté for 30 seconds. Put the chicken in the pan and sauté within 10 minutes. Add lemon zest and lemon juice and bring to boil. Remove from heat and season with pepper and salt. Serve and enjoy.

Nutrition:

Calories: 439

Fat: 27.8g

Protein: 42.9g

Carbs: 4.9g

Sodium 306 mg

Steamed Chicken with Mushroom and Ginger

Preparation time: 10 minutes

Cooking time: 10 minutes

Servings: 3

Ingredients:

4 x 150g chicken breasts

2 teaspoons extra-virgin olive oil

1 1/2 tablespoons balsamic vinegar

8cm piece ginger, cut into matchsticks

1 bunch broccoli

1 bunch carrots, diced

6 small dried shiitake mushrooms, chopped

Spring onion, sliced

Fresh coriander leaves,

Directions:

In a bowl, combine sliced chicken with salt, vinegar, and pepper; let marinate for at least 10 minutes.

Transfer the chicken to a baking dish and scatter with mushrooms and ginger; cook in a preheated oven at 350 degrees for about 15 minutes; place chopped broccoli and carrots on top of the chicken and return to the oven.

Cook for another 3 minutes or until chicken is tender.

Divide the chicken, broccoli, and carrots on serving plates and drizzle each with olive oil and top with coriander and red onions. Enjoy!

Nutrition: Calories: 200, Fat: 6.0g, Total Carbs: 32.4g, Sugars: 15.3g, Protein: 11.7g

Chicken Breast & Zucchini Linguine

Preparation time: 10 minutes

Cooking time: 10 minutes

Servings: 3

Ingredients:

450g chicken breast fillets, halved

1 tablespoon olive oil

2 garlic cloves, crushed

3 cups zucchini noodles

1/2 cup coconut cream

1/3 cup homemade chicken broth

1 tablespoon fresh dill leaves

2 tablespoons fresh chives, chopped

1 cup baby spinach

½ cup toasted chopped cashews

Directions:

Coat a pan with oil and set over medium high heat; season chicken with salt and pepper and cook in the pan for about 3 minutes per side or until cooked through; transfer to a plate and keep warm.

Add oil to the pan and sauté garlic until fragrant; stir in zucchini noodles and cook for about 2 minutes; stir in coconut cream and chicken broth and simmer for about 2 minutes or until tender.

Slice the chicken and add to the zucchini sauce along with chives and dill. Divide among serving bowls and top each with spinach and toasted cashews.

Enjoy!

Nutrition: Calories: 200, Fat: 6.0g, Total Carbs: 32.4g, Sugars: 15.3g, Protein: 11.7g

Detox Salad with Grilled White Fish

Preparation time: 10 minutes

Cooking time: 0 minutes

Servings: 3

Ingredients:

For the Salad:

2 (150g each) pre-grilled white fish

½ cup snap peas, sliced

1 cup baby spinach

1 cup chopped Romaine lettuce

½ cup avocado, sliced

½ cup blueberries

2 green onions, sliced

½ cup shredded carrot

1 large cucumber, chopped

1 tablespoon chia seeds

For the Dressing:

¼ teaspoon oregano

1 clove garlic, minced

1 tablespoon tahini

1 teaspoon honey

1 tablespoon rice wine vinegar

1 tablespoon lemon juice

1 teaspoon sesame oil

1/8 teaspoon red pepper flakes

¼ teaspoon black pepper

Directions:

In a large bowl, combine all salad ingredients, except fish.

Whisk together the ingredients for your dressing until well blended; pour over the salad and toss until well blended. Top each serving with the grilled white fish and enjoy!

Nutrition: Calories: 200, Fat: 6.0g, Total Carbs: 32.4g, Sugars: 15.3g, Protein: 11.7g

Chicken & Veggies with Toasted Walnuts

Preparation time: 10 minutes

Cooking time: 15minutes

Servings: 3

Ingredients:

4 (about 250g) chicken tenderloins

1 teaspoon extra virgin olive oil

1 small zucchini, sliced

2 cups drained and rinsed cannellini beans

1 cup chopped green beans

1/4 cup pitted and halved green olives

1 tablespoon fresh lemon juice

2 garlic cloves, sliced

400g can cherry tomatoes

1 teaspoon harissa paste

1 teaspoon smoked paprika

Fresh parsley sprigs

1 cup toasted walnuts, chopped

Directions:

In a plastic container, mix together lemon juice, garlic, harissa, and paprika until well combined; add in chicken and shake to coat well. Let sit a few minutes.

Heat oil in a skillet and add in the chicken along with the marinade; cook for about 2 minutes per side or until golden browned.

Stir in the veggies and simmer for about 10 minutes or until tender. Divide among serving plates and serve topped with fresh parsley and toasted walnuts.

Nutrition: Calories: 200, Fat: 6.0g, Total Carbs: 32.4g, Sugars: 15.3g, Protein: 11.7g

Lemon-Pepper Tuna Bake

Preparation time: 10 minutes

Cooking time: 35 minutes

Servings: 4

Ingredients:

4 (140g each) tuna fillets

1 bunch asparagus, trimmed

3 cups baby potatoes, diced

250g cherry tomatoes, diced

1 tablespoon extra-virgin olive oil

2 lemons, plus lemon zest to serve

8 sprigs fresh lemon thyme

1/4 teaspoon cracked pepper

Directions:

Preheat your oven to 400 degrees and line a greased baking tray with baking paper. On the preparation ared tray, toss together lemon juice, potatoes, half of thyme, lemon wedges and two teaspoons of oil until well coated.

Roast for about 15 minutes and then add in tomatoes; continue cooking for another 10 minutes; place the asparagus and tuna over the veggies and drizzle with the remaining oil.

Continue roasting for another 8 minutes. serve topped with lemon zest and thyme. Enjoy!

Nutrition: Calories: 250, Fat: 15.5g, Total Carbs: 11.5g, Sugars: 3.7g, Protein: 19.2g

Chicken Meatballs with Stir-Fried Greens

Preparation time: 10 minutes

Cooking time: 30 minutes

Servings: 3

Ingredients:

500g chicken mince

2 green onions, chopped

2 garlic cloves, crushed

1 medium zucchini, grated

1/4 cup oyster sauce

1/2 cup frozen peas

2 tablespoons canola oil

Stir-fried greens

1/2 cup dried gluten-free breadcrumbs

Directions:

Preheat your oven to 400 degrees and line a greased baking tray with baking paper.

In a bowl, mix together peas, oyster sauce, zucchini, garlic, red onion, gluten-free breadcrumbs, pepper and mince until well combined. Shape into meat balls.

Heat oil in a skillet and in batches, cook in the meat balls for about 4 minutes per side or until golden brown.

Transfer the balls on the preparation ared tray and bake for about 20 minutes until cooked through. Serve the meat balls with stir fried greens.

Nutrition: Calories: 250, Fat: 15.5g, Total Carbs: 11.5g, Sugars: 3.7g, Protein: 19.2g

Sesame Chicken with Black Rice, Broccoli & Snap Peas

Preparation time: 10 minutes

Cooking time: 25 minutes

Servings: 3

Ingredients:

2/3 cup black rice

2 (200g each) chicken breast fillets

2 cups chopped broccoli

200g snap peas, trimmed

1 1/2 cups picked watercress leaves

1 1/2 tablespoon salt-reduced tamari

1 tablespoon sesame seeds

2 tablespoons tahini

1/2 teaspoon raw honey

Directions:

Boil rice in a saucepan for about 15 minutes or until al dente; drain.

Coat chicken fillets with sesame seeds and cook in hot oil in a skillet set over medium high heat for about 5 minutes per side or until cooked through.

Let cool and slice. In the meantime, steam broccoli and peas until tender.

In a small bowl, whisk together tahini, tamari and raw honey until very smooth. Divide cooked black rice among serving bowls and top each with broccoli and peas. Top with chicken and watercress; drizzle each serving with tahini dressing. Enjoy!

Nutrition: Calories: 250, Fat: 15.5g, Total Carbs: 11.5g, Sugars: 3.7g, Protein: 19.2g

Clean Eating Lemon Grilled Tuna & Avocado Vegetable Salad

Preparation time: 10 minutes

Cooking time: 0 minutes

Servings: 3

Ingredients:

3 (150g each) tuna fillet

¼ cup freshly squeezed lemon juice

A pinch of sea salt

A pinch of pepper

1 small red onion, sliced into thin rings

1 cup watercress, rinsed

1 zucchini, shaved

1 small broccoli head, rinsed and cut in small florets

1 avocado, diced

2 tablespoon s fresh lemon juice

1 tablespoon extra-virgin olive oil

½ teaspoon Dijon mustard

½ teaspoon sea salt

¼ cup crushed toasted almonds

1 tablespoon chia seeds

Directions:

In a bowl, mix lemon juice, salt and pepper until well combined; smear on the fish fillets until well coated and grill on a preheated charcoal grill for about 7 minutes per side or until browned and cooked to your liking.

In another bowl, mix together the veggies until well combined.

In a small bowl, whisk together lemon juice, olive oil, mustard and salt until well blended; pour over the salad and toss until well coated. Add almonds and chia seeds and toss to combine. Set the salad aside for at least 5 minutes for flavors to combine before serving.

Serve the salad drizzled with the dressing and topped with the grilled tuna for a satisfying meal.

Nutrition: Calories: 250, Fat: 15.5g, Total Carbs: 11.5g, Sugars: 3.7g, Protein: 19.2g

Lemon & Garlic Barbecued Ocean Trout with Green Salad

Preparation time: 10 minutes

Cooking time: 10 minutes

Servings: 3

Ingredients:

1.5kg piece trout fillet

2 tablespoons lemon juice

4 garlic cloves, sliced

1 long red chilli, sliced

2 tablespoons chopped capers

1/2 cup fresh parsley

1/2 cup olive oil

Lemon wedges

Salad greens for serving

Directions:

Brush the trout with 2 tablespoons of oil and then place it, skin-side up on a barbecue plate.

Cook over the preheated barbecue on high for about 5 minutes and then turn it over. Close the hood and cook on medium heat for another 15 minutes or until cooked through. Transfer to a plate.

In a pan, heat the remaining oil and then sauté garlic until lightly browned. Remove from heat and stir in chili, capers and fresh lemon juice; drizzle over the fish and then sprinkle with parsley. Serve garnished with fresh lemon wedges.

Nutrition: Calories: 250, Fat: 15.5g, Total Carbs: 11.5g, Sugars: 3.7g, Protein: 19.2g

Gingery Lemon Roasted Chicken with Steamed Greens

Preparation time: 10 minutes

Cooking time: 30 minutes

Servings: 3

Ingredients:

1 tablespoon extra-virgin olive oil

½ cup fresh lemon juice

2 tablespoons fresh lemon zest

3 cloves garlic, minced

2-3 tablespoons minced ginger

3 pound whole chicken

1 pound chopped carrots

handful of rosemary

Pinch of sea salt

Pinch of pepper

Steamed greens for serving

Directions:

Preheat oven to 400°F. Place chicken in a baking dish. In a bowl, whisk together olive oil, lemon juice, lemon zest, garlic, and ginger until well combined; pour over the chicken and top with carrots and rosemary.

Sprinkle with salt and pepper and roast for about 1 ½ hours or until chicken is cooked through. Serve warm over a bowl of steamed greens.

Nutrition: Calories: 381, Fat: 28.5g, Total Carbs: 30.8g, Sugars: 17.4g, Protein: 6.4g

Grilled Chicken with Rainbow Salad Bowl

Preparation time: 10 minutes

Cooking time: 0 minutes

Servings: 3

Ingredients:

300g grilled skinless chicken, shredded

2 cups mixed salad leaves

4 radishes, thinly sliced

1 cup chopped tomatoes

1 cup shredded carrot

1 cup podded edamame

4 tablespoons almond butter

2 tablespoons freshly squeezed lemon juice

2 tablespoons freshly squeezed lime juice

½ teaspoon sea salt

Directions:

Blanch edamame in boiling water for about 2 minutes and then drain; transfer to a serving bowl and add in salad leaves, radish, tomatoes, carrots and chicken.

In a bowl, whisk together fresh lemon juice, lime juice, almond butter, and sea salt until smooth; drizzle over the salad and serve.

Nutrition: Calories: 381, Fat: 28.5g, Total Carbs: 30.8g, Sugars: 17.4g, Protein: 6.4g

Pepper Chicken and Lettuce Wraps

Preparation time: 10 minutes

Cooking time: 5 minutes

Servings: 3

Ingredients:

450g lean diced chicken

1 tablespoon extra-virgin olive oil

1 teaspoon black pepper

1 teaspoon white pepper

1 teaspoon salt

1 cup bean sprouts, trimmed

16 baby cos lettuce leaves

1 large red onion, diced

12 fresh lemon wedges

16 large fresh mint leaves

Directions:

Preheat your pan over medium high heat; in a bowl, mix together oil, white pepper, salt and black pepper until well combined; add in chicken and toss to coat well. Grill for about 5 minutes per side or until cooked through. Let rest for at least 5 minutes.

Arrange lettuce leaves on serving plates and top each mint and bean sprouts. Serve topped with sliced beef and garnished with lemon wedges.

Nutrition: Calories: 381, Fat: 28.5g, Total Carbs: 30.8g, Sugars: 17.4g, Protein: 6.4g

Chicken Lettuce Wraps

Preparation time: 10 minutes

Cooking time: 30 minutes

Servings: 3

Ingredients:

500g chicken breast, minced

2 teaspoons extra-virgin olive oil

2 cups shredded cabbage

1 large carrot, grated

1 celery stick, chopped

2 garlic cloves, chopped

1/2 red onion, chopped

2 spring onions, sliced

2 tablespoons chopped coriander

1 iceberg lettuce, halved, cored

Directions:

Heat a skillet over medium high heat; cook in chicken mince, stirring to break up the chicken with a spoon for about 5 minutes or until cooked through. Transfer to a dish.

Add oil to the pan and sauté red onions and garlic until fragrant and then stir in celery for about 3 minutes. return the chicken and cook for about 1 minute or until flavors blend; stir in carrots, cabbage, spring onions, and pepper and then remove the pan from the heat.

Divide the lettuce leaves among four serving plates and spoon the chicken mixture onto each serving. Top each with coriander and the remaining spring onions. Enjoy!

Nutrition: Calories: 381, Fat: 28.5g, Total Carbs: 30.8g, Sugars: 17.4g, Protein: 6.4g

Pan-Seared Tuna with Crunchy Cabbage Slaw & Toasted Macadamias

Preparation time: 10 minutes

Cooking time: 10 minutes

Servings: 7

Ingredients:

4 x 180g tuna skin-on

1 1/2 tablespoons olive oil

4 cups thinly sliced cabbage

2 teaspoons raw honey

1/4 cup fresh lime juice

2 spring onions, chopped

1 yellow capsicum, thinly sliced

200g seedless white grapes, halved

1/2 cup fresh mint leaves

1/2 cup fresh coriander leaves

1/2 cup chopped toasted macadamias

Lime wedges

Directions:

Heat half tablespoon of oil in a skillet over medium heat; place in tuna, skin side down and cook for about 5 minutes or until the skin is crisp; turn over to cook the other side for about 3 minutes or until cooked through.

In the meantime, whisk together raw honey, lime juice, lime zest, salt and the remaining oil until well blended; add in grapes, cabbage, spring onions, capsicum, mint and coriander.

Stir in salt and pepper. Divide the cabbage slaw among serving plates and to each serving with tuna.

Sprinkle with toasted macadamia and garnish with lime wedges. Enjoy!

Nutrition: Calories: 381, Fat: 28.5g, Total Carbs: 30.8g, Sugars: 17.4g, Protein: 6.4g

Brazilian Inspired Shrimp Stew

Preparation time: 10 minutes

Cooking time: 20 minutes

Servings: 5

Ingredients:

1 ½ pounds jumbo shrimp, peeled and deveined

2 cloves garlic, minced

¼ cup olive oil

1 small yellow onion, diced

¼ cup fresh cilantro, chopped

¼ cup roasted red peppers, diced

1 (14 ounce) can chopped tomatoes with chilies

2 tablespoons Sambal Oelek – check in the Asian food section in the supermarket or food store

1 cup full-fat coconut milk

Juice of 1 lime

Freshly ground pepper and sea salt to taste

Directions:

Pour the olive oil in a saucepan over medium to high heat and sauté the onions until tender.

Stir in the roasted peppers and garlic and cook until fragrant, careful not to burn the garlic.

Stir in the shrimp, tomatoes and three quarter of the cilantro. Cook until the shrimp turns opaque for 5-8 minutes.

Stir in the Sambal Oelek and pour in the coconut milk. Reduce heat to low and cook for 5 minutes then add the lime juice and season well with pepper and salt.

Turn of the heat and garnish with the extra cilantro and serve hot.

Pan-Seared Tuna Salad with Snow Peas & Grapefruit

Preparation time: 10 minutes

Cooking time: 0 minutes

Servings: 4

Ingredients:

4 (100g) skin-on tuna fillets

1/8 teaspoon sea salt

2 teaspoons extra virgin olive oil

4 cups arugula

8 leaves Boston lettuce, washed and dried

1 cup snow peas, cooked

2 avocados, diced

For Grapefruit-Dill Dressing:

1/4 cup grapefruit juice

1/4 cup extra virgin olive oil

1 teaspoon raw honey

1 tablespoon Dijon mustard

1 tablespoon chopped fresh dill

2 garlic cloves, minced

1/2 teaspoon salt

Directions:

Sprinkle fish with about 1/8 teaspoon salt and cook in 2 teaspoons of olive oil over medium heat for about 4 minutes per side or until golden.

In a small bowl, whisk together al dressing ingredients and set aside. Divide arugula and lettuce among four serving plates.

Divide lettuce and arugula among 4 plates and add the remaining salad ingredients; top each with seared tuna and drizzle with dressing. Enjoy!

Chicken Cacciatore

Preparation Time: 5 minutes

Cooking Time: 45 minutes

Servings: 6

Ingredients:

2 tablespoons extra virgin olive oil

6 chicken thighs

1 sweet onion, chopped

2 garlic cloves, minced

2 red bell peppers, cored and diced

2 carrots, diced

1 rosemary sprig

1 thyme sprig

4 tomatoes, peeled and diced

½ cup tomato juice

¼ cup dry white wine

1 cup chicken stock

1 bay leaf

Salt and pepper to taste

Directions:

Heat the oil in a heavy saucepan.

Cook chicken on all sides until golden.

Stir in the onion and garlic and cook for 2 minutes.

Stir in the rest of the ingredients and season with salt and pepper.

Cook on low heat for 30 minutes.

Serve the chicken cacciatore warm and fresh.

Nutrition:

Calories: 363

Fat: 14g

Protein: 42g

Carbohydrates: 9g

Fennel Wild Rice Risotto

Preparation Time: 5 minutes

Cooking Time: 35 minutes

Servings: 6

Ingredients:

2 tablespoons extra virgin olive oil

1 shallot, chopped

2 garlic cloves, minced

1 fennel bulb, chopped

1 cup wild rice

¼ cup dry white wine

2 cups chicken stock

1 teaspoon grated orange zest

Salt and pepper to taste

Directions:

Heat the oil in a heavy saucepan.

Add the garlic, shallot and fennel and cook for a few minutes until softened.

Stir in the rice and cook for 2 additional minutes then add the wine, stock and orange zest, with salt and pepper to taste.

Cook on low heat for 20 minutes.

Serve the risotto warm and fresh.

Nutrition:

Calories: 162

Fat: 2g

Protein: 8g

Carbohydrates: 20g

Wild Rice Prawn Salad

Preparation Time: 5 minutes

Cooking Time: 35 minutes

Servings: 6

Ingredients:

¾ cup wild rice

1¾ cups chicken stock

1 pound prawns

Salt and pepper to taste

2 tablespoons lemon juice

2 tablespoons extra virgin olive oil

2 cups arugula

Directions:

Combine the rice and chicken stock in a saucepan and cook until the liquid has been absorbed entirely.

Transfer the rice in a salad bowl.

Season the prawns with salt and pepper and drizzle them with lemon juice and oil.

Heat a grill pan over medium flame.

Place the prawns on the hot pan and cook on each side for 2-3 minutes.

For the salad, combine the rice with arugula and prawns and mix well.

Serve the salad fresh.

Nutrition:

Calories: 207

Fat: 4g

Protein: 20.6g

Carbohydrates: 17g

Fragrant Asian Hotpot

Preparation Time: 10 minutes

Cooking Time: 15 minutes

Servings: 2

Ingredients:

1 tsp tomato purée

1 star anise, squashed (or 1/4 tsp ground anise)

Little bunch (10g) parsley, stalks finely cleaved

Little bunch (10g) coriander, stalks finely cleaved

Juice of 1/2 lime

500ml chicken stock, new or made with 1 solid shape

1/2 carrot, stripped and cut into matchsticks

50g broccoli, cut into little florets

50g beansprouts

100 g crude tiger prawns

100 g firm tofu, slashed

50g rice noodles, cooked according to parcel directions

50g cooked water chestnuts, depleted

20g sushi ginger, slashed

1 tbsp. great quality miso glue

Directions:

Spot the tomato purée, star anise, parsley stalks, coriander stalks, lime juice and chicken stock in an enormous container and bring to a stew for 10 minutes.

Include the carrot, broccoli, prawns, tofu, noodles and water chestnuts and stew tenderly until the prawns are cooked through.

Expel from the warmth and mix in the sushi ginger and miso glue. Serve sprinkled with the parsley and coriander leaves.

Nutrition:

Calories 434

Fat: 2 g

Carbohydrates: 12 g

Protein: 12 g

Fiber: 0 g

Chicken Fry with Peanut Sauce

Preparation Time: 10 minutes

Cooking Time: 15 minutes

Servings: 4

Ingredients

Meat from 4 chicken thighs, cut into bite-size pieces

2 tbsp. + ¼ cup peanut oil

½ cup peanut butter

3 tbsp. toasted sesame oil

2 tbsp. soy sauce

1 tbsp. lime juice

1 clove garlic, minced

1 tsp. powdered ginger

1-2 tsp. hot sauce, if desired

2 red bell peppers, chopped

2 tbsp. toasted sesame seeds

4 green onions, thinly sliced

Directions:

Heat 2 tbsp. peanut oil in a large frying pan.

Add the chicken and cook for about 10 minutes, until no pink remains.

Meanwhile, mix together the peanut butter, ¼ cup peanut oil, sesame oil, soy sauce, lime juice, garlic, ginger, and hot sauce.

Add more water if needed to achieve a smooth consistency.

When the chicken is done, add the red pepper and cook for 1 minutes more.

Divide the chicken and peppers between four plates and top with peanut sauce, toasted sesame seeds, and green onions.

Nutrition:

Calories: 426.9

Sugars: 4.8 g

Total Carbohydrate: 16.9 g

Protein: 38.7 g

Stewed Chicken Greek Style

Preparation time: 10 minutes

Cooking time: 60 minutes

Servings: 9

Ingredients:

½ cup red wine

1 ½ cups chicken stock or more if needed

1 cup olive oil

1 cup tomato sauce

1 pc, 4lbs whole chicken cut into pieces

1 pinch dried oregano or to taste

10 small shallots, peeled

2 bay leaves

2 cloves garlic, finely chopped

2 tbsp chopped fresh parsley

2 tsps butter

Salt and ground black pepper to taste

Directions:

Bring to a boil a large pot of lightly salted water. Mix in the shallots and let boil uncovered until tender for around three minutes. Then drain the shallots and dip in cold water until no longer warm.

In another large pot over medium fire, heat butter and olive oil until bubbling and melted. Then sauté in the chicken and shallots for 15 minutes or until chicken is cooked and shallots are soft and translucent. Then add the chopped garlic and cook for three mins more.

Then add bay leaves, oregano, salt and pepper, parsley, tomato sauce and the red wine and let simmer for a minute before adding the chicken stock. Stir before covering and let cook for 50 minutes on medium-low fire or until chicken is tender.

Nutrition: Calories per Serving: 644.8; Carbs: 8.2g; Protein: 62.1g; Fat: 40.4g

Hot Pork Meatballs

Preparation time: 10 minutes

Cooking time: 10 minutes

Servings: 3

Ingredients:

4 oz pork loin, grinded

½ teaspoon garlic powder

¼ teaspoon chili powder

¼ teaspoon cayenne pepper

¼ teaspoon ground black pepper

¼ teaspoon white pepper

1 tablespoon water

1 teaspoon olive oil

Directions:

Mix up together grinded meat, garlic powder, cayenne pepper, ground black pepper, white pepper, and water.

With the help of the fingertips make the small meatballs.

Heat up olive oil in the skillet.

Arrange the kofte in the oil and cook them for 10 minutes totally. Flip the kofte on another side from time to time.

Nutrition: :calories 162, fat 10.3, fiber 0.3, carbs 1, protein 15.7

Beef And Zucchini Skillet

Preparation time: 10 minutes

Cooking time: 30 minutes

Servings: 3

Ingredients:

2 oz ground beef

½ onion, sliced

½ bell pepper, sliced

1 tablespoon butter

½ teaspoon salt

1 tablespoon tomato sauce

1 small zucchini, chopped

½ teaspoon dried oregano

Directions:

Place the ground beef in the skillet.

Add salt, butter, and dried oregano.

Mix up the meat mixture and cook it for 10 minutes.

After this, transfer the cooked ground beef in the bowl.

Place zucchini, bell pepper, and onion in the skillet (where the ground meat was cooking) and roast the vegetables for 7 minutes over the medium heat or until they are tender.

Then add cooked ground beef and tomato sauce. Mix up well.

Cook the beef toss for 2-3 minutes over the medium heat.

Nutrition: :calories 182, fat 8.7, fiber 0.1, carbs 0.3, protein 24.1

Greek Chicken Stew

Preparation time: 10 minutes

Cooking time: 60 minutes

Servings: 3

Ingredients:

10 smalls shallots, peeled

1 cup olive oil

2 teaspoons butter

1 (4 pound) whole chicken, cut into pieces

2 cloves garlic, finely chopped

½ cup red wine

1 cup tomato sauce

2 tablespoons chopped fresh parsley

salt and ground black pepper to taste

1 pinch dried oregano, or to taste

2 bay leaves

1 ½ cups chicken stock, or more if needed

Directions:

In a large pot, fill half full of water and bring to a boil. Lightly salt the water and once boiling add shallots and boil uncovered for 3 minutes. Drain and quickly place on an ice bath for 5 minutes. Drain well.

In same pot, heat for 3 minutes and add oil and butter. Heat for 3 minutes.

Add chicken and shallots. Cook 15 minutes.

Add chopped garlic and cook for another 3 minutes or until garlic starts to turn golden.

Add red wine and tomato sauce. Deglaze pot.

Stir in bay leaves, oregano, pepper, salt, and parsley. Cook for 3 minutes.

Stir in chicken stock.

Cover and simmer for 40 minutes while occasionally stirring pot.

Serve and enjoy while hot with a side of rice if desired.

Nutrition: Calories per Serving: 574; Carbs: 6.8g; Protein: 31.8g; Fats: 45.3g

Meatloaf

Preparation time: 10 minutes

Cooking time: 35 minutes

Servings: 7

Ingredients:

2 lbs ground beef

2 eggs, lightly beaten

1/4 tsp dried basil

3 tbsp olive oil

1/2 tsp dried sage

1 1/2 tsp dried parsley

1 tsp oregano

2 tsp thyme

1 tsp rosemary

Pepper

Salt

Directions:

Pour 1 1/2 cups of water into the instant pot then place the trivet in the pot.

Spray loaf pan with cooking spray.

Add all ingredients into the mixing bowl and mix until well combined.

Transfer meat mixture into the preparation ared loaf pan and place loaf pan on top of the trivet in the pot.

Seal pot with lid and cook on high for 35 minutes.

Once done, allow to release pressure naturally for 10 minutes then release remaining using quick release. Remove lid.

Serve and enjoy.

Nutrition: Calories 365 Fat 18 g Carbohydrates 0.7 g Sugar 0.1 g Protein 47.8 g Cholesterol 190 mg

Tasty Lamb Ribs

Preparation time: 10 minutes

Cooking time: 30 minutes

Servings: 4

Ingredients:

2 garlic cloves, minced

¼ cup shallot, chopped

2 tablespoons fish sauce

½ cup veggie stock

2 tablespoons olive oil

1 and ½ tablespoons lemon juice

1 tablespoon coriander seeds, ground

1 tablespoon ginger, grated

Salt and black pepper to the taste

2 pounds lamb ribs

Directions:

In a roasting pan, combine the lamb with the garlic, shallots and the rest of the ingredients, toss, introduce in the oven at 300 degrees F and cook for 2 hours.

Divide the lamb between plates and serve with a side salad.

Nutrition: calories 293, fat 9.1, fiber 9.6, carbs 16.7, protein 24.2

Peas And Ham Thick Soup

Preparation time: 10 minutes

Cooking time: 30 minutes

Servings: 3

Ingredients:

Pepper and salt to taste

1 lb. ham, coarsely chopped

24 oz frozen sweet peas

4 cup ham stock

¼ cup white wine

1 carrot, chopped coarsely

1 onion, chopped coarsely

2 tbsp butter, divided

Directions:

On medium fireplace a medium pot and heat oil. Sauté for 6 minutes the onion or until soft and translucent.

Add wine and cook for 4 minutes or until nearly evaporated.

Add ham stock and bring to a simmer and simmer continuously while covered for 4 minutes.

Add peas and cook for 7 minutes or until tender.

Meanwhile, in a nonstick fry pan, cook to a browned crisp the ham in 1 tbsp butter, around 6 minutes. Remove from fire and set aside.

When peas are soft, transfer to a blender and puree. Return to pot, continue cooking while seasoning with pepper, salt and ½ of crisped ham. Once soup is to your desired taste, turn off fire.

Transfer to 4 serving bowls and garnish evenly with crisped ham.

Nutrition: Calories per Serving: 403; Carbs: 32.5g; Protein: 37.3g; Fat: 12.5g

Bell Peppers On Chicken Breasts

Preparation time: 10 minutes

Cooking time: 30 minutes

Servings: 6

Ingredients:

¼ tsp freshly ground black pepper

½ tsp salt

1 large red bell pepper, cut into ¼-inch strips

1 large yellow bell pepper, cut into ¼-inch strips

1 tbsp olive oil

1 tsp chopped fresh oregano

2 1/3 cups coarsely chopped tomato

2 tbsp finely chopped fresh flat-leaf parsley

20 Kalamata olives

3 cups onion sliced crosswise

6 4-oz skinless, boneless chicken breast halves, cut in half horizontally

Cooking spray

Directions:

On medium high fire, place a large nonstick fry pan and heat oil. Once oil is hot, sauté onions until soft and translucent, around 6 to 8 minutes.

Add bell peppers and sauté for another 10 minutes or until tender.

Add black pepper, salt and tomato. Cook until tomato juice has evaporated, around 7 minutes.

Add olives, oregano and parsley, cook until heated through around 1 to 2 minutes. Transfer to a bowl and keep warm.

Wipe pan with paper towel and grease with cooking spray. Return to fire and place chicken breasts. Cook for three minutes per side or until desired doneness is reached. If needed, cook chicken in batches.

When cooking the last batch of chicken is done, add back the previous batch of chicken and the onion-bell pepper mixture and cook for a minute or two while tossing chicken to coat well in the onion-bell pepper mixture.

Serve and enjoy.

Nutrition: Calories per Serving: 261.8; Carbs: 11.0g; Protein: 36.0g; Fat: 8.2g

Yummy Turkey Meatballs

Preparation time: 10 minutes

Cooking time: 30 minutes

Servings: 3

Ingredients:

¼ yellow onion, finely diced

1 14-oz can of artichoke hearts, diced

1 lb. ground turkey

1 tsp dried parsley

1 tsp oil

4 tbsp fresh basil, finely chopped

Pepper and salt to taste

Directions:

Grease a cookie sheet and preheat oven to 350oF.

On medium fire, place a nonstick medium saucepan and sauté artichoke hearts and diced onions for 5 minutes or until onions are soft.

Remove from fire and let cool.

Meanwhile, in a big bowl, mix with hands parsley, basil and ground turkey. Season to taste.

Once onion mixture has cooled add into the bowl and mix thoroughly.

With an ice cream scooper, scoop ground turkey and form into balls, makes around 6 balls.

Place on preparation ped cookie sheet, pop in the oven and bake until cooked through around 15-20 minutes.

Remove from pan, serve and enjoy.

Nutrition: Calories per Serving: 328; Carbs: 11.8g; Protein: 33.5g; Fat: 16.3g

Garlic Caper Beef Roast

Preparation time: 10 minutes

Cooking time: 40 minutes

Servings: 3

Ingredients:

2 lbs beef roast, cubed

1 tbsp fresh parsley, chopped

1 tbsp capers, chopped

1 tbsp garlic, minced

1 cup chicken stock

1/2 tsp dried rosemary

1/2 tsp ground cumin

1 onion, chopped

1 tbsp olive oil

Pepper

Salt

Directions:

Add oil into the instant pot and set the pot on sauté mode.

Add garlic and onion and sauté for 5 minutes.

Add meat and cook until brown.

Add remaining ingredients and stir well.

Seal pot with lid and cook on high for 30 minutes.

Once done, allow to release pressure naturally. Remove lid.

Stir well and serve.

Nutrition: Calories 470 Fat 17.9 g Carbohydrates 3.9 g Sugar 1.4 g Protein 69.5 g Cholesterol 203 mg

Olive Oil Drenched Lemon Chicken

Preparation time: 10 minutes

Cooking time: 60 minutes

Servings: 3

Ingredients:

1 lemon, thinly sliced

1 red bell pepper, cut into 1-inch wide strips

1 red onion, cut into 1-inch wedges

1 tablespoon dried oregano

1/2 teaspoon coarsely ground black pepper

1/4 cup olive oil

2 tablespoons fresh lemon juice

2 tablespoons fresh lemon zest

3/4 teaspoon salt

4 large cloves garlic, pressed

4 skinless, boneless chicken breast halves

8 baby red potatoes, halved

Directions:

Preheat oven to 400oF.

In a bowl, mix well pepper, salt, oregano, garlic, lemon zest, lemon juice, and olive oil.

In a 9 x 13-inch casserole dish, evenly spread chicken in a single layer. Brush lemon juice mixture over chicken.

In a bowl mix well lemon slices, red onion, bell pepper, and potatoes. Drizzle remaining olive oil sauce and toss well to coat. Arrange vegetables and lemon slices around chicken breasts in baking dish.

Bake for 50 minutes; brush chicken and vegetables with pan drippings halfway through cooking time.

Let chicken rest for ten minutes before serving.

Nutrition: Calories per Serving: 517; Carbs: 65.1g; Protein: 30.8g; Fats: 16.7g

Beef Spread

Preparation time: 10 minutes

Cooking time: 25 minutes

Servings: 3

Ingredients:

8 oz beef liver

½ onion, peeled

½ carrot, peeled

½ teaspoon peppercorns

1 bay leaf

½ teaspoon salt

1/3 cup water

1 teaspoon ground black pepper

Directions:

Chop the beef liver and put it in the saucepan.

Add onion, carrot, peppercorns, bay leaf, salt, and ground black pepper.

Add water and close the lid.

Boil the beef liver for 25 minutes or until all ingredients are tender.

Transfer the cooked mixture in the blender and blend it until smooth.

Then place the cooked pate in the serving bowl and flatten the surface of it.

Refrigerate the pate for 20-30 minutes before serving.

Nutrition: :calories 109, fat 2.7, fiber 0.6, carbs 5.3, protein 15.3

Pork Chops And Relish

Preparation time: 10 minutes

Cooking time: 14 minutes

Servings: 3

Ingredients:

6 pork chops, boneless

7 ounces marinated artichoke hearts, chopped and their liquid reserved

A pinch of salt and black pepper

1 teaspoon hot pepper sauce

1 and ½ cups tomatoes, cubed

1 jalapeno pepper, chopped

½ cup roasted bell peppers, chopped

½ cup black olives, pitted and sliced

Directions:

In a bowl, mix the chops with the pepper sauce, reserved liquid from the artichokes, cover and keep in the fridge for 15 minutes.

Heat up a grill over medium-high heat, add the pork chops and cook for 7 minutes on each side.

In a bowl, combine the artichokes with the peppers and the remaining ingredients, toss, divide on top of the chops and serve.

Nutrition: calories 215, fat 6, fiber 1, carbs 6, protein 35

Tasty Beef Goulash

Preparation time: 10 minutes

Cooking time: 30 minutes

Servings: 3

Ingredients:

1/2 lb beef stew meat, cubed

1 tbsp olive oil

1/2 onion, chopped

1/2 cup sun-dried tomatoes, chopped

1/4 zucchini, chopped

1/2 cabbage, sliced

1 1/2 tbsp olive oil

2 cups chicken broth

Pepper

Salt

Directions:

Add oil into the instant pot and set the pot on sauté mode.

Add onion and sauté for 3-5 minutes.

Add tomatoes and cook for 5 minutes.

Add remaining ingredients and stir well.

Seal pot with lid and cook on high for 20 minutes.

Once done, allow to release pressure naturally for 10 minutes then release remaining using quick release. Remove lid.

Stir well and serve.

Nutrition: Calories 389 Fat 15.8 g Carbohydrates 19.3 g Sugar 10.7 g Protein 43.2 g Cholesterol 101 mg

Beef And Grape Sauce

Preparation time: 10 minutes

Cooking time: 30 minutes

Servings: 3

Ingredients:

1-pound beef sirloin

1 teaspoon molasses

1 tablespoon lemon zest, grated

1 teaspoon soy sauce

1 chili pepper, chopped

¼ teaspoon fresh ginger, minced

1 cup grape juice

½ teaspoon salt

1 tablespoon butter

Directions:

Sprinkle the beef sirloin with salt and minced ginger.

Heat up butter in the saucepan and add meat.

Roast it for 5 minutes from each side over the medium heat.

After this, add soy sauce, chili pepper, and grape juice.

Then add lemon zest and simmer the meat for 10 minutes.

Add molasses and mix up meat well.

Close the lid and cook meat for 5 minutes.

Serve the cooked beef with grape juice sauce.

Nutrition: :calories 267, fat 10, fiber 0.2, carbs 7.4, protein 34.9

Lamb And Tomato Sauce

Preparation time: 10 minutes

Cooking time: 55 minutes

Servings: 3

Ingredients:

9 oz lamb shanks

1 onion, diced

1 carrot, diced

1 tablespoon olive oil

1 teaspoon salt

1 teaspoon ground black pepper

1 ½ cup chicken stock

1 tablespoon tomato paste

Directions:

Sprinkle the lamb shanks with salt and ground black pepper.

Heat up olive oil in the saucepan.

Add lamb shanks and roast them for 5 minutes from each side.

Transfer meat in the plate.

After this, add onion and carrot in the saucepan.

Roast the vegetables for 3 minutes.

Add tomato paste and mix up well.

Then add chicken stock and bring the liquid to boil.

Add lamb shanks, stir well, and close the lid.

Cook the meat for 40 minutes over the medium-low heat.

Nutrition: :calories 232, fat 11.3, fiber 1.7, carbs 7.3, protein 25.1

Shrimp Fried 'Rice'

Preparation Time: 10 minutes

Cooking Time: 15 minutes

Servings: 4

Ingredients

2 + 2 tbsp. coconut oil

3 cups grated cauliflower

2 bell peppers, chopped

6 green onions, thinly sliced

1 lb. shrimp

4 eggs, lightly beaten

1 tbsp. soy sauce

2 tbsp. toasted sesame oil

Directions:

Heat 2 tbsp. of coconut oil in a large skillet over high heat. Add shrimp and cook for 2-4 minutes until opaque and pink.

Remove from pan and set aside.

Add 2 tbsp. coconut oil and add the cauliflower, peppers, and green onions.

Sautee for 4-5 minutes, stirring frequently.

Add the eggs and soy sauce to the pan and stir continuously until the eggs are firm.

Add the toasted sesame oil and stir, then toss with the shrimp and serve.

Nutrition:

Calories 482

Carbs 44.5g

Protein 29.5g

Fat 15g

Toasted Sardines with Parsley

Preparation Time: 10 minutes

Cooking Time: 15 minutes

Servings: 4

Ingredients:

400 g fresh sardines already cleaned

2 lemons zest

Salt

50 g chopped parsley

1 teaspoon black pepper

1 crushed clove garlic

2 tbsp. white wine

1 tablespoon extra-virgin olive oil

Directions:

Preparation are the sauce by blending the parsley, pepper, garlic clove and thinly grated lemon zest. Also add the white wine, lemon juice and oil.

Cook the sardines in a non-stick pan (or grill) for one minute per side.

When serving, pour a little sauce on the plate, lay the sardines on top and season with other sauce. Complete with a pinch of salt and lemon zest cut into strips.

Nutrition:

Calories: 300

Fat: 16.9g

Protein: 20.3g

Carbohydrate: 6.9g

Fiber: 0.9g

Tuscan Bean Stew

Preparation Time: 15 minutes

Cooking Time: 40 minutes

Servings: 1

Ingredients

1 tbsp. additional virgin olive oil

50g red onion, finely hacked

30g carrot, stripped and finely chopped

30g celery, cut and finely hacked

1 garlic clove, finely hacked

½ 10,000 foot bean stew, finely slashed (discretionary)

1 tsp herbs de Provence

200ml vegetable stock

1 x 400g tin hacked Italian tomatoes

1 tsp tomato purée

200g tinned blended beans

50g kale, generally hacked

1 tbsp. generally hacked parsley

40g buckwheat

Directions

Spot the oil in a medium pot over a low–medium warmth and delicately fry the onion, carrot, celery, garlic, chili (if utilizing) and herbs, until the onion is delicate yet not shaded.

Include the stock, tomatoes and tomato purée and bring to the bubble. Include the beans and stew for 30 minutes.

Include the kale and cook for another 5–10 minutes, until delicate, then include the parsley. In the interim, cook the buckwheat according to the bundle Directions, deplete, and afterward present with the stew.

Nutrition:

Calories 289

Fat: 2 g

Carbohydrates: 10 g

Protein: 12 g

Fiber: 0 g

Vegetable Lover's Chicken Soup

Preparation time: 10 minutes

Cooking time: 20 minutes

Servings: 3

Ingredients:

1 ½ cups baby spinach

2 tbsp orzo (tiny pasta)

¼ cup dry white wine

1 14oz low sodium chicken broth

2 plum tomatoes, chopped

1/8 tsp salt

½ tsp Italian seasoning

1 large shallot, chopped

1 small zucchini, diced

8-oz chicken tenders

1 tbsp extra virgin olive oil

Directions:

In a large saucepan, heat oil over medium heat and add the chicken. Stir occasionally for 8 minutes until browned. Transfer in a plate. Set aside.

In the same saucepan, add the zucchini, Italian seasoning, shallot and salt and stir often until the vegetables are softened, around 4 minutes.

Add the tomatoes, wine, broth and orzo and increase the heat to high to bring the mixture to boil. Reduce the heat and simmer.

Add the cooked chicken and stir in the spinach last.

Serve hot.

Nutrition: Calories per Serving: 207; Carbs: 14.8g; Protein: 12.2g; Fat: 11.4g

Lemony Lamb And Potatoes

Preparation time: 10 minutes

Cooking time: 30 minutes

Servings: 3

Ingredients:

2 pound lamb meat, cubed

2 tablespoons olive oil

2 springs rosemary, chopped

2 tablespoons parsley, chopped

1 tablespoon lemon rind, grated

3 garlic cloves, minced

2 tablespoons lemon juice

2 pounds baby potatoes, scrubbed and halved

1 cup veggie stock

Directions:

In a roasting pan, combine the meat with the oil and the rest of the ingredients, introduce in the oven and bake at 400 degrees F for 2 hours and 10 minutes.

Divide the mix between plates and serve.

Nutrition: calories 302, fat 15.2, fiber 10.6, carbs 23.3, protein 15.2

Cumin Lamb Mix

Preparation time: 10 minutes

Cooking time: 30 minutes

Servings: 3

Ingredients:

2 lamb chops (3.5 oz each)

1 tablespoon olive oil

1 teaspoon ground cumin

½ teaspoon salt

Directions:

Rub the lamb chops with ground cumin and salt.

Then sprinkle them with olive oil.

Let the meat marinate for 10 minutes.

After this, preheat the skillet well.

Place the lamb chops in the skillet and roast them for 10 minutes. Flip the meat on another side from time to time to avoid burning.

Nutrition: :calories 384, fat 33.2, fiber 0.1, carbs 0.5, protein 19.2

Almond Lamb Chops

Preparation time: 10 minutes

Cooking time: 20 minutes

Servings: 3

Ingredients:

1 teaspoon almond butter

2 teaspoons minced garlic

1 teaspoon butter, softened

½ teaspoon salt

½ teaspoon chili flakes

½ teaspoon ground paprika

12 oz lamb chop

Directions:

Churn together minced garlic, butter, salt, chili flakes, and ground paprika.

Carefully rub every lamb chop with the garlic mixture.

Toss almond butter in the skillet and melt it.

Place the lamb chops in the melted almond butter and roast them for 20 minutes (for 10 minutes from each side) over the medium-low heat.

Nutrition: :calories 194, fat 9.5, fiber 0.5, carbs 1.4, protein 24.9

Pork And Figs Mix

Preparation time: 10 minutes

Cooking time: 30 minutes

Servings: 3

Ingredients:

3 tablespoons avocado oil

1 and ½ pounds pork stew meat, roughly cubed

Salt and black pepper to the taste

1 cup red onions, chopped

1 cup figs, dried and chopped

1 tablespoon ginger, grated

1 tablespoon garlic, minced

1 cup canned tomatoes, crushed

2 tablespoons parsley, chopped

Directions:

Heat up a pot with the oil over medium-high heat, add the meat and brown for 5 minutes.

Add the onions and sauté for 5 minutes more.

Add the rest of the ingredients, bring to a simmer and cook over medium heat for 30 minutes more.

Divide the mix between plates and serve.

Nutrition: calories 309, fat 16, fiber 10.4, carbs 21.1, protein 34.2

Lamb Chops

Preparation time: 10 minutes

Cooking time: 6 minutes

Servings: 3

Ingredients:

6 (3/4-in.-thick) lamb chops

2 TB. fresh rosemary, finely chopped

3 TB. minced garlic

1 tsp. salt

1 tsp. ground black pepper

3 TB. extra-virgin olive oil

Directions:

In a large bowl, combine lamb chops, rosemary, garlic, salt, black pepper, and extra-virgin olive oil until chops are evenly coated. Let chops marinate at room temperature for at least 25 minutes.

Preheat a grill to medium heat.

Place chops on the grill, and cook for 3 minutes per side for medium well.

Serve warm.

Chicken Quinoa Pilaf

Preparation time: 10 minutes

Cooking time: 30 minutes

Servings: 3

Ingredients:

2 (8-oz.) boneless, skinless chicken breasts, cut into 1/2-in. cubes

3 TB. extra-virgin olive oil

1 medium red onion, finely chopped

1 TB. minced garlic

1 (16-oz.) can diced tomatoes, with juice

2 cups water

2 tsp. salt

1 TB. dried oregano

1 TB. turmeric

1 tsp. paprika

1 tsp. ground black pepper

2 cups red or yellow quinoa

1/2 cup fresh parsley, chopped

Directions:

In a large, 3-quart pot over medium heat, heat extra-virgin olive oil. Add chicken, and cook for 5 minutes.

Add red onion and garlic, stir, and cook for 5 minutes.

Add tomatoes with juice, water, salt, oregano, turmeric, paprika, and black pepper. Stir, and simmer for 5 minutes.

Add red quinoa, and stir. Cover, reduce heat to low, and cook for 20 minutes. Remove from heat.

Fluff with a fork, cover again, and let sit for 10 minutes.

Serve warm.

Greek Styled Lamb Chops

Preparation time: 10 minutes

Cooking time: 4 minutes

Servings: 3

Ingredients:

¼ tsp black pepper

½ tsp salt

1 tbsp bottled minced garlic

1 tbsp dried oregano

2 tbsp lemon juice

8 pcs of lamb loin chops, around 4 oz

Cooking spray

Directions:

Preheat broiler.

In a big bowl or dish, combine the black pepper, salt, minced garlic, lemon juice and oregano. Then rub it equally on all sides of the lamb chops.

Then coat a broiler pan with the cooking spray before placing the lamb chops on the pan and broiling until desired doneness is reached or for four minutes.

Nutrition: Calories per Serving: 131.9; Carbs: 2.6g; Protein: 17.1g; Fat: 5.9g

Bulgur And Chicken Skillet

Preparation time: 10 minutes

Cooking time: 40 minutes

Servings: 3

Ingredients:

4 (6-oz.) skinless, boneless chicken breasts

1 tablespoon olive oil, divided

1 cup thinly sliced red onion

1 tablespoon thinly sliced garlic

1 cup unsalted chicken stock

1 tablespoon coarsely chopped fresh dill

1/2 teaspoon freshly ground black pepper, divided

1/2 cup uncooked bulgur

2 teaspoons chopped fresh or 1/2 tsp. dried oregano

4 cups chopped fresh kale (about 2 1/2 oz.)

1/2 cup thinly sliced bottled roasted red bell peppers

2 ounces feta cheese, crumbled (about 1/2 cup)

3/4 teaspoon kosher salt, divided

Directions:

Place a cast iron skillet on medium high fire and heat for 5 minutes. Add oil and heat for 2 minutes.

Season chicken with pepper and salt to taste.

Brown chicken for 4 minutes per side and transfer to a plate.

In same skillet, sauté garlic and onion for 3 minutes. Stir in oregano and bulgur and toast for 2 minutes.

Stir in kale and bell pepper, cook for 2 minutes. Pour in stock and season well with pepper and salt.

Return chicken to skillet and turn off fire. Pop in a preheated 400oF oven and bake for 15 minutes.

Remove form oven, fluff bulgur and turn over chicken. Let it stand for 5 minutes.

Serve and enjoy with a sprinkle of feta cheese.

Nutrition: Calories per Serving: 369; Carbs: 21.0g; Protein: 45.0g; Fats: 11.3g

Kibbeh With Yogurt

Preparation time: 10 minutes

Cooking time: 30 minutes

Servings: 3

Ingredients:

1/2 cup bulgur wheat, grind #1

4 cups water

1 large yellow onion, chopped

2 fresh basil leaves

1 lb. lean ground chuck beef

2 tsp. salt

1 tsp. ground black pepper

1/2 tsp. ground allspice

1/2 tsp. ground coriander

1/2 tsp. ground cumin

1/2 tsp. ground nutmeg

1/2 tsp. ground cloves

1/2 tsp. ground cinnamon

1/2 tsp. dried sage

1/4 cup long-grain rice

1/2 lb. ground beef

3 TB. extra-virgin olive oil

1/2 cup pine nuts

1 tsp. seven spices

4 cups Greek yogurt

2 TB. minced garlic

1 tsp. dried mint

Directions:

In a small bowl, soak bulgur wheat in 1 cup water for 30 minutes.

In a food processor fitted with a chopping blade, blend 1/2 of yellow onion and basil for 30 seconds. Add bulgur, and blend for 30 more seconds.

Add ground chuck, 11/2 teaspoons salt, black pepper, allspice, coriander, cumin, nutmeg, cloves, cinnamon, and sage, and blend for 1 minute.

Transfer mixture to a large bowl, and knead for 3 minutes.

In a large pot, combine long-grain rice and remaining 3 cups water, and cook for 30 minutes.

In a medium skillet over medium heat, brown beef for 5 minutes, breaking up chunks with a wooden spoon.

Add remaining 1/2 of yellow onion, extra-virgin olive oil, remaining 1/2 teaspoon salt, pine nuts, and seven spices, and cook for 7 minutes. Set aside to cool.

Whisk Greek yogurt into cooked rice, add garlic and mint, reduce heat to low, and cook for 5 minutes.

Form meat-bulgur mixture into 12 equal-size balls. Create a groove in center of each ball, fill with beef and onion mixture, and seal groove.

Carefully drop balls into yogurt sauce, and cook for 15 minutes. Serve warm.

Nutrition: Calories 476, Fat 40, Fiber 9, Carbs 33, Protein 6

Mustard Chops With Apricot-basil Relish

Preparation time: 10 minutes

Cooking time: 30 minutes

Servings: 3

Ingredients:

¼ cup basil, finely shredded

¼ cup olive oil

½ cup mustard

¾ lb. fresh apricots, stone removed, and fruit diced

1 shallot, diced small

1 tsp ground cardamom

3 tbsp raspberry vinegar

4 pork chops

Pepper and salt

Directions:

Make sure that pork chops are defrosted well. Season with pepper and salt. Slather both sides of each pork chop with mustard. Preheat grill to medium-high fire.

In a medium bowl, mix cardamom, olive oil, vinegar, basil, shallot, and apricots. Toss to combine and season with pepper and salt, mixing once again.

Grill chops for 5 to 6 minutes per side. As you flip, baste with mustard.

Serve pork chops with the Apricot-Basil relish and enjoy.

Nutrition: Calories per Serving: 486.5; Carbs: 7.3g; Protein: 42.1g; Fat: 32.1g

Pork And Peas

Preparation time: 10 minutes

Cooking time: 30 minutes

Servings: 3

Ingredients:

4 ounces snow peas

2 tablespoons avocado oil

1 pound pork loin, boneless and cubed

¾ cup beef stock

½ cup red onion, chopped

Salt and white pepper to the taste

Directions:

Heat up a pan with the oil over medium-high heat, add the pork and brown for 5 minutes.

Add the peas and the rest of the ingredients, toss, bring to a simmer and cook over medium heat for 15 minutes.

Divide the mix between plates and serve right away.

Nutrition: calories 332, fat 16.5, fiber 10.3, carbs 20.7, protein 26.5

Paprika And Feta Cheese On Chicken Skillet

Preparation time: 10 minutes

Cooking time: 30 minutes

Servings: 3

Ingredients:

¼ cup black olives, sliced in circles

½ teaspoon coriander

½ teaspoon paprika

1 ½ cups diced tomatoes with the juice

1 cup yellow onion, chopped

1 teaspoon onion powder

2 garlic cloves, peeled and minced

2 lb. free range organic boneless skinless chicken breasts

2 tablespoons feta cheese

2 tablespoons ghee or olive oil

Crushed red pepper to taste

Salt and black pepper to taste

Directions:

Preheat oven to 400oF.

Place a cast-iron pan on medium high fire and heat for 5 minutes. Add oil and heat for 2 minutes more.

Meanwhile in a large dish, mix well pepper, salt, crushed red pepper, paprika, coriander, and onion powder. Add chicken and coat well in seasoning.

Add chicken to pan and brown sides for 4 minutes per side. Increase fire to high.

Stir in garlic and onions. Lower fire to medium and mix well.

Pop pan in oven and bake for 15 minutes.

Remove from oven, turnover chicken and let it stand for 5 minutes before serving.

Nutrition: Calories per Serving: 232; Carbs: 5.0g; Protein: 33.0g; Fats: 8.0g

Jalapeno Beef Chili

Preparation time: 10 minutes

Cooking time: 30 minutes

Servings: 3

Ingredients:

1 lb ground beef

1 tsp garlic powder

1 jalapeno pepper, chopped

1 tbsp ground cumin

1 tbsp chili powder

1 lb ground pork

4 tomatillos, chopped

1/2 onion, chopped

5 oz tomato paste

Pepper

Salt

Directions:

Add oil into the instant pot and set the pot on sauté mode.

Add beef and pork and cook until brown.

Add remaining ingredients and stir well.

Seal pot with lid and cook on high for 35 minutes.

Once done, allow to release pressure naturally. Remove lid.

Stir well and serve.

Nutrition: Calories 217 Fat 6.1 g Carbohydrates 6.2 g Sugar 2.7 g Protein 33.4 g Cholesterol 92 mg

Kibbeh In A Pan

Preparation time: 10 minutes

Cooking time: 30 minutes

Servings: 3

Ingredients:

1/2 cup bulgur wheat, grind #1

1 cup water

1 large yellow onion, chopped

2 fresh basil leaves

1 lb. lean ground chuck beef

2 tsp. salt

1 tsp. ground black pepper

1/2 tsp. ground allspice

1/2 tsp. ground coriander

1/2 tsp. ground cumin

1/2 tsp. ground nutmeg

1/2 tsp. ground cloves

1/2 tsp. ground cinnamon

1/2 tsp. dried sage

1/2 lb. ground beef

4 TB. extra-virgin olive oil

1/2 cup pine nuts

1 tsp. seven spices

Directions:

In a small bowl, soak bulgur wheat in water for 30 minutes.

In a food processor fitted with a chopping blade, blend 1/2 of yellow onion and basil for 30 seconds. Add bulgur, and blend for 30 more seconds.

Add ground chuck, 11/2 teaspoons salt, black pepper, allspice, coriander, cumin, nutmeg, cloves, cinnamon, and sage, and blend for 1 minute.

Transfer mixture to a large bowl, and knead for 3 minutes.

In a medium skillet over medium heat, brown beef for 5 minutes, breaking up chunks with a wooden spoon.

Add remaining 1/2 of yellow onion, 2 tablespoons extra-virgin olive oil, remaining 1/2 teaspoon salt, pine nuts, and seven spices, and cook for 7 minutes.

Preheat the oven to 450ºF. Grease an 8×8-inch baking dish with extra-virgin olive oil.

Divide kibbeh dough in half, spread a layer of dough on bottom of the preparation ared baking dish, add a layer of sautéed vegetables, and top with remaining kibbeh dough.

Paint top of kibbeh with remaining 2 tablespoons extra-virgin olive oil, and cut kibbeh into 12 equal-size pieces. Bake for 25 minutes.

Let kibbeh rest for 15 minutes before serving.

Nutrition: Calories 476, Fat 40, Fiber 9, Carbs 33, Protein 6

Saffron Beef

Preparation time: 10 minutes

Cooking time: 15 minutes

Servings: 3

Ingredients:

¾ teaspoon saffron

¾ teaspoon dried thyme

¾ teaspoon ground coriander

¼ teaspoon ground cinnamon

1 tablespoon butter

1/3 teaspoon salt

9 oz beef sirloin

Directions:

Rub the beef sirloin with dried thyme, ground coriander, saffron, ground cinnamon, and salt.

Leave the meat for at least 10 minutes to soak all the spices.

Then preheat the grill to 395F.

Place the beef sirloin in the grill and cook it for 5 minutes.

Then spread the meat with butter carefully and cook for 10 minutes more. Flip it on another side from time to time.

Nutrition: :calories 291, fat 13.8, fiber 0.3, carbs 0.6, protein 38.8

Cayenne Pork

Preparation time: 10 minutes

Cooking time: 30 minutes

Servings: 3

Ingredients:

8 oz beef sirloin

1 poblano pepper, grinded

1 teaspoon minced garlic

½ cup of water

1 tablespoon butter

1 teaspoon ground black pepper

1 teaspoon salt

½ teaspoon paprika

1 teaspoon cayenne pepper

Directions:

Toss the butter in the saucepan and melt it.

Meanwhile rub the beef sirloin with minced garlic, salt, ground black pepper, paprika, and cayenne pepper.

Put the meat in the hot butter and roast for 5 minutes from each side over the medium heat.

After this, add water and poblano pepper.

Cook the meat for 50 minutes over the medium heat.

Then transfer the beef sirloin on the cutting board and shred it with the help of the fork.

Nutrition: :calories 97, fat 5.5, fiber 0.5, carbs 3, protein 9.5

Basil And Shrimp Quinoa

Preparation time: 10 minutes

Cooking time: 20 minutes

Servings: 3

Ingredients:

3 TB. extra-virgin olive oil

2 TB. minced garlic

1 cup fresh broccoli florets

3 stalks asparagus, chopped (1 cup)

4 cups chicken or vegetable broth

1 1/2 tsp. salt

1 tsp. ground black pepper

1 TB. lemon zest

2 cups red quinoa

1/2 cup fresh basil, chopped

Directions:

1/2 lb. medium raw shrimp (18 to 20), shells and veins removed

In a 2-quart pot over low heat, heat extra-virgin olive oil. Add garlic, and cook for 3 minutes.

Increase heat to medium, add broccoli and asparagus, and cook for 2 minutes.

Add chicken broth, salt, black pepper, and lemon zest, and bring to a boil. Stir in red quinoa, cover, and cook for 15 minutes.

Fold in basil and shrimp, cover, and cook for 10 minutes.

Remove from heat, fluff with a fork, cover, and set aside for 10 minutes. Serve warm.

Nutrition: Calories 476, Fat 40, Fiber 9, Carbs 33, Protein 6

Kefta Burgers

Preparation time: 10 minutes

Cooking time: 10 minutes

Servings: 3

Ingredients:

1 lb. ground beef

1 cup fresh parsley, finely chopped

1 tsp. seven spices

1 1/2 tsp. salt

1 large yellow onion, finely sliced

1 TB. sumac

1/2 cup mayonnaise

3 TB. tahini paste

2 TB. balsamic vinegar

1/2 tsp. ground black pepper

4 (4-in.) pitas

1 medium tomato, sliced

Directions:

In a large bowl, combine beef, 1/2 cup parsley, seven spices, 1 teaspoon salt. Form mixture into 4 patties.

In a medium bowl, combine remaining 1/2 cup parsley, yellow onion, and sumac.

In a small bowl, whisk together mayonnaise, tahini paste, remaining 1/2 teaspoon salt, balsamic vinegar, and black pepper.

Preheat a large skillet over medium-high heat. Place patties in the skillet, and cook for 5 minutes per side.

To assemble burgers, open each pita into a pocket, and spread both sides with tahini mayonnaise. Add 1 burger patty, some parsley mixture, and a few tomato slices, and serve.

Nutrition: Calories 476, Fat 40, Fiber 9, Carbs 33, Protein 6

Beef Dish

Preparation time: 10 minutes

Cooking time: 20 minutes

Servings: 3

Ingredients:

1 lb. skirt steak

2 TB. minced garlic

1/4 cup fresh lemon juice

2 TB. apple cider vinegar

3 TB. extra-virgin olive oil

1 tsp. salt

1/2 tsp. ground black pepper

1/4 tsp. ground cinnamon

1/4 tsp. ground cardamom

1 tsp. seven spices

Directions:

Using a sharp knife, cut skirt steak into thin, 1/4-inch strips. Place strips in a large bowl.

Add garlic, lemon juice, apple cider vinegar, extra-virgin olive oil, salt, black pepper, cinnamon, cardamom, and seven spices, and mix well.

Place steak in the refrigerator and marinate for at least 20 minutes and up to 24 hours.

Preheat a large skillet over medium heat. Add meat and marinade, and cook for 20 minutes or until meat is tender and marinade has evaporated.

Serve warm with pita bread and tahini sauce.

Nutrition: Calories 476, Fat 40, Fiber 9, Carbs 33, Protein 6

Tasty Beef Stew

Preparation time: 10 minutes

Cooking time: 30 minutes

Servings: 3

Ingredients:

2 1/2 lbs beef roast, cut into chunks

1 cup beef broth

1/2 cup balsamic vinegar

1 tbsp honey

1/2 tsp red pepper flakes

1 tbsp garlic, minced

Pepper

Salt

Directions:

Add all ingredients into the inner pot of instant pot and stir well.

Seal pot with lid and cook on high for 30 minutes.

Once done, allow to release pressure naturally. Remove lid.

Stir well and serve.

Nutrition: Calories 562 Fat 18.1 g Carbohydrates 5.7 g Sugar 4.6 g Protein 87.4 g Cholesterol 253 mg

Pork And Sage Couscous

Preparation time: 10 minutes

Cooking time: 8 Hours

Servings: 3

Ingredients:

2 pounds pork loin boneless and sliced

¾ cup veggie stock

2 tablespoons olive oil

½ tablespoon chili powder

2 teaspoon sage, dried

½ tablespoon garlic powder

Salt and black pepper to the taste

2 cups couscous, cooked

Directions:

In a slow cooker, combine the pork with the stock, the oil and the other ingredients except the couscous, put the lid on and cook on Low for 7 hours.

Divide the mix between plates, add the couscous on the side, sprinkle the sage on top and serve.

Nutrition: calories 272, fat 14.5, fiber 9.1, carbs 16.3, protein 14.3

Chicken Burgers With Brussel Sprouts Slaw

Preparation 10 minutes

Cooking time: 15 minutes

Servings: 3

Ingredients:

¼ cup apple, diced

¼ cup green onion, diced

½ avocado, cubed

½ pound Brussels sprouts, shredded

1 garlic clove, minced

1 tablespoon Dijon mustard

1/3 cup apple, sliced into strips

1/8 teaspoon red pepper flakes, optional

1-pound cooked ground chicken

3 slices bacon, cooked and diced

Salt and pepper to taste

Directions:

In a mixing bowl, combine together chicken, green onion, Dijon mustard, garlic, apple, bacon and pepper flakes. Season with salt and pepper to taste. Mix the ingredients then form 4 burger patties.

Heat a grill pan over medium-high flame and grill the burgers. Cook for five minutes on side. Set aside.

In another bowl, toss the Brussels sprouts and apples.

In a small pan, heat coconut oil and add the Brussels sprouts mixture until everything is slightly wilted. Season with salt and pepper to taste.

Serve burger patties with the Brussels sprouts slaw.

Nutrition: Calories per Serving: 325.1; Carbs: 11.5g; Protein: 32.2g; Fat: 16.7g

Sautéed Cabbage

Preparation time: 10 minutes

Cooking time: 30 minutes

Servings: 3

Ingredients:

1/2 head red cabbage, chopped

3 tablespoons olive oil

1 small red bell pepper, chopped

1 small yellow bell pepper, chopped

1/2 onion, chopped

low sodium salt and ground black pepper to taste

Directions:

Set your oil on high heat in a skillet to get hot.

Stir in your bell peppers, cabbage, and onion. Cook, pausing to stir every 30 seconds until tender (about 7 minutes).

Season to taste. Enjoy!

Nutrition: Calories 476, Fat 40, Fiber 9, Carbs 33, Protein 6

Sautéed Cauliflower Delight

Preparation time: 10 minutes

Cooking time: 30 minutes

Servings: 3

Ingredients:

1 head cauliflower, cut into florets

1/4 teaspoon red pepper flakes

1/4 cup olive oil

1 cup cherry tomatoes, halved, or more to taste

1 red onion, chopped

1 teaspoon natural sweetener as per your taste (raw honey or maple syrup are good options)

2 tablespoons raisins

1 clove garlic, minced

1 teaspoon dried parsley

1 tablespoon fresh lemon juice, or to taste (optional)

Directions:

Set your oil on medium heat to get hot.

Cook and stir onion until tender (5 to 10 minutes).

Add raisins, cauliflower, sweetener and cherry tomatoes; cover and cook until tender (about 5 minutes), stirring occasionally.

Add in your red pepper flakes, parsley and garlic. Switch to high heat and sauté until cauliflower is browned (about 2 minutes).

Drizzle lemon juice over cauliflower.

Nutrition: Calories 476, Fat 40, Fiber 9, Carbs 33, Protein 6

Simple Sautéed Spinach

Preparation time: 10 minutes

Cooking time: 30 minutes

Servings: 3

Ingredients:

1/4 teaspoon crushed red pepper

4 cloves garlic, thinly sliced

2 tablespoons extra-virgin olive oil

20 ounces fresh spinach

1/4 teaspoon low sodium salt

1 tablespoon lemon juice

Directions:

Set your oil to get hot on medium heat in a Dutch oven.

Add in your garlic then cook until lightly brown (about 1minutes).

Stir in your spinach to coat. Cover then cook until the spinach wilts1 (about 5 minutes).

Remove from the heat and add in salt, crushed red pepper and lemon juice.

Toss and serve immediately.

Chapter 8: Drinks Recipes and Smoothie Recipes

Clean Liver Green Juice

Preparation time: 10 minutes

Cooking time: 0 minutes

Servings: 2

Ingredients

2½ C. fresh spinach

2 large celery stalks

2 large green apples, cored and sliced

1 medium orange, peeled, seeded and sectioned

1 tbsp. fresh lime juice

1 tbsp. fresh lemon juice

Directions

In a juicer, add all ingredients and extract the juice according to manufacturer's directions.

Transfer into 2 serving glasses and stir in lime and lemon juices.

Serve immediately.

Nutrition: Calories 476, Fat 40, Fiber 9, Carbs 33, Protein 6

Green Tea Purifying Smoothie

Preparation time: 10 minutes

Cooking time: 0 minutes

Servings: 2

Ingredients

2 C. fresh baby spinach

3 C. frozen green grapes

1 medium ripe avocado peeled, pitted and chopped

2 tsp. organic honey

1½ C. strong brewed green tea

Directions

a high-speed blender, add all ingredients and pulse until smooth.

Transfer into serving glasses and serve immediately.

Nutrition: Calories 476, Fat 40, Fiber 9, Carbs 33, Protein 6

PP cleansing smoothie

Preparation time: 10 minutes

Cooking time: 0 minutes

Servings: 2

Ingredients:

1 cup water

½ cup papaya chunks

¼ cup organic pineapple chunks

1 teaspoon anti parasitic coconut oil

1 teaspoon raw pumpkin seeds

A pinch of garlic paste

Directions:

Mix all the ingredients in a blender and blend well till mixed well, add ice if needed and you can also add more water if consistency is thick to drink easily.

Nutrition: Calories 476, Fat 40, Fiber 9, Carbs 33, Protein 6

Blue Breeze shake

Preparation time: 10 minutes

Cooking time: 0 minutes

Servings: 2

Ingredients:

½ cup blueberries

1 small banana

1 cup chilled unsweetened vanilla almond milk

Water as needed

1 scoop unflavored protein powder

Directions:

Mix in a blender for 40-50 seconds and serve as ready.

Nutrition: Calories 476, Fat 40, Fiber 9, Carbs 33, Protein 6

Coconut breezy shake dose

This shake is a dose of 20 grams of protein with refreshing and sweet natural coconut.

Ingredients:

1 cup skimmed milk (chilled)

1 cup pineapple chunks

4 tablespoons shredded coconut

Water as needed

½ scoop of vanilla protein powder

Directions:
 Mix all the ingredients in a mixer and shake well for 20 seconds, serve when smooth texture is seen. Pour in a large glass, use water to make proper smoothness only.

Nutrition: Calories 476, Fat 40, Fiber 9, Carbs 33, Protein 6

Triple C shake

Preparation time: 10 minutes

Cooking time: 0 minutes

Servings: 2

Ingredients:

¼ cup raw spinach

1 tablespoon cacao nibs

1 cup skimmed chocolate nut milk

¾ cup black or blue berries

A dash of red pepper flakes

A scoop of chocolate whey powder

Water as needed

6 crushed ice cubes

A handful of nuts

A pinch of cinnamon powder

Directions:

Put all the ingredients in a blender and shake well till smooth. Serve chilled in a large glass and enjoy.

Nutrition: Calories 476, Fat 40, Fiber 9, Carbs 33, Protein 6

Buttery banana shake

Preparation time: 10 minutes

Cooking time: 0 minutes

Servings: 2

Ingredients:

1 tablespoon raw peanut butter

1 cup almond milk

1 scoop protein powder any flavor

¼ cup greek yogurt

1 teaspoon basil

1 teaspoon ginger paste

1 teaspoon vanilla extract

1 teaspoon sesame seeds

Directions:

Mix and blend all ingredients in a blender and shake for a whole minute to drink a smooth shake in the morning or evening during workouts.

Nutrition: Calories 170, Fat 3, Fiber 6, Carbs 8, Protein 5

Fats burning & water based smoothies

. Preparation time: 10 minutes

Cooking time: 0 minutes

Servings: 2

Ingredients:

¾ cup water

Ice as needed

4 big strawberries

1 small piece of banana or an apple slice with peel

¼ teaspoon of cinnamon powder

1 teaspoon honey

Directions:

Take a blender and add water, remove stems from the berries and add in the blender, put cinnamon powder, honey, crushed ice cubes and remaining fruit. Mix and serve.

Nutrition: Calories 170, Fat 3, Fiber 6, Carbs 8, Protein 5

Grapefruit smoothie with cinnamon

Preparation time: 10 minutes

Cooking time: 0 minutes

Servings: 2

Ingredients:

1 cup grapefruit juice, use pulp for fiber (optional)

Ice cubes in crushed form as needed (2-3)

1 cinnamon stick

1 sliced banana

1 teaspoon brown sugar

Directions:

Mix all ingredients in a blender and mix for 30 seconds to blend well, when done, serve.

Nutrition: Calories 170, Fat 3, Fiber 6, Carbs 8, Protein 5

BB Citric Blast smoothie

Preparation time: 10 minutes

Cooking time: 0 minutes

Servings: 2

Ingredients:

½ cup strawberries without stems and raspberries mixed

1 cup chilled fresh orange juice

1 teaspoon honey

A pinch of lemon zest

Directions:

Take a mixer and add all the ingredients, fruits and juice in it to mix for few seconds and serve chilled.

Nutrition: Calories 170, Fat 3, Fiber 6, Carbs 8, Protein 5

Lemon and garlic smoothie

Preparation time: 10 minutes

Cooking time: 0 minutes

Servings: 2

Ingredients:

1 lemon juice

1 small clove of fresh garlic

1 glass water

Few mint leaves

1 teaspoon brown sugar

Directions:

Chop, slice or crush garlic clove and add in an electric mixer with water, lemon juice, sugar and mint leaves to blend and serve immediately. It is better to serve warm.

Nutrition: Calories 170, Fat 3, Fiber 6, Carbs 8, Protein 5

Smoothie with ginger and cucumber

Preparation time: 10 minutes

Cooking time: 0 minutes

Servings: 2

Ingredients:

1 cup chilled water

2 slices of cucumber

1 tablespoon lime juice

Couple of mint leaves

1 small piece of ginger fresh

Directions:

Add chilled cup of water in an electric mixer, grate ginger piece. Mix with cucumber slices, lime juice and mint leaves to serve.

Nutrition: Calories 170, Fat 3, Fiber 6, Carbs 8, Protein 5

Oatmeal blast with fruit

Preparation time: 10 minutes

Cooking time: 0 minutes

Servings: 2

Ingredients:

½ cup oats (steel cut)

A pinch of ground cinnamon

Ice cubes as needed

1 cup water

½ cup pineapple chunks

Directions:

Throw oats in a blender and slightly blend with water, add the fruit and other ingredients afterwards and blend again.

Nutrition: Calories 150, Fat 3, Fiber 2, Carbs 6, Protein 8

White bean smoothie to burn fats

Preparation time: 10 minutes

Cooking time: 0 minutes

Servings: 2

Ingredients:

1 cup unsweetened rice milk (chilled)

¼ cup peach slices

¼ cup white beans cooked

A pinch of cinnamon powder

A pinch of nutmeg

Directions:

Pour milk in the blender and add other ingredients to blend till smooth enough to serve and drink.

Nutrition: Calories 150, Fat 3, Fiber 2, Carbs 6, Protein 8

Meal replacement smoothie with banana

Preparation time: 10 minutes

Cooking time: 0 minutes

Servings: 2

Ingredients:

1 large banana (ripped or green)

1 cup coconut milk

A drop of vanilla extract

1 tablespoon of natural peanut powder

1 teaspoon carob powder

Ice as needed

4 small fresh berries without stems

Preparation

Mix all foods and condiments in milk and shake them all well in an electric machine.

Nutrition: Calories 150, Fat 3, Fiber 2, Carbs 6, Protein 8

Coconut cherry smoothie

Preparation time: 10 minutes

Cooking time: 0 minutes

Servings: 2

Ingredients:

1 cup nondairy coconut milk

4 Ice cubes as needed

1 cup mixed berries (blueberries, blackberries and cherries)

½ plantains

A handful of mixed chopped fruits- pear/peach/guava

2 tablespoons plain soy yogurt

Directions:

Toss in the berries, milk and other ingredients in a blender, shake well to make a smooth drink.

Nutrition: Calories 150, Fat 3, Fiber 2, Carbs 6, Protein 8

Grapes and peach smoothie

Preparation time: 10 minutes

Cooking time: 0 minutes

Servings: 2

Ingredients:

1 cup red grapes juice

3 tablespoon shredded coconut

½ scoop protein powder

A handful of chopped pistachios

1 small guava and peach chopped

Ice as required

Directions:

Use natural juice to add in the smoothie, mix all the foods in a blender and shake to make it a smooth drink.

Nutrition: Calories 150, Fat 3, Fiber 2, Carbs 6, Protein 8

Twin berry smoothie

Preparation time: 10 minutes

Cooking time: 0 minutes

Servings: 2

Ingredients:

½ cup peach chunks

¾ cup almond milk

A handful of cranberries and raspberries

Peel of an orange

1 scoop protein powder (whey)

Ice cubes as required

Directions:

Chop berries well, use natural orange peel, add all foods in a blender and shake to serve.

Nutrition: Calories 150, Fat 3, Fiber 2, Carbs 6, Protein 8

Light fiber smoothie

Preparation time: 10 minutes

Cooking time: 0 minutes

Servings: 2

Ingredients:

2 teaspoons nutmeg

1 ½ scoop vanilla protein powder mix

1½ cup soy milk

½ cup low fat egg nog

A pinch of cinnamon

4-5 crushed ice cubes

1 lemon zest

Directions:

Grab the ingredients, measure and add them all in a blender to mix for a drink.

Nutrition: Calories 150, Fat 3, Fiber 2, Carbs 6, Protein 8

Creamy milk smoothie as meal replacement

Preparation time: 10 minutes

Cooking time: 0 minutes

Servings: 2

Ingredients:

½ teaspoon cinnamon powder

½ teaspoon ground ginger

1 cup almond milk

¼ cup plain soy yogurt

1 tablespoon whey protein vanilla

Spearmint to toss in

Directions:

Shake this creamy smoothie with a blending machine and pour in a glass to drink.

Nutrition: Calories 191, Fat 10, Fiber 3, Carbs 13, Protein 1

Melon and nuts smoothie

Preparation time: 10 minutes

Cooking time: 0 minutes

Servings: 2

Ingredients:

1 cup water melon chunks

¼ cup mixed nuts

1 cup soy milk

½ cup tofu

Chilled water as needed

1 scoop of chocolate whey protein powder

Directions:

Blend all ingredients greatly to attain a smooth and soft drink.

Nutrition: Calories 191, Fat 10, Fiber 3, Carbs 13, Protein 1

Peach and kiwi smoothie

Preparation time: 10 minutes

Cooking time: 0 minutes

Servings: 2

Ingredients:

1 cup plain low fat yogurt

½ cup peach chunks

1 tablespoon protein powder

Water as needed

½ cup kiwi fruit

Directions:

Blend powder and fruits finely in liquid, serve chilled when smooth.

Carrot drink

Preparation time: 10 minutes

Cooking time: 0 minutes

Servings: 2

Ingredients

2 cups carrots

1 cup apple

½ tsp brown sugar

Directions

In a blender place all ingredients and blend until smooth

Pour smoothie in a glass and serve

Nutrition: Calories 140, Fat 4, Fiber 2, Carbs 7, Protein 8

Watermelon drink

Preparation time: 10 minutes

Cooking time: 0 minutes

Servings: 2

Ingredients

2 cups watermelon

¼ cup tomatoes

¼ cup apples

¼ cup pears

Directions

In a blender place all ingredients and blend until smooth

Pour smoothie in a glass and serve

Nutrition: Calories 140, Fat 4, Fiber 2, Carbs 7, Protein 8

Muskmelon juice

Preparation time: 10 minutes

Cooking time: 0 minutes

Servings: 2

Ingredients

2 cups muskmelon

2 cups pineapple

1 cup ice

Directions

In a blender place all ingredients and blend until smooth

Pour smoothie in a glass and serve

Nutrition: Calories 191, Fat 10, Fiber 3, Carbs 13, Protein 1

Beetroot & parsley smoothie

Preparation time: 10 minutes

Cooking time: 0 minutes

Servings: 2

Ingredients

1 cup carrot

1 cup beetroot

1 tablespoon parsley

1 tablespoon celery

1 cup ice

Directions

In a blender place all ingredients and blend until smooth

Pour smoothie in a glass and serve

Nutrition: Calories 100, Fat 1, Fiber 2, Carbs 2, Protein 6

Ginger melon juice

Preparation time: 10 minutes

Cooking time: 0 minutes

Servings: 2

Ingredients

1 cup watermelon

1-piece ginger

1 cup ice

1 cup melon

Directions

In a blender place all ingredients and blend until smooth

Pour smoothie in a glass and serve

Nutrition: Calories 69, Fat 6.5 g, Fiber 2.6 g, Carbs 10.6 g, Protein 9.4 g

Papaya juice

Preparation time: 10 minutes

Cooking time: 0 minutes

Servings: 2

Ingredients

½ cup papaya cubes

½ cup coconut

½ cup coconut water

1 cup ice

Directions

In a blender place all ingredients and blend until smooth

Pour smoothie in a glass and serve

Nutrition: Calories 191, Fat 10, Fiber 3, Carbs 13, Protein 1

Red capsicum juice

Preparation time: 10 minutes

Cooking time: 0 minutes

Servings: 2

Ingredients

1 cup red capsicum

1 cup carrot

1 cup apple

1 cup ice

Directions

In a blender place all ingredients and blend until smooth

Pour smoothie in a glass and serve

Nutrition: Calories 69, Fat 6.5 g, Fiber 2.6 g, Carbs 10.6 g, Protein 9.4 g

Blueberry smoothie

Preparation time: 10 minutes

Cooking time: 0 minutes

Servings: 2

Ingredients

½ cup blueberries

1 cup milk

1 tsp honey

1 fresh mint

ice cubes

Directions

In a blender place all ingredients and blend until smooth

Pour smoothie in a glass and serve

Nutrition: Calories 69, Fat 6.5 g, Fiber 2.6 g, Carbs 10.6 g, Protein 9.4 g

Cashew boost smoothie

Preparation time: 10 minutes

Cooking time: 0 minutes

Servings: 2

Ingredients:

2/4 cup raw cashews

1 cup chilled almond milk

¼ cup mixed fruit

Directions:

Grind all ingredients mixed and serve.

Nutrition: Calories 191, Fat 10, Fiber 3, Carbs 13, Protein 1

Heavy metal cleansing smoothie

Preparation time: 10 minutes

Cooking time: 0 minutes

Servings: 2

Ingredients:

1 cup soy milk

A pinch of turmeric

A pinch of freshly crushed ginger

1 teaspoon cinnamon powder

1 tablespoon maple syrup

A big date without pit

Directions:

Take a blender and combine all ingredients to mix and serve when smooth. Serve at room temperature or slightly warm as you like.

Nutrition: Calories 69, Fat 6.5 g, Fiber 2.6 g, Carbs 10.6 g, Protein 9.4 g

Power detox smoothie

Preparation time: 10 minutes

Cooking time: 0 minutes

Servings: 2

Ingredients:

1 tablespoon honey

1 cup almond milk (unsweetened)

1 teaspoon ginger paste

A pinch of flaxseeds

¼ cup cherries without pits

Ice to chill

Few drops lemon juice

Directions:

Blend milk with cherries first and then add the rest of the ingredients with ice. Serve chilled.

Nutrition: Calories 69, Fat 6.5 g, Fiber 2.6 g, Carbs 10.6 g, Protein 9.4 g

Detox action super green smoothie

Preparation time: 10 minutes

Cooking time: 0 minutes

Servings: 2

Ingredients:

1 cup chilled mango juice

¼ cup chopped flat leaf parsley

¼ cup chilled tangerine

1 Medium ribs celery

½ cup orange pulp without seeds

Directions:

Blend all the above listed ingredients in an electric blender and serve immediately. Fresh smoothie is the best to consume.

Nutrition: Calories 69, Fat 6.5 g, Fiber 2.6 g, Carbs 10.6 g, Protein 9.4 g

Kale batch detox smoothie

Preparation time: 10 minutes

Cooking time: 0 minutes

Servings: 2

Ingredients:

¼ cup kale

1 cup chilled coconut water

2 pear slices

¼ cup avocado

A handful of cilantro

Directions:

Blend all the ingredients in a blender for a minute and serve fresh.

Nutrition: Calories 191, Fat 10, Fiber 3, Carbs 13, Protein 1

Smoothie with a spirit

Preparation time: 10 minutes

Cooking time: 0 minutes

Servings: 2

Ingredients:

¼ cup greek yogurt

½ of a banana

1 teaspoon spirulina

¼ cup blueberries

½ cup chilled almond milk

¼ cup peach chunks

Directions:

Mix all the ingredients in a mixing blender and serve as soon as it becomes smooth.

Nutrition: Calories 69, Fat 6.5 g, Fiber 2.6 g, Carbs 10.6 g, Protein 9.4 g

Alkaline green bliss smoothie

Preparation time: 10 minutes

Cooking time: 0 minutes

Servings: 2

Ingredients:

¼ cup spinach

¼ pear slices

1 cup chilled water

A pinch of pumpkin seeds

Preparation

Just mix all ingredients in water and transfer in a glass to drink.

Nutrition: Calories 69, Fat 6.5 g, Fiber 2.6 g, Carbs 10.6 g, Protein 9.4 g

Soothing smoothie for stomach

Preparation time: 10 minutes

Cooking time: 0 minutes

Servings: 2

Ingredients:

1 teaspoon brown sugar

1 teaspoon lime juice

1 cup lite coconut milk

¾ cup papaya

Preparation

Pour a cup of the milk in an electric blender and mix in the lime juice, papaya and sugar then mix and serve, add ice if you want to in crushed form only 2-3 cubes.

Nutrition: Calories 191, Fat 10, Fiber 3, Carbs 13, Protein 1

Smooth root green cleansing smoothie

Preparation time: 10 minutes

Cooking time: 0 minutes

Servings: 2

Ingredients:

½ cup fresh lettuce leaves

¼ green apple chunks

A handful of cilantro

¼ lime juice

Couple of cucumber slices

1 date without pit

1 cup chilled water

Directions:

Wash apple and leaves well before use, do not peel apple just remove seeds and inedible parts, mix all the ingredients blend and serve.

Nutrition: Calories 140, Fat 4, Fiber 2, Carbs 7, Protein 8

Glory smoothie

Preparation time: 10 minutes

Cooking time: 0 minutes

Servings: 2

Ingredients:

¼ cup kale

A handful of romaine

A handful of broccoli stems

A celery stalk

1cup juice of green apple

2 big cucumber slices

½ of a lemon juice and zest both

Directions:

This smoothie is preparation ared by combining all ingredients listed above with juice and shake well to form a smooth drink to serve. Use ice or chilled juice to get drink chilled.

Nutrition: Calories 69, Fat 6.5 g, Fiber 2.6 g, Carbs 10.6 g, Protein 9.4 g

Smoothie for detoxification

Preparation time: 10 minutes

Cooking time: 0 minutes

Servings: 2

Ingredients:

1 cup unsweetened chilled coconut water

1 teaspoon cinnamon powder

¼ cup kale

A handful of blackberries

Slices of a small banana

Directions:

Chop kale and add in coconut water with berries and cinnamon powder to blend and serve when smooth.

Nutrition: Calories 69, Fat 6.5 g, Fiber 2.6 g, Carbs 10.6 g, Protein 9.4 g

Strawberry nutty smoothie

Preparation time: 10 minutes

Cooking time: 0 minutes

Servings: 2

Ingredients:

½ cup strawberries

1 cup nut milk

1 tablespoon honey

2 slices of orange

2 drops of lemon juice

½ of a banana slices

¼ cup spinach

Directions:

You can also use any skimmed milk, remove stems of strawberries and after washing all foods, chop and mix them in a blender to shake and serve in a glass.

Nutrition: Calories 69, Fat 6.5 g, Fiber 2.6 g, Carbs 10.6 g, Protein 9.4 g

Berries Almond shake

Preparation time: 10 minutes

Cooking time: 0 minutes

Servings: 2

Ingredients

½ C. frozen blackberries

½ C. frozen strawberries

½ C. frozen blueberries

3 Medjool dates, pitted and chopped

1 C. unsweetened almond milk

Directions

In a high-speed blender, add all ingredients and pulse until smooth.

Transfer into serving glasses and serve immediately.

Nutrition: Calories 140, Fat 4, Fiber 2, Carbs 7, Protein 8

Fresh Ginger Lemonade

Preparation time: 10 minutes

Cooking time: 0 minutes

Servings: 2

Ingredients

2 medium fresh rosemary sprigs

2 tbsp. fresh ginger root, peeled and grated

4 large lemon peel strips

1/3 C. organic honey

8 C. water, divided

Fresh juice of 4 lemons

Ice cubes, as required

Lemon slices, for garnishing

Directions

In a pan, add rosemary sprigs, ginger, lemon peel strips, honey and 2 c. of the water and bring to a boil.

Reduce the heat to low and simmer for about 10 minutes, stirring continuously.

Remove from the heat and keep aside to cool for about 15 minutes.

Through a strainer, strain the mixture into large pitcher, discarding the solids.

Add remaining water and lemon juice and stir to blend well.

Transfer the lemonade into glasses over ice.

Garnish with lemon slices and serve.

Nutrition: Calories 140, Fat 4, Fiber 2, Carbs 7, Protein 8

Citrus Mocktail

Preparation time: 10 minutes

Cooking time: 0 minutes

Servings: 2

Ingredients

3 lime slices

11-12 fresh mint leaves plus more for garnishing

6 oz. lime flavored seltzer water

1 tbsp. organic honey

Ice cubes, as required

Directions

In a tall glass, place lime slices and mint leaves and with a spoon, muddle for about 1 minute.

Add seltzer water, honey and ice and stir to blend well.

Garnish with mint leaves and serve.

Nutrition: Calories 69, Fat 6.5 g, Fiber 2.6 g, Carbs 10.6 g, Protein 9.4 g

Tropical Green Tea

Preparation time: 10 minutes

Cooking time: 0 minutes

Servings: 2

Ingredients

7 C. boiling water

¼ C. fresh ginger, chopped

5 green tea bags

¼ C. frozen pineapple, peeled and cubed

¼ C. frozen mango, peeled, pitted and cubed

1 orange, seeded and cut into rings

1 lemon, seeded and cut into rings

Directions

In a pan, add water and ginger and bring to a boil.

Remove from the heat and stir in the tea bags.

Cover the pan tightly and steep for about 15 minutes.

Through a strainer, strain the mixture into a large glass pitcher.

Stir in remaining ingredients and keep aside at the room temperature to cool completely.

Refrigerate to chill before serving.

Nutrition: Calories 140, Fat 4, Fiber 2, Carbs 7, Protein 8

Pumpkin Vanilla Cappuccino

Preparation time: 10 minutes

Cooking time: 0 minutes

Servings: 2

Ingredients

1 C. fresh spinach

½ C. chilled coffee

¼ C. unsweetened almond milk

¼ C. sugar-free pumpkin puree

1 scoop unsweetened vanilla protein powder

½ tsp. organic vanilla extract

¼ tsp. ground ginger

¼ tsp. ground cinnamon

1/8 tsp. ground nutmeg

4-5 drops vanilla stevia

Ice cubes, as required

Chia seeds, for sprinkling

Directions

In a blender, add all ingredients and pulse until smooth.

Transfer the cappuccino into glasses over ice.

Sprinkle with chia seeds and serve.

Nutrition: Calories 69, Fat 6.5 g, Fiber 2.6 g, Carbs 10.6 g, Protein 9.4 g

Iced Coffee

Preparation time: 10 minutes

Cooking time: 0 minutes

Servings: 2

Ingredients

6 C. water

1 C. ground coffee beans

Ice cubes, as required

Unsweetened almond milk, as required

Honey, to taste

Directions

In a large container, add water and coffee beans and stir to combine.

Keep aside, covered at room temperature for at least 8 hours to overnight.

Through a cheese cloth lined fine mesh strainer, strain the mixture into a pitcher.

Refrigerate to chill completely.

Fill serving glasses with ice cubes.

Fill each glass with coffee about 2/3 of full.

Add almond milk and honey and stir to combine.

Serve immediately.

Nutrition: Calories 69, Fat 6.5 g, Fiber 2.6 g, Carbs 10.6 g, Protein 9.4 g

Old Spice Ginger Tea

Preparation time: 10 minutes

Cooking time: 0 minutes

Servings: 2

Ingredients

8 C. water

1 (4-inch) piece fresh ginger, chopped

4 lemons, sliced

6 cardamom pods, bruised

1 cinnamon stick

1 whole star anise pod

3 tbsp. organic honey

Directions

In a pan, add water over medium-high heat and bring to a boil.

Add ginger, lemon slices and spices and stir to combine.

Reduce the heat to medium-low and simmer for about 5-10 minutes.

Through a strainer, strain the tea into a pitcher, discarding the solids.

Stir in honey and serve.

Nutrition: Calories 69, Fat 6.5 g, Fiber 2.6 g, Carbs 10.6 g, Protein 9.4 g

Pumpkin Ginger Latte

Preparation time: 10 minutes

Cooking time: 0 minutes

Servings: 2

Ingredients

6 C. water

½ of lemon, seeded and chopped roughly

1 (1-inch) piece fresh ginger, chopped

2 tbsp. maple syrup

1/8 tsp. ground turmeric

Pinch of ground cinnamon

Directions

In a pan, add all ingredients over medium-high heat and bring to a boil.

Reduce the heat to medium-low and simmer for about 10-12 minutes.

Through a strainer, strain into mug and serve hot.

Nutrition: Calories 140, Fat 4, Fiber 2, Carbs 7, Protein 8

Ginger Citrus Liver Detox Drink

Preparation Time: 10 minutes

Cooking Time: 0 minutes

Servings: 1

Ingredients

1 lemon, peeled

1-inch knob fresh ginger root, finely grated

1 orange, peeled

1 grapefruit, peeled

A pinch of cayenne pepper

Directions

Juice all the ingredients in a juicer, except cayenne pepper; stir in cayenne pepper and serve.

Nutrition:

Calories: 11;

Total Fat: 0 g;

Carbs: 0 g;

Dietary Fiber: 0 g;

Sugars: 1 g;

Protein: 5 g;

Cholesterol: 0 mg;

Sodium: 2 mg

Ginger, Pineapple & Kale Detox Juice

Preparation Time: 10 minutes

Cooking Time: 0 minutes

Servings: 1

Ingredients

1/4 medium pineapple

1 lemon, peeled

1-inch fresh ginger

2 large cucumbers

1 cup chopped kale

½ cup fresh mint

Directions

Juice all the ingredients, one at a time, in a juicer and serve.

Nutrition:

Calories: 125;

Total Fat: 0.8 g;

Carbs: 30.2 g;

Dietary Fiber: 7.4 g;

Sugars: 10.5 g;

Protein: 5.1 g;

Cholesterol: 0 mg;

Sodium: 46 mg

Beet Citrus Cleanser

Preparation Time: 10 minutes

Cooking Time: 0 minutes

Servings: 2

Ingredients

2 beets

1 tangerine

1 orange

1 lime

2 carrots

2 cups dandelion greens

2-inch knob ginger

Directions

Add all ingredients to the juicer and juice. Enjoy!

Nutritional info per Serving:

Calories: 173;

Total Fat: 0.9 g;

Carbs: 41.6 g;

Dietary Fiber: 9.4 g;

Sugars: 25.1 g;

Protein: 5.2 g;

Cholesterol: 0 mg;

Sodium: 163 mg

Super Detox Green Juice

Preparation Time: 10 minutes

Cooking Time: 0 minutes

Servings: 1

Ingredients

1 apple, seeded, cored, chopped

1 lemon peeled

1 cup spinach

2 kale leaves

1 cucumber, chopped

2 celery stalks, chopped

Handful of fresh parsley or cilantro

2 teaspoons chia seeds

Directions

Add all ingredients, except chia seed, to the juicer and juice; stir in the chia seeds and drink.

Nutrition:

Calories: 158;

Total Fat: 1 g;

Carbs: 39 g;

Dietary Fiber: 9 g;

Sugars: 20 g;

Protein: 5 g;

Cholesterol: 0 mg;

Sodium: 112 mg

Refreshing Carrot Detoxifier

Preparation Time: 10 minutes

Cooking Time: 0 minutes

Servings: 2

Ingredients

4 carrots

1 cup sprouts

1-cm fresh ginger

1 kiwi fruit

1 lemon

1 green apple

1 cucumber

2 stalks celery

1 cup parsley

Directions

Add all ingredients to the juicer and juice. Enjoy!

Nutrition:

Calories: 173;

Total Fat: 0.8 g;

Carbs: 42.3 g;

Dietary Fiber: 9.5 g;

Sugars: 23.8 g;

Protein: 1.4 g;

Cholesterol: 0 mg;

Sodium: 126 mg

Super Cleanser Juice

Preparation Time: 10 minutes

Cooking Time: 0 minutes

Servings: 1

Ingredients

¼ cup fresh aloe vera juice

1 lemon, peeled

5 asparagus spears

1 cucumber

10 stalks celery

Handful of cilantro

Handful of parsley

Directions

Add all ingredients to the juicer and juice. Enjoy!

Nutrition:

Calories: 113;

Total Fat: 0.9 g;

Carbs: 26.1 g;

Dietary Fiber: 8.4 g;

Sugars: 11 g;

Protein: 6.4 g;

Cholesterol: 0 mg;

Sodium: 160 mg

Ginger, Pineapple & Cabbage Detoxifier

Preparation Time: 10 minutes

Cooking Time: 0 minutes

Servings: 1

Ingredients

1/4 medium pineapple

1 lemon, peeled

1-inch fresh ginger

2 large cucumbers

1 cup chopped cabbage

½ cup fresh mint

Directions

Juice all the ingredients, one at a time, in a juicer and serve.

Nutrition:

Calories: 125;

Total Fat: 0.8 g;

Carbs: 30.2 g;

Dietary Fiber: 7.4 g;

Sugars: 10.5 g;

Protein: 5.1 g;

Cholesterol: 0 mg;

Sodium: 46 mg

Chilled Toxin Flush Detox Drink

Preparation Time: 15 minutes

Cooking Time: 15 minutes

Servings: 6

Ingredients

6 tea bags

1/2 cup fresh mint leaves

3 lemons, sliced

3 limes, sliced

3 oranges, sliced

6 cups water

1 teaspoon liquid stevia

1 handful ice cubes

Directions

Mix lemon slices, lime slices, orange slices, mint leaves and water in a large teapot; bring to a rolling boil and simmer for about 10 minutes; let cool and strain the mixture through a fine mesh and stir in stevia. Serve over ice.

Nutrition:

Calories: 24;

Total Fat: 0 g;

Carbs: 4.2 g;

Dietary Fiber: 0.5 g;

Sugars: 1.6 g;

Protein: 0 g;

Cholesterol: 0 mg;

Sodium: 7 mg

Liver Detox Juice

Preparation Time: 10 minutes

Cooking Time: 0 minutes

Servings: 1

Ingredients

1 orange, peeled

1 cucumber

1 cup watercress leaves

2 garlic cloves

6 leaves kale

5 stalks celery

1-inch fresh ginger

Dash of cayenne

Directions

Add all ingredients to the juicer and juice. Enjoy!

Nutrition:

Calories: 206;

Total Fat: 0.3 g;

Carbs: 47.4 g;

Dietary Fiber: 11.2 g;

Sugars: 25.9 g;

Protein: 9.3 g;

Cholesterol: 0 mg;

Sodium: 160 mg

Ginger Radish Zinger

Preparation Time: 10 minutes

Cooking Time: 0 minutes

Servings: 1

Ingredients

1 lemon

1/2 green apple

1 cups spinach

1 radish

2 stalks celery

1.5-cm ginger

½ cup parsley

Directions

Add all ingredients to the juicer and juice. Enjoy!

Nutrition:

Calories: 150;

Total Fat: 0.2 g;

Carbs: 36.7 g;

Dietary Fiber: 8.7 g;

Sugars: 9.1 g;

Protein: 5.7 g;

Cholesterol: 0 mg;

Sodium: 100 mg

Ginger Pineapple Drink

Preparation Time: 5 minutes

Cooking Time: 0 minutes

Servings: 2

Ingredients

1-inch piece fresh ginger

1/2 cup pineapple chunks

2 tablespoons lime juice

1 apple, diced

1/2 cup mango chunks

Directions

Blend together all ingredients until smooth. Serve over ice.

Nutrition:

Calories: 186;

Total Fat: 0.8 g;

Carbs: 47.2 g;

Dietary Fiber: 6.6 g;

Protein: 1.8 g;

Cholesterol: 0 mg;

Sodium: 6 mg;

Sugars: 28.7 g

Detoxifying Turmeric Tea

Preparation Time: 10 minutes

Cooking Time: 0 minutes

Servings: 1

Ingredients

1 ½ cups boiling water

1 bag of chamomile tea

1 bag of peppermint tea

½ teaspoon vanilla extract

1 teaspoon turmeric

1 teaspoon ginger

1/4 teaspoon pepper

1 teaspoon raw honey

Directions

In a large mug, combine hot water, chamomile and peppermint teas and let steep for at least 3 minutes; stir in the remaining ingredients and serve hot!

Nutrition:

Calories: 116;

Total Fat: 7 g;

Carbs: 13 g;

Dietary Fiber: 1 g;

Sugars: 2 g

Protein: 17 g;

Cholesterol: 0 mg;

Sodium: 13 mg

Lemon Ginger Detox Juice

Preparation Time: 10 minutes

Cooking Time: 0 minutes

Servings: 1

Ingredients

1 lemon, peeled

1-inch knob fresh ginger root, finely grated

1 orange, peeled

1 grapefruit, peeled

1 garlic clove

A pinch of cayenne pepper

Directions

Juice all the ingredients in a juicer, except cayenne pepper; stir in cayenne pepper and serve.

Nutrition:

Calories: 11;

Total Fat: 0 g;

Carbs: 0 g;

Dietary Fiber: 0 g;

Sugars: 1 g;

Protein: 5 g;

Cholesterol: 0 mg;

Sodium: 2 mg

Ginger Pineapple Detox Drink

Preparation Time: 10 minutes

Cooking Time: 0 minutes

Servings: 1

Ingredients

1 pineapple center

1-inch ginger root

2 carrots

3 celery stalks

Handful mint leaves

Small handful of cilantro

Directions

Juice all the ingredients in a juicer and serve.

Nutrition:

Calories: 152;

Total Fat: 0.5 g;

Carbs: 37.2 g;

Dietary Fiber: 6.8 g;

Sugars: 23.3 g;

Protein: 2.8 g;

Cholesterol: 0 mg;

Sodium: 137 mg

Chilled Ginger Citrus Drink

Preparation Time: 10 minutes

Cooking Time: 0 minutes

Servings: 1

Ingredients

1 knob fresh ginger

1 large grapefruit

1 orange

1 lemon

Directions

Juice ginger and red grapefruit and orange; set aside. Squeeze in the lemon juice and stir to combine well. Refrigerate until chilled before serving.

Nutrition:

Calories: 193;

Total Fat: 0.6 g;

Carbs: 48.6g;

Dietary Fiber: 8.1g;

Protein: 3.8g;

Cholesterol: 0mg;

Sodium: 0mg;

Sugars: 40.4g

Healthy Vacation Peach Drink

Preparation 5 minutes

Cooking time 5 minutes

Servings: 4-5

Ingredients:

2 fresh lemon juice

Ice cubes

10 tbsp of sweetener of choice

5 cups of water

8 peeled peaches, cut into slices

For garnish:

Mint leaves

Peach slices

Directions

Add peach slices, sweetener of choice, lemon juice, ice cubes and water in the bowl of your blender and blend on medium speed. Blend another time until smooth.

Pour peach drink over ice in glass and garnish with mint leaves and peach slice, if desired.

Nutrition: Calories 69, Fat 6.5 g, Fiber 2.6 g, Carbs 10.6 g, Protein 9.4 g

Easy Pumpkin Spice Latte

Preparation 5 minutes

Cooking time 5 minutes

Servings: 2

Ingredients:

1 tsp of vanilla, alcohol-free

Pinch of cinnamon

16 ounces of fresh-brewed coffee

4-6 drops of liquid stevia

1 cup of vanilla almond milk, unsweetened

2 tsp of pumpkin pie spice

6 tbsp of pumpkin puree

Directions

Combine pumpkin and almond milk together in a saucepan, and cook over medium heat until hot (not boiling) or place in the microwave for 30 to 45 seconds.

Stir in spices, vanilla, and sweetener.

Transfer the mix to a blender and blend until foamy, about 30 seconds.

Add the milk mixture into coffee, and top with cinnamon.

Nutrition: Calories 69, Fat 6.5 g, Fiber 2.6 g, Carbs 10.6 g, Protein 9.4 g

Pineapple, Watermelon Smoothie

Preparation 5 minutes

Cooking time 0 minutes

Servings: 6

Ingredients:

1 1/2 cup of coconut milk

2 1/2 teaspoon honey (optional)

5 teaspoons of freshly grated turmeric

5 cups of cubed frozen watermelon

3 1/2 cups of cubed frozen coconut water

1 1/2 orange, peeled, seeded removed

5 cups of fresh cubed frozen pineapple

2 1/2 teaspoon of fresh ginger, grated

Directions

Add together all the ingredients in the bowl of your blender and blend until a smooth mixture emerges.

Add honey if using, blend and serve.

Nutrition: Calories 69, Fat 6.5 g, Fiber 2.6 g, Carbs 10.6 g, Protein 9.4 g

Ginger Honey Lemonade

Preparation 2 minutes

Cooking time 0 minutes

Servings: 4

Ingredients:

Lemon slices for garnish, if desired

1 medium sprigs of fresh rosemary

Ice cubes

1/6 cup of honey

1/2 large sprig of fresh rosemary for garnish, if desired

2 large strips of lemon peel

1 tbsp of fresh ginger root, grated

Juice of 2 lemons

Directions

Combine together sprigs of fresh rosemary, lemon peel, ginger, honey and add 1 cups of water in a small pot.

Bring mixture to a boil then simmer on low heat for about 10 minutes, stirring frequently.

Let cool about 15 minutes then strain mixture into large pitcher. Discard the rosemary and ginger.

Add in the 2 lemon juice and three cups of cold water to pitcher, mix to combine.

To serve, pour over ice along with lemon slice and little piece of fresh rosemary as garnish, if desired.

Nutrition: Calories 69, Fat 6.5 g, Fiber 2.6 g, Carbs 10.6 g, Protein 9.4 g

Perfect "Shamrock" Shake

Preparation 2 minutes

Cooking time 0 minutes

Servings: 4

Ingredients:

2 scoop of Ultra Nourish

1 teaspoon of mint extract, alcohol-free

3 cups of vanilla almond milk

4 cups of vanilla frozen yogurt

Directions

Combine every ingredient in a blender and blend to have a smooth mixture. Enjoy!

Nutrition: Calories 100, Fat 1, Fiber 2, Carbs 2, Protein 6

Green Pumpkin Spice Smoothie

Preparation 4 minutes

Cooking time 2 minutes

Servings: 2

Ingredients:

1/2 teaspoon of ground ginger

Pinch of ground nutmeg

2 handfuls of ice cubes

Pinch of ground cloves

2 cup sweetened, vanilla almond milk

Pinch of allspice

1/2 teaspoon of ground cinnamon

2 tablespoon honey

1 cup of canned pumpkin

1 ripe banana, peeled

2 scoop of Ultra Nourish

Directions

Combine together the entire ingredient in a blender and blend to have a smooth mixture.

Adjust spice and sweetness to taste, serve and enjoy!

Nutrition: Calories 100, Fat 1, Fiber 2, Carbs 2, Protein 6

Summer OatBerry Smoothie

Preparation 4 minutes

Cooking time 0 minutes

Servings: 3

Ingredients:

3 cup of almond milk

3 cup of mixed frozen berries (blackberries, blueberries, raspberries, strawberries)

3 tbsp of your preferred nut butter

3/4 cup of oats

3 scoop of Ultra Nourish

Directions

Pour the oats in the bowl of your food processor and process to make a powder.

Pour in the rest ingredients, blend to have a smooth mixture. Serve and enjoy.

Nutrition: Calories 100, Fat 1, Fiber 2, Carbs 2, Protein 6

Sweet Berry Banana Yogurt Smoothie

Preparation 2 minutes

Cooking time 5 minutes

Servings: 3

Ingredients:

3 (15 ounces) container of Greek yogurt

3 scoop of Ultra Nourish

3 cup of unsweetened juice of your choice

3 bananas cut into small sizes

3/4 cup of blueberries

Several strawberries, halved

1 cup of ice

Directions

Combine together the entire ingredient in a blender and blend to have a smooth mixture. Enjoy!

Nutrition: Calories 69, Fat 6.5 g, Fiber 2.6 g, Carbs 10.6 g, Protein 9.4 g

Banana Apple Smoothie

Preparation 5 minutes

Cooking time 5 minutes

Servings: 4

Directions

2 cup (8 oz.) almond milk

2 tbsp of or almond butter or natural peanut butter

2 scoop Ultra Nourish

1 frozen banana, cut into small sizes

2 cored and sliced apple

Directions

Whisk together the entire ingredient in a blender and blend to have a smooth mixture.

Note: frozen bananas will make the texture thicker and won't require ice to chill the smoothie.

Nutrition: Calories 69, Fat 6.5 g, Fiber 2.6 g, Carbs 10.6 g, Protein 9.4 g

Eastertide Nectarine Smoothie

Preparation 5 minutes

Cooking time 0 minutes

Servings: 2

Ingredients:

4 tbsp of whey protein powder

2 tbsp of ground flaxseeds

3 cups of water

4 tbsp of canned coconut cream

2 large nectarines

Directions

Combine the entire ingredient in a blender and blend to have a smooth mixture.

Nutrition: Calories 100, Fat 1, Fiber 2, Carbs 2, Protein 6

Ginger Citrus Liver Detox Drink

Preparation 2 minutes

Cooking time 0 minutes

Servings: 4

Ingredients:

1 lemon, peeled

1-inch knob fresh ginger root, finely grated

1 orange, peeled

1 grapefruit, peeled

A pinch of cayenne pepper

Directions:

Juice all the ingredients in a juicer, except cayenne pepper; stir in cayenne pepper and serve.

Nutrition: Calories 100, Fat 1, Fiber 2, Carbs 2, Protein 6

Beet Citrus Cleanser

Preparation 2 minutes

Cooking time 0 minutes

Servings: 4

Ingredients:

2 beets

1 tangerine

1 orange

1 lime

2 carrots

2 cups dandelion greens

2-inch knob ginger

Directions:

Add all ingredients to the juicer and juice. Enjoy!

Nutrition: Calories 69, Fat 6.5 g, Fiber 2.6 g, Carbs 10.6 g, Protein 9.4 g

Super Detox Green Juice

Preparation 2 minutes

Cooking time 0 minutes

Servings: 4

Ingredients:

1 apple, seeded, cored, chopped

1 lemon peeled

1 cup spinach

2 kale leaves

1 cucumber, chopped

2 celery stalks, chopped

Handful of fresh parsley or cilantro

2 teaspoons chia seeds

Directions:

Add all ingredients, except chia seed, to the juicer and juice; stir in the chia seeds and drink.

Nutrition: Calories 100, Fat 1, Fiber 2, Carbs 2, Protein 6

Super Green Detox Juice

Preparation 2 minutes

Cooking time 0 minutes

Servings: 4

Ingredients:

1 apple

1 cup seedless grapes

1 lemon

2-inch ginger root

1 cup apple

1 cucumber

1/2 cup parsley

2 mint sprigs

Directions:

Add all ingredients to the juicer and juice. Enjoy!

Nutrition: Calories 69, Fat 6.5 g, Fiber 2.6 g, Carbs 10.6 g, Protein 9.4 g

Ginger, Apple & Kale Detox Juice

Preparation 2 minutes

Cooking time 0 minutes

Servings: 4

Ingredients:

1/4 medium apple

1 lemon, peeled

1-inch fresh ginger

2 large cucumbers

1 cup chopped kale

½ cup fresh mint

Directions:

Juice all the ingredients, one at a time, in a juicer and serve.

Nutrition: Calories 69, Fat 6.5 g, Fiber 2.6 g, Carbs 10.6 g, Protein 9.4 g

Refreshing Carrot Detoxifier

Preparation 2 minutes

Cooking time 0 minutes

Servings: 4

Ingredients:

4 carrots

1 cup sprouts

1-cm fresh ginger

1 kiwi fruit

1 lemon

1 green apple

1 cucumber

2 stalks celery

1 cup parsley

Directions:

Add all ingredients to the juicer and juice. Enjoy!

Nutrition: Calories 100, Fat 1, Fiber 2, Carbs 2, Protein 6

Super Cleanser Juice

Preparation 2 minutes

Cooking time 0 minutes

Servings: 4

Ingredients:

¼ cup fresh aloe vera juice

1 lemon, peeled

5 asparagus spears

1 cucumber

10 stalks celery

Handful of cilantro

Handful of parsley

Directions:

Add all ingredients to the juicer and juice. Enjoy!

Nutrition: Calories 69, Fat 6.5 g, Fiber 2.6 g, Carbs 10.6 g, Protein 9.4 g

Ginger, Apple & Cabbage Detoxifier

Preparation 2 minutes

Cooking time 0 minutes

Servings: 4

Ingredients:

1/4 medium apple

1 lemon, peeled

1-inch fresh ginger

2 large cucumbers

1 cup chopped cabbage

½ cup fresh mint

Directions:

Juice all the ingredients, one at a time, in a juicer and serve.

Nutrition: Calories 69, Fat 6.5 g, Fiber 2.6 g, Carbs 10.6 g, Protein 9.4 g

Ultimate Toxin Flush Shot

Preparation 2 minutes

Cooking time 0 minutes

Servings: 4

Ingredients:

1 knob of ginger

1 cup water

2 tablespoons fresh lemon juice

½ teaspoon cayenne pepper

1 teaspoon turmeric

½ teaspoon pepper

1 teaspoon raw honey

ice

Directions:

Juice ginger through a juicer; stir in water, fresh lemon juice, cayenne, turmeric, black pepper, raw honey, and ice. Enjoy!

Nutrition: Calories 100, Fat 1, Fiber 2, Carbs 2, Protein 6

Detoxifying Vegetable Juice

Preparation 2 minutes

Cooking time 0 minutes

Servings: 4

Ingredients:

1/2 cup chopped kale

1/2 cup baby spinach

1 cucumber

1-inch ginger

2 carrots

1 pear

1/2 apple

2 celery stalks

Directions:

Add all ingredients to the juicer and juice. Enjoy!

Nutrition: Calories 69, Fat 6.5 g, Fiber 2.6 g, Carbs 10.6 g, Protein 9.4 g

Hot Golden Elixir

Preparation 2 minutes

Cooking time 0 minutes

Servings: 4

Ingredients:

¼ cup fresh lemon juice

1 cup hot water

raw honey, 1 teaspoon

¼ teaspoon cayenne pepper

1/8 teaspoon ground ginger

1/8 teaspoon turmeric

Directions:

In a mug, stir everything together until well blended. Enjoy!

Nutrition: Calories 100, Fat 1, Fiber 2, Carbs 2, Protein 6

Ultimate Liver Detox Juice

Preparation 2 minutes

Cooking time 0 minutes

Servings: 4

Ingredients:

3 carrots, peeled

1 beet, peeled

2 red apples, chopped

½ lemon, peeled

½ inch ginger root

6 kale leaves

1 cup chopped cabbage

Directions:

Place all the ingredients in a juicer and juice. Stir to mix well and serve with ice cubes.

Nutrition: Calories 100, Fat 1, Fiber 2, Carbs 2, Protein 6

Charcoal Black Lemonade

Preparation 2 minutes

Cooking time 0 minutes

Servings: 4

Ingredients:

1 capsule activated charcoal

¼ cup fresh lemon juice

4 cups filtered water

2 tablespoons raw honey

Directions:

In a large bowl, whisk all the ingredients together until well blended. Serve over ice.

Nutrition: Calories 69, Fat 6.5 g, Fiber 2.6 g, Carbs 10.6 g, Protein 9.4 g

Magical Liver Elixir

Preparation 2 minutes

Cooking time 0 minutes

Servings: 4

Ingredients:
2 knobs of fresh turmeric

2-inch piece of fresh ginger root

2 garlic cloves

2 red onions

1 cup spinach

4 celery stalks

1 carrot

Directions:

Wash and run all ingredients through a juicer. Serve right away.

Nutrition: Calories 100, Fat 1, Fiber 2, Carbs 2, Protein 6

Chilled Toxin Flush Detox Drink

Preparation 2 minutes

Cooking time 0 minutes

Servings: 4

Ingredients:

6 tea bags

1/2 cup fresh mint leaves

3 lemons, sliced

3 limes, sliced

3 oranges, sliced

6 cups water

1 teaspoon liquid stevia

1 handful ice cubes

Directions:

Mix lemon slices, lime slices, orange slices, mint leaves and water in a large teapot; bring to a rolling boil and simmer for about 10 minutes; let cool and strain the mixture through a fine mesh and stir in stevia. Serve over ice.

Nutrition: Calories 100, Fat 1, Fiber 2, Carbs 2, Protein 6

Liver Detox Juice

Preparation 2 minutes

Cooking time 0 minutes

Servings: 4

Ingredients:

1 orange, peeled

1 cucumber

1 cup watercress leaves

2 garlic cloves

6 leaves kale

5 stalks celery

1-inch fresh ginger

Dash of cayenne

Directions:

Add all ingredients to the juicer and juice. Enjoy!

Nutrition: Calories 100, Fat 1, Fiber 2, Carbs 2, Protein 6

Ginger Radish Zinger

Preparation 2 minutes

Cooking time 0 minutes

Servings: 4

Ingredients:

1 lemon

1/2 green apple

1 cups spinach

1 radish

2 stalks celery

1.5-cm ginger

½ cup parsley

Directions:

Add all ingredients to the juicer and juice. Enjoy!

Nutrition: Calories 100, Fat 1, Fiber 2, Carbs 2, Protein 6

Ginger Apple Drink

Preparation 2 minutes

Cooking time 0 minutes

Servings: 4

Ingredients:

1-inch piece fresh ginger

1/2 cup apple chunks

2 tablespoons lime juice

1 apple, diced

1/2 cup mango chunks

Directions:

Blend together all ingredients until smooth. Serve over ice.

Nutrition: Calories 140, Fat 4, Fiber 2, Carbs 7, Protein 8

Detoxifying Turmeric Tea

Preparation 2 minutes

Cooking time 0 minutes

Servings: 4

Ingredients:

1 ½ cups boiling water

1 bag of chamomile tea

1 bag of peppermint tea

½ teaspoon vanilla extract

1 teaspoon turmeric

1 teaspoon ginger

1/4 teaspoon pepper

1 teaspoon raw honey

Directions:

In a large mug, combine hot water, chamomile and peppermint teas and let steep for at least 3 minutes; stir in the remaining ingredients and serve hot!

Nutrition: Calories 100, Fat 1, Fiber 2, Carbs 2, Protein 6

Lemon Ginger Detox Juice

Preparation 2 minutes

Cooking time 0 minutes

Servings: 4

Ingredients:

1 lemon, peeled

1-inch knob fresh ginger root, finely grated

1 orange, peeled

1 grapefruit, peeled

1 garlic clove

A pinch of cayenne pepper

Directions:

Juice all the ingredients in a juicer, except cayenne pepper; stir in cayenne pepper and serve.

Nutrition: Calories 69, Fat 6.5 g, Fiber 2.6 g, Carbs 10.6 g, Protein 9.4 g

Ginger Apple Detox Drink

Preparation 2 minutes

Cooking time 0 minutes

Servings: 4

Ingredients:

1 apple center

1-inch ginger root

2 carrots

3 celery stalks

Handful mint leaves

Small handful of cilantro

Directions:

Juice all the ingredients in a juicer and serve.

Nutrition: Calories 140, Fat 4, Fiber 2, Carbs 7, Protein 8

Chilled Ginger Citrus Drink

Preparation 2 minutes

Cooking time 0 minutes

Servings: 4

Ingredients:

1 knob fresh ginger

1 large grapefruit

1 orange

1 lemon

Directions:

Juice ginger and red grapefruit and orange; set aside. Squeeze in the lemon juice and stir to combine well. Refrigerate until chilled before serving.

Nutrition: Calories 69, Fat 6.5 g, Fiber 2.6 g, Carbs 10.6 g, Protein 9.4 g

Simple Lemon Herb Chicken

Preparation 2 minutes

Cooking time 0 minutes

Servings: 4

Ingredients:

2 chicken breast halves, skinless, boneless

1 pinch dried oregano

1 lemon, juiced

low sodium salt, to taste

1 tablespoon olive oil

pepper to taste

2 sprigs fresh parsley, for garnish

Directions:

Add ½ your lemon juice on your chicken the season to taste and allow to rest for about 15 minutes.

Set oil over medium heat to get hot.

Add in your chicken and sauté, add with the rest of your lemon juice and oregano. Season to your liking.

Continue to cook until the juices run clear (about 10 minutes).

Garnish and serve.

Nutrition: Calories 100, Fat 1, Fiber 2, Carbs 2, Protein 6

Grilled Lemon Chicken

Preparation 2 minutes

Cooking time 0 minutes

Servings: 4

Ingredients:

2 tablespoons red bell pepper, finely chopped

1/4 cup olive oil

1 tablespoon dijon mustard

1/2 teaspoon low sodium salt

1/3 cup lemon juice

1/4 teaspoon ground black pepper

4 skinless, boneless chicken breast halves

2 large cloves garlic, finely chopped

Directions:

Combine your Dijon mustard, olive oil, lemon juice, pepper, red bell pepper, garlic and salt to create a baste and marinade. A quarter of this will be used as a baste so set this aside.

Coat chicken well with your mixture then refrigerate for at least 20 minutes.

Set your grill to preheat on high and lightly grease grate.

Drain and discard marinade from the bowl, and place chicken on the grill.

Cook 6 to 8 minutes on each side, until juices run clear, basting occasionally with the reserved marinade.

Nutrition: Calories 140, Fat 4, Fiber 2, Carbs 7, Protein 8

Chapter 9: Salad Recipes and soups

Pumpkin Cream Soup

Preparation Time: 10 minutes

Cooking Time: 20 minutes

Servings: 2

Ingredients:

1-pound pumpkin, chopped

1 teaspoon ground cumin

½ cup cauliflower, chopped

4 cups of water

1 teaspoon ground turmeric

½ teaspoon ground nutmeg

1 tablespoon fresh dill, chopped

1 teaspoon olive oil

½ cup skim milk

Directions:

Roast the pumpkin with olive oil in the saucepan for 3 minutes.

Then stir well and add cauliflower, cumin, turmeric, nutmeg, and water.

Close the lid and cook the soup on medium mode for 15 minutes or until the pumpkin is soft.

Then blend the mixture until smooth and add skim milk. Remove the soup from heat and top with dill.

Nutrition:

56 calories,

2.2g protein,

10g carbohydrates,

1.4g fat,

3.1g fiber,

0mg cholesterol,

28mg sodium,

Zucchini Noodles Soup

Preparation Time: 10 minutes

Cooking Time: 15 minutes

Servings: 2

Ingredients:

2 zucchinis, trimmed

4 cups low-sodium chicken stock

2 oz fresh parsley, chopped

½ teaspoon chili flakes

1 oz carrot, shredded

1 teaspoon canola oil

Directions:

Roast the carrot with canola oil in the saucepan for 5 minutes over the medium-low heat.

Stir it well and add chicken stock. Bring the mixture to boil.

Meanwhile, make the noodles from the zucchini with the help of the spiralizer.

Add them in the boiling soup liquid.

Add parsley and chili flakes. Bring the soup to boil and remove it from the heat.

Leave for 10 minutes to rest.

Nutrition:

39 calories,

2.7g protein,

4.9g carbohydrates,

1.5g fat,

1.7g fiber,

0mg cholesterol,

158mg sodium,

Chicken Oatmeal Soup

Preparation Time: 10 minutes

Cooking Time: 15 minutes

Servings: 2

Ingredients:

1 cup oats

4 cups of water

1 oz fresh dill, chopped

10 oz chicken fillet, chopped

1 teaspoon ground black pepper

1 teaspoon potato starch

½ carrot, diced

Directions:

Put the chopped chicken in the saucepan, add water and bring it to boil. Simmer the chicken for 10 minutes.

Add dill, ground black pepper, oats, and diced carrot.

Bring the soup to boil and add potato starch. Stir it until soup starts to thicken. Simmer the soup for 5 minutes on the low heat.

Nutrition:

192 calories,

19.8g protein,

16.1g carbohydrates,

5.5g fat,

2.7g fiber,

50mg cholesterol,

72mg sodium,

Celery Cream Soup

Preparation Time: 10 minutes

Cooking Time: 25 minutes

Servings: 1

Ingredients:

2 cups celery stalk, chopped

1 shallot, chopped

1 potato, chopped

4 cups low-sodium vegetable stock

1 tablespoon margarine

1 teaspoon white pepper

Directions:

Melt the margarine in the saucepan, add shallot, and celery stalk. Cook the vegetables for 5 minutes. Stir them occasionally.

After this, add vegetable stock and potato.

Simmer the soup for 15 minutes.

Blend the soup tilly ou get the creamy texture and sprinkle with white pepper.

Simmer it for 5 minutes more.

Nutrition:

88 calories,

2.3g protein,

13.3g carbohydrates,

3g fat,

2.9g fiber,

0mg cholesterol,

217mg sodium,

449mg potassium.

Cauliflower Soup

Preparation Time: 10 minutes

Cooking Time: 20 minutes

Servings: 2

Ingredients:

1 cup cauliflower, chopped

¼ cup potato, chopped

1 cup skim milk

1 cup of water

1 teaspoon ground coriander

1 teaspoon margarine

Directions:

Put cauliflower and potato in the saucepan.

Add water and boil the ingredients for 15 minutes.

Then add ground coriander and margarine.

With the help of the immersion blender, blend the soup until smooth.

Add skim milk and stir well.

Nutrition:

82 calories,

5.2g protein,

10.3g carbohydrates,

2g fat,

1.5g fiber,

2mg cholesterol,

106mg sodium,

Buckwheat Soup

Preparation Time: 10 minutes

Cooking Time: 25 minutes

Servings: 2

Ingredients:

½ cup buckwheat

1 carrot, chopped

1 yellow onion, diced

1 tablespoon avocado oil

1 tablespoon fresh dill, chopped

1-pound chicken breast, chopped

1 teaspoon ground black pepper

6 cups of water

Directions:

Saute the onion, carrot, and avocado oil in the saucepan for 5 minutes. Stir them from time to time.

Then add buckwheat, chicken breast, and ground black pepper.

Add water and close the lid.

Simmer the soup for 20 minutes.

After this, add dill and remove the soup from the heat. Leave it for 10 minutes to rest.

Nutrition:

152 calories,

18.4g protein,

13.5g carbohydrates,

2.7g fat,

2.3g fiber,

48mg cholesterol,

48mg sodium,

Spring Greens Salad

Preparation Time: 5 minutes

Cooking Time: 0 minutes

Servings: 2

Ingredients:

½ cup radish, sliced

1 cup fresh spinach, chopped

½ cup green peas, cooked

½ lemon

1 cup arugula, chopped

1 tablespoon avocado oil

½ teaspoon dried sage

Directions:

In the salad bowl, mix up radish, spinach, green peas, arugula, and dried sage.

Then squeeze the lemon over the salad.

Add avocado oil and shake the salad.

Nutrition:

54 calories,

3.1g protein,

9g carbohydrates,

1.3g fat,

3.6g fiber,

0mg cholesterol,

28mg sodium,

Tuna Salad

Preparation Time: 7 minutes

Cooking Time: 0 minutes

Servings: 2

Ingredients:

½ cup low-fat Greek yogurt

8 oz tuna, canned

½ cup fresh parsley, chopped

1 cup corn kernels, cooked

½ teaspoon ground black pepper

Directions:

Mix up tuna, parsley, kernels, and ground black pepper.

Then add yogurt and stir the salad until it is homogenous.

Nutrition:

172 calories,

17.8g protein,

13.6g carbohydrates,

5.5g fat,

1.4g fiber,

19mg cholesterol,

55mg sodium,

Fish Salad

Preparation Time: 5 minutes

Cooking Time: 0 minutes

Servings: 2

Ingredients:

7 oz canned salmon, shredded

1 tablespoon lime juice

1 tablespoon low-fat yogurt

1 cup baby spinach, chopped

1 teaspoon capers, drained and chopped

Directions:

Mix up all ingredients together and transfer them in the salad bowl.

Nutrition:

71 calories,

10.1g protein,

0.8g carbohydrates,

3.2g fat,

0.2g fiber,

22mg cholesterol,

52mg sodium,

Grilled Tomatoes Soup

Preparation Time: 10 minutes

Cooking Time: 20 minutes

Servings: 1

Ingredients:

2-pounds tomatoes

½ cup shallot, chopped

1 tablespoon avocado oil

½ teaspoon ground black pepper

¼ teaspoon minced garlic

1 tablespoon dried basil

3 cups low-sodium chicken broth

Directions:

Cut the tomatoes into halves and grill them in the preheated to 390F grill for 1 minute from each side.

After this, transfer the grilled tomatoes in the blender and blend until smooth.

Place the shallot and avocado oil in the saucepan and roast it until light brown.

Add blended grilled tomatoes, ground black pepper, and minced garlic.

Bring the soup to boil and sprinkle with dried basil.

Simmer the soup for 2 minutes more.

Nutrition:

72 calories,

4.1g protein,

13.4g carbohydrates,

0.9g fat,

3g fiber,

0mg cholesterol,

98mg sodium,

Salmon Salad

Preparation Time: 10 minutes

Cooking Time: 0 minutes

Servings: 2

Ingredients:

4 oz canned salmon, flaked

1 tablespoon lemon juice

2 tablespoons red bell pepper, chopped

1 tablespoon red onion, chopped

1 teaspoon dill, chopped

1 tablespoon olive oil

Directions:

Mix up all ingredients in the salad bowl.

Nutrition:

119 calories,

8.3g protein,

6.6g carbohydrates,

7.3g fat,

1.2g fiber,

17mg cholesterol,

21mg sodium,

Arugula Salad with Shallot

Preparation Time: 10 minutes

Cooking Time: 0 minutes

Servings: 2

Ingredients:

1 cup cucumber, chopped

1 tablespoon lemon juice

1 tablespoon avocado oil

2 shallots, chopped

½ cup black olives, sliced

3 cups arugula, chopped

Directions:

Mix up all ingredients from the list above in the salad bowl and refrigerate in the fridge for 5 minutes.

Nutrition:

33 calories,

0.8g protein,

2.9g carbohydrates,

2.4g fat,

1.1g fiber,

0mg cholesterol,

152mg sodium,

Watercress Salad

Preparation Time: 10 minutes

Cooking Time: 4 minutes

Servings: 2

Ingredients:

2 cups asparagus, chopped

16 ounces shrimp, cooked

4 cups watercress, torn

1 tablespoon apple cider vinegar

¼ cup olive oil

Directions:

In the mixing bowl mix up asparagus, shrimps, watercress, and olive oil.

Nutrition:

264 calories,

28.3g protein,

4.5g carbohydrates,

14.8g fat,

1.8g fiber,

239mg cholesterol,

300mg sodium,

Pumpkin Cream Soup

Preparation Time: 10 minutes

Cooking Time: 20 minutes

Servings: 2

Ingredients:

1-pound pumpkin, chopped

1 teaspoon ground cumin

½ cup cauliflower, chopped

4 cups of water

1 teaspoon ground turmeric

½ teaspoon ground nutmeg

1 tablespoon fresh dill, chopped

1 teaspoon olive oil

½ cup skim milk

Directions:

Roast the pumpkin with olive oil in the saucepan for 3 minutes.

Then stir well and add cauliflower, cumin, turmeric, nutmeg, and water.

Close the lid and cook the soup on medium mode for 15 minutes or until the pumpkin is soft.

Then blend the mixture until smooth and add skim milk. Remove the soup from heat and top with dill.

Nutrition:

56 calories,

2.2g protein,

10g carbohydrates,

1.4g fat,

3.1g fiber,

0mg cholesterol,

28mg sodium,

Zucchini Noodles Soup

Preparation Time: 10 minutes

Cooking Time: 15 minutes

Servings: 2

Ingredients:

2 zucchinis, trimmed

4 cups low-sodium chicken stock

2 oz fresh parsley, chopped

½ teaspoon chili flakes

1 oz carrot, shredded

1 teaspoon canola oil

Directions:

Roast the carrot with canola oil in the saucepan for 5 minutes over the medium-low heat.

Stir it well and add chicken stock. Bring the mixture to boil.

Meanwhile, make the noodles from the zucchini with the help of the spiralizer.

Add them in the boiling soup liquid.

Add parsley and chili flakes. Bring the soup to boil and remove it from the heat.

Leave for 10 minutes to rest.

Nutrition:

39 calories,

2.7g protein,

4.9g carbohydrates,

1.5g fat,

1.7g fiber,

0mg cholesterol,

158mg sodium,

Grilled Tomatoes Soup

Preparation Time: 10 minutes

Cooking Time: 20 minutes

Servings: 1

Ingredients:

2-pounds tomatoes

½ cup shallot, chopped

1 tablespoon avocado oil

½ teaspoon ground black pepper

¼ teaspoon minced garlic

1 tablespoon dried basil

3 cups low-sodium chicken broth

Directions:

Cut the tomatoes into halves and grill them in the preheated to 390F grill for 1 minute from each side.

After this, transfer the grilled tomatoes in the blender and blend until smooth.

Place the shallot and avocado oil in the saucepan and roast it until light brown.

Add blended grilled tomatoes, ground black pepper, and minced garlic.

Bring the soup to boil and sprinkle with dried basil.

Simmer the soup for 2 minutes more.

Nutrition:

72 calories,

4.1g protein,

13.4g carbohydrates,

0.9g fat,

3g fiber,

0mg cholesterol,

98mg sodium,

Sliced Mushrooms Salad

Preparation Time: 10 minutes

Cooking Time: 20 minutes

Servings: 2

Ingredients:

1 cup mushrooms, sliced

1 tablespoon margarine

1 cup lettuce, chopped

1 teaspoon lemon juice

1 tablespoon fresh dill, chopped

1 teaspoon cumin seeds

Directions:

Melt the margarine in the skillet.

Add mushrooms and lemon juice. Saute the vegetables for 20 minutes over the medium heat.

Then transfer the cooked mushrooms in the salad bowl, add lettuce, dill, and cumin seeds.

Stir the salad well.

Nutrition:

35 calories,

0.9g protein,

1.7g carbohydrates,

3.1g fat,

0.5g fiber,

0mg cholesterol,

38mg sodium,

Tender Green Beans Salad

Preparation Time: 5 minutes

Cooking Time: 5 minutes

Servings: 2

Ingredients:

2 cups green beans, trimmed, chopped, cooked

2 tablespoons olive oil

2 pounds shrimp, cooked, peeled

1 cup tomato, chopped

¼ cup apple cider vinegar

Directions:

Mix up all ingredients together.

Then transfer the salad in the salad bowl.

Nutrition:

179 calories,

26.5g protein,

4.6g carbohydrates,

5.5g fat,

1.2g fiber,

239mg cholesterol,

280mg sodium,

Crispy Fennel Salad

Preparation Time: 5 minutes

Cooking Time: 15 minutes

Servings: 2

Ingredients:

1 fennel bulb, finely sliced

1 grapefruit, cut into segments

1 orange, cut into segments

2 tablespoons almond slices, toasted

1 teaspoon chopped mint

1 tablespoon chopped dill

Salt and pepper to taste

1 tablespoon grape seed oil

Directions:

Mix the fennel bulb with the grapefruit and orange segments on a platter.

Top with almond slices, mint and dill then drizzle with the oil and season with salt and pepper.

Serve the salad as fresh as possible.

Nutrition: Per Serving:Calories:104 Fat:0.5g Protein:3.1g Carbohydrates:25.5g

Red Beet Feta Salad

Preparation Time: 5 minutes

Cooking Time: 10 minutes

Servings: 2

Ingredients:

6 red beets, cooked and peeled

3 oz. feta cheese, cubed

2 tablespoons extra virgin olive oil

2 tablespoons balsamic vinegar

Directions:

Combine the beets and feta cheese on a platter.

Drizzle with oil and vinegar and serve right away.

Nutrition: Per Serving:Calories: 230 Fat: 12.0g Protein: 7.3g Carbohydrates: 26.3g

Cheesy Potato Mash

Preparation Time: 5 minutes

Cooking Time: 20 minutes

Servings: 2

Ingredients:

2 pounds gold potatoes, peeled and cubed

1 and ½ cup cream cheese, soft

Sea salt and black pepper to the taste

½ cup almond milk

2 tablespoons chives, chopped

Directions:

Put potatoes in a pot, add water to cover, add a pinch of salt, bring to a simmer over medium heat, cook for 20 minutes, drain and mash them.

Add the rest of the ingredients except the chives and whisk well.

Add the chives, stir, divide between plates and serve as a side dish.

Nutrition: calories 243, fat 14.2, fiber 1.4, carbs 3.5, protein 1.4

Provencal Summer Salad

Preparation Time: 5 minutes

Cooking Time: 25 minutes

Servings: 2

Ingredients:

1 zucchini, sliced

1 eggplant, sliced

2 red onions, sliced

2 tomatoes, sliced

1 teaspoon dried mint

2 garlic cloves, minced

2 tablespoons balsamic vinegar

Salt and pepper to taste

Directions:

Season the zucchini, eggplant, onions and tomatoes with salt and pepper. Cook the vegetable slices on the grill until browned.

Transfer the vegetables in a salad bowl then add the mint, garlic and vinegar.

Serve the salad right away.

Nutrition: Per Serving:Calories: 74 Fat: 0.5g Protein: 3.0g Carbohydrates: 16.5g

Sunflower Seeds And Arugula Garden Salad

Preparation Time: 5 minutes

Cooking Time: 10 minutes

Servings: 2

Ingredients:

¼ tsp black pepper

¼ tsp salt

1 tsp fresh thyme, chopped

2 tbsp sunflower seeds, toasted

2 cups red grapes, halved

7 cups baby arugula, loosely packed

1 tbsp coconut oil

2 tsp honey

3 tbsp red wine vinegar

½ tsp stone-ground mustard

Directions:

In a small bowl, whisk together mustard, honey and vinegar. Slowly pour oil as you whisk.

In a large salad bowl, mix thyme, seeds, grapes and arugula.

Drizzle with dressing and serve.

Nutrition: Calories per serving: 86.7; Protein: 1.6g; Carbs: 13.1g; Fat: 3.1g

Ginger Pumpkin Mash

Preparation Time: 5 minutes

Cooking Time: 30 minutes

Servings: 2

Ingredients:

10 oz pumpkin, peeled

½ teaspoon butter

¾ teaspoon ground ginger

1/3 teaspoon salt

Directions:

Chop the pumpkin into the cubes and bake in the preheated to the 360F oven for 30 minutes or until the pumpkin is soft.

After this, transfer the pumpkin cubes in the food processor.

Add butter, salt, and ground ginger.

Blend the vegetable until you get puree or use the potato masher for this step.

Nutrition: :calories 30, fat 0.7, fiber 2.1, carbs 6, protein 0.8

Yogurt Peppers Mix

Preparation Time: 5 minutes

Cooking Time: 10 minutes

Servings: 2

Ingredients:

2 red bell peppers, cut into thick strips

2 tablespoons olive oil

3 shallots, chopped

3 garlic cloves, minced

Salt and black pepper to the taste

½ cup Greek yogurt

1 tablespoon cilantro, chopped

Directions:

Heat up a pan with the oil over medium heat, add the shallots and garlic, stir and cook for 5 minutes.

Add the rest of the ingredients, toss, cook for 10 minutes more, divide the mix between plates and serve as a side dish.

Nutrition: calories 274, fat 11, fiber 3.5, protein 13.3, carbs 6.5

Lemony Carrots

Preparation Time: 5 minutes

Cooking Time: 40 minutes

Servings: 2

Ingredients:

3 tablespoons olive oil

2 pounds baby carrots, trimmed

Salt and black pepper to the taste

½ teaspoon lemon zest, grated

1 tablespoon lemon juice

1/3 cup Greek yogurt

1 garlic clove, minced

1 teaspoon cumin, ground

1 tablespoon dill, chopped

Directions:

In a roasting pan, combine the carrots with the oil, salt, pepper and the rest of the ingredients except the dill, toss and bake at 400 degrees F for 20 minutes.

Reduce the temperature to 375 degrees F and cook for 20 minutes more.

Divide the mix between plates, sprinkle the dill on top and serve.

Nutrition: calories 192, fat 5.4, fiber 3.4, carbs 7.3, protein 5.6

Roasted Vegetable Salad

Servings: 6

Cooking Time: 30 Minutes

Ingredients:

½ pound baby carrots

2 red onions, sliced

1 zucchini, sliced

2 eggplants, cubed

1 cauliflower, cut into florets

1 sweet potato, peeled and cubed

1 endive, sliced

3 tablespoons extra virgin olive oil

1 teaspoon dried basil

Salt and pepper to taste

1 lemon, juiced

1 tablespoon balsamic vinegar

Directions:

Combine the vegetables with the oil, basil, salt and pepper in a deep dish baking pan and cook in the preheated oven at 350F for 25-30 minutes.

When done, transfer in a salad bowl and add the lemon juice and vinegar.

Serve the salad fresh.

Nutrition: Per Serving:Calories:164 Fat:7.6g Protein:3.7g Carbohydrates:24.2g

Chicken Kale Soup

Preparation Time: 5 minutes

Cooking Time: 10 minutes

Servings: 2

Ingredients:

2poundschicken breast, skinless

1/3cuponion

1tablespoonolive oil

14ounceschicken bone broth

½ cup olive oil

4 cups chicken stock

¼ cup lemon juice

5ouncesbaby kale leaves

Salt, to taste

Directions:

Season chicken with salt and black pepper.

Heat olive oil over medium heat in a large skillet and add seasoned chicken.

Reduce the temperature and cook for about 15 minutes.

Shred the chicken and place in the crock pot.

Process the chicken broth and onions in a blender and blend until smooth.

Pour into crock pot and stir in the remaining ingredients.

Cook on low for about 6 hours, stirring once while cooking.

Nutrition: Calories: 261 Carbs: 2g Fats: 21g Proteins: 14.1g Sodium: 264mg Sugar: 0.3g

Mozzarella Pasta Mix

Preparation Time: 5 minutes

Cooking Time: 15 minutes

Servings: 2

Ingredients:

2 oz whole grain elbow macaroni

1 tablespoon fresh basil

¼ cup cherry size Mozzarella

½ cup cherry tomatoes, halved

1 tablespoon olive oil

1 teaspoon dried marjoram

1 cup water, for cooking

Directions:

Boil elbow macaroni in water for 15 minutes. Drain water and chill macaroni little.

Chop fresh basil roughly and place it in the salad bowl.

Add Mozzarella, cherry tomatoes, dried marjoram, olive oil, amd macaroni.

Mix up salad well.

Nutrition: :calories 170, fat 9.7, fiber 1.1, carbs 15, protein 6

Quinoa Salad

Preparation Time: 5 minutes

Cooking Time: 20 minutes

Servings: 2

Ingredients:

2 cups red quinoa

4 cups water

1 (15-oz.) can chickpeas, drained

1 medium red onion, chopped (1/2 cup)

3 TB. fresh mint leaves, finely chopped

1/4 cup extra-virgin olive oil

3 TB. fresh lemon juice

1/2 tsp. salt

1/2 tsp. fresh ground black pepper

Directions:

In a medium saucepan over medium-high heat, bring red quinoa and water to a boil. Cover, reduce heat to low, and cook for 20 minutes or until water is absorbed and quinoa is tender. Let cool.

In a large bowl, add quinoa, chickpeas, red onion, and mint.

In a small bowl, whisk together extra-virgin olive oil, lemon juice, salt, and black pepper.

Pour dressing over quinoa mixture, and stir well to combine.

Serve immediately, or refrigerate and enjoy for up to 2 or 3 days.

Couscous And Toasted Almonds

Preparation Time: 5 minutes

Cooking Time: 10 minutes

Servings: 2

Ingredients:

1 cup (about 200 g) whole-grain couscous

400 ml boiling water

1 tablespoon extra-virgin olive oil

1/2 red onion, chopped

1/2 teaspoon ground ginger,

1/2 teaspoon ground cinnamon and

1/2 teaspoon ground coriander

2 tablespoons blanched almonds, toasted, and chopped

Directions:

Preheat the oven to 110C.

In a casserole, toss the couscous with the olive oil, onion, spices, salt and pepper. Stir in the boiling water, cover, and bake for 10 minutes. Fluff using a fork. Scatter the nuts over the top and then serve. Pair with harira.

Nutrition: :261.23 cal,8 g total fat (1 g sat. fat), 37 g carb, 7 g protein, 1 g sugar, and 6.85 mg sodium.

Spanish Tomato Salad

Preparation Time: 5 minutes

Cooking Time: 10 minutes

Servings: 2

Ingredients:

1 pound tomatoes, cubed

2 cucumbers, cubed

2 garlic cloves, chopped

1 red onion, sliced

2 anchovy fillets

1 tablespoon balsamic vinegar

1 pinch chili powder

Salt and pepper to taste

Directions:

Combine the tomatoes, cucumbers, garlic and red onion in a bowl.

In a mortar, mix the anchovy fillets, vinegar, chili powder, salt and pepper.

Drizzle the mixture over the salad and mix well.

Serve the salad fresh.

Nutrition: Per Serving:Calories: 61 Fat: 0.6g Protein: 3.0g Carbohydrates: 13.0g

Chickpeas And Beets Mix

Preparation Time: 5 minutes

Cooking Time: 25 minutes

Servings: 2

Ingredients:

3 tablespoons capers, drained and chopped

Juice of 1 lemon

Zest of 1 lemon, grated

1 red onion, chopped

3 tablespoons olive oil

14 ounces canned chickpeas, drained

8 ounces beets, peeled and cubed

1 tablespoon parsley, chopped

Salt and pepper to the taste

Directions:

Heat up a pan with the oil over medium heat, add the onion, lemon zest, lemon juice and the capers and sauté fro 5 minutes.

Add the rest of the ingredients, stir and cook over medium-low heat for 20 minutes more.

Divide the mix between plates and serve as a side dish.

Nutrition: calories 199, fat 4.5, fiber 2.3, carbs 6.5, protein 3.3

Roasted Bell Pepper Salad With Anchovy Dressing

Preparation Time: 5 minutes

Cooking Time: 20 minutes

Servings: 2

Ingredients:

8 roasted red bell peppers, sliced

2 tablespoons pine nuts

1 cup cherry tomatoes, halved

2 tablespoons chopped parsley

4 anchovy fillets

1 lemon, juiced

1 garlic clove

1 tablespoon extra-virgin olive oil

Salt and pepper to taste

Directions:

Combine the anchovy fillets, lemon juice, garlic and olive oil in a mortar and mix them well.

Mix the rest of the ingredients in a salad bowl then drizzle in the dressing.

Serve the salad as fresh as possible.

Nutrition: Per Serving: Calories: 81 Fat: 7.0g Protein: 2.4g Carbohydrates: 4.0g

Warm Shrimp And Arugula Salad

Preparation Time: 5 minutes

Cooking Time: 20 minutes

Servings: 2

Ingredients:

2 tablespoons extra virgin olive oil

2 garlic cloves, minced

1 red pepper, sliced

1 pound fresh shrimps, peeled and deveined

1 orange, juiced

Salt and pepper to taste

3 cups arugula

Directions:

Heat the oil in a frying pan and stir in the garlic and red pepper. Cook for 1 minute then add the shrimps.

Cook for 5 minutes then add the orange juice and cook for another 5 more minutes.

When done, spoon the shrimps and the sauce over the arugula.

Serve the salad fresh.

Nutrition: Per Serving:Calories:232 Fat:9.2g Protein:27.0g Carbohydrates:10.0g

Cheesy Tomato Salad

Preparation Time: 5 minutes

Cooking Time: 0 minutes

Servings: 2

Ingredients:

2 pounds tomatoes, sliced

1 red onion, chopped

Sea salt and black pepper to the taste

4 ounces feta cheese, crumbled

2 tablespoons mint, chopped

A drizzle of olive oil

Directions:

In a salad bowl, mix the tomatoes with the onion and the rest of the ingredients, toss and serve as a side salad.

Nutrition: calories 190, fat 4.5, fiber 3.4, carbs 8.7, protein 3.3

Garlic Cucumber Mix

Preparation Time: 5 minutes

Cooking Time: 10 minutes

Servings: 2

Ingredients:

2 cucumbers, sliced

2 spring onions, chopped

2 tablespoons olive oil

3 garlic cloves, grated

1 tablespoon thyme, chopped

Salt and black pepper to the taste

3 and ½ ounces goat cheese, crumbled

Directions:

In a salad bowl, mix the cucumbers with the onions and the rest of the ingredients, toss and serve after keeping it in the fridge for 15 minutes.

Nutrition: calories 140, fat 5.4, fiber 4.3, carbs 6.5, protein 4.8

Cucumber Salad Japanese Style

Preparation Time: 5 minutes

Cooking Time: 10 minutes

Servings: 2

Ingredients:

1 ½ tsp minced fresh ginger root

1 tsp salt

1/3 cup rice vinegar

2 large cucumbers, ribbon cut

4 tsp white sugar

Directions:

Mix well ginger, salt, sugar and vinegar in a small bowl.

Add ribbon cut cucumbers and mix well.

Let stand for at least one hour in the ref before serving.

Nutrition: Calories per Serving: 29; Fat: .2g; Protein: .7g; Carbs: 6.1g

Cheesy Keto Zucchini Soup

Preparation Time: 5 minutes

Cooking Time: 10 minutes

Servings: 2

Ingredients:

½ medium onion, peeled and chopped

1 cup bone broth

1 tablespoon coconut oil

1½ zucchinis, cut into chunks

½ tablespoon nutrition al yeast

Dash of black pepper

½ tablespoon parsley, chopped, for garnish

½ tablespoon coconut cream, for garnish

Directions:

Melt the coconut oil in a large pan over medium heat and add onions.

Sauté for about 3 minutes and add zucchinis and bone broth.

Reduce the heat to simmer for about 15 minutes and cover the pan.

Add nutrition al yeast and transfer to an immersion blender.

Blend until smooth and season with black pepper.

Top with coconut cream and parsley to serve.

Nutrition: Calories: 154 Carbs: 8.9g Fats: 8.1g Proteins: 13.4g Sodium: 93mg Sugar: 3.9g

Grilled Salmon Summer Salad

Preparation Time: 5 minutes

Cooking Time: 30 minutes

Servings: 2

Ingredients:

Salmon fillets - 2

Salt and pepper - to taste

Vegetable stock - 2 cups

Bulgur - 1 2 cup

Cherry tomatoes - 1 cup, halved

Sweet corn - 1 2 cup

Lemon - 1, juiced

Green olives - 1 2 cup, sliced

Cucumber - 1, cubed

Green onion - 1, chopped

Red pepper - 1, chopped

Red bell pepper - 1, cored and diced

Directions:

Heat a grill pan on medium and then place salmon on, seasoning with salt and pepper. Grill both sides of salmon until brown and set aside.

Heat stock in sauce pan until hot and then add in bulgur and cook until liquid is completely soaked into bulgur.

Mix salmon, bulgur and all other Ingredients in a salad bowl and again add salt and pepper, if desired, to suit your taste.

Serve salad as soon as completed.

Nutrition: Calories 69, Fat 6.5 g, Fiber 2.6 g, Carbs 10.6 g, Protein 9.4 g

Dill Beets Salad

Preparation Time: 5 minutes

Cooking Time: 0 minutes

Servings: 2

Ingredients:

2 pounds beets, cooked, peeled and cubed

2 tablespoons olive oil

1 tablespoon lemon juice

2 tablespoons balsamic vinegar

1 cup feta cheese, crumbled

3 small garlic cloves, minced

4 green onions, chopped

5 tablespoons parsley, chopped

Salt and black pepper to the taste

Directions:

In a bowl, mix the beets with the oil, lemon juice and the rest of the ingredients, toss and serve as a side dish.

Nutrition: calories 268, fat 15.5, fiber 5.1, carbs 25.7, protein 9.6

Green Couscous With Broad Beans, Pistachio, And Dill

Preparation Time: 5 minutes

Cooking Time: 10 minutes

Servings: 2

Ingredients:

200 g fresh or frozen broad beans, podded

2 teaspoons ground ginger

2 tablespoons spring onion, thinly sliced

2 tablespoons pistachio kernels, roughly chopped

2 tablespoons lemon juice, and wedges to serve

Dill, chopped - 1/4 cup

Olive oil, extra-virgin - 1/4 cup (about 60 ml)

1/2 onion, thinly sliced

Watercress, leaves picked - 1/2 bunch

1/2 avocado, chopped

1 green bell pepper, thinly sliced

1 garlic clove, crushed

1 cup (about 200 g) whole-grain couscous

1 1/2 cups boiling water

Directions:

In a heat-safe bowl, toss the couscous with the ginger and the onion. Stir in the boiling water, cover and let stand for 5 minutes.

Meanwhile, cook the beans for about 3 minutes in boiling salted water, drain, and refresh under running cold water; discard the outer skins.

With a fork, fluff the couscous. Add the beans, avocado, bell pepper, spring onion, and dill.

In a bowl, whisk the olive oil, lemon juice, and garlic; toss with the couscous. Scatter the pistachio over the mix, serve with cress and the lemon wedges.

Nutrition: :608 cal, 25.40 g total fat (4 g sat. fat), 51.50 g carb, 18.10 g protein, 45 mg sodium, and 11 g fiber.

Bell Peppers Salad

Preparation Time: 5 minutes

Cooking Time: 10 minutes

Servings: 2

Ingredients:

2 green bell peppers, cut into thick strips

2 red bell peppers, cut into thick strips

2 tablespoons olive oil

1 garlic clove, minced

½ cup goat cheese, crumbled

A pinch of salt and black pepper

Directions:

In a bowl, mix the bell peppers with the garlic and the other ingredients, toss and serve.

Nutrition: calories 193, fat 4.5, fiber 2, carbs 4.3, protein 3

Thyme Corn And Cheese Mix

Preparation Time: 5 minutes

Cooking Time: 10 minutes

Servings: 2

Ingredients:

1 tablespoon olive oil

1 teaspoon thyme, chopped

1 cup scallions, sliced

2 cups corn

Salt and black pepper to the taste

2 tablespoons blue cheese, crumbled

1 tablespoon chives, chopped

Directions:

In a salad bowl, combine the corn with scallions, thyme and the rest of the ingredients, toss, divide between plates and serve.

Nutrition: calories 183, fat 5.5, fiber 7.5, carbs 14.5

Garden Salad With Oranges And Olives

Preparation Time: 5 minutes

Cooking Time: 10 minutes

Servings: 2

Ingredients:

½ cup red wine vinegar

1 tbsp extra virgin olive oil

1 tbsp finely chopped celery

1 tbsp finely chopped red onion

16 large ripe black olives

2 garlic cloves

2 navel oranges, peeled and segmented

4 boneless, skinless chicken breasts, 4-oz each

4 garlic cloves, minced

8 cups leaf lettuce, washed and dried

Cracked black pepper to taste

Directions:

Preparation are the dressing by mixing pepper, celery, onion, olive oil, garlic and vinegar in a small bowl. Whisk well to combine.

Lightly grease grate and preheat grill to high.

Rub chicken with the garlic cloves and discard garlic.

Grill chicken for 5 minutes per side or until cooked through.

Remove from grill and let it stand for 5 minutes before cutting into ½-inch strips.

In 4 serving plates, evenly arrange two cups lettuce, ¼ of the sliced oranges and 4 olives per plate.

Top each plate with ¼ serving of grilled chicken, evenly drizzle with dressing, serve and enjoy.

Nutrition: Calories per serving: 259.8; Protein: 48.9g; Carbs: 12.9g; Fat: 1.4g

Smoked Salmon Lentil Salad

Preparation Time: 5 minutes

Cooking Time: 10 minutes

Servings: 2

Ingredients:

1 cup green lentils, rinsed

2 cups vegetable stock

½ cup chopped parsley

2 tablespoons chopped cilantro

1 red pepper, chopped

1 red onion, chopped

Salt and pepper to taste

4 oz. smoked salmon, shredded

1 lemon, juiced

Directions:

Combine the lentils and stock in a saucepan. Cook on low heat for 15-20 minutes or until all the liquid has been absorbed completely.

Transfer the lentils in a salad bowl and add the parsley, cilantro, red pepper and onion. Season with salt and pepper.

Add the smoked salmon and lemon juice and mix well.

Serve the salad fresh.

Nutrition: Per Serving:Calories:233 Fat:2.0g Protein:18.7g Carbohydrates:35.5g

Salmon & Arugula Salad

Preparation Time: 5 minutes

Cooking Time: 10 minutes

Servings: 2

Ingredients:

¼ cup red onion, sliced thinly

1 ½ tbsp fresh lemon juice

1 ½ tbsp olive oil

1 tbsp extra-virgin olive oil

1 tbsp red-wine vinegar

2 center cut salmon fillets (6-oz each)

2/3 cup cherry tomatoes, halved

3 cups baby arugula leaves

Pepper and salt to taste

Directions:

In a shallow bowl, mix pepper, salt, 1 ½ tbsp olive oil and lemon juice. Toss in salmon fillets and rub with the marinade. Allow to marinate for at least 15 minutes.

Grease a baking sheet and preheat oven to 350oF.

Bake marinated salmon fillet for 10 to 12 minutes or until flaky with skin side touching the baking sheet.

Meanwhile, in a salad bowl mix onion, tomatoes and arugula.

Season with pepper and salt. Drizzle with vinegar and oil. Toss to combine and serve right away with baked salmon on the side.

Nutrition: Calories per serving: 400; Protein: 36.6g; Carbs: 5.8g; Fat: 25.6g

Keto Bbq Chicken Pizza Soup

Preparation Time: 5 minutes

Cooking Time: 1 Hour 10 minutes

Servings: 2

Ingredients:

6 chicken legs

1 medium red onion, diced

4 garlic cloves

1 large tomato, unsweetened

4 cups green beans

¾ cup BBQ Sauce

1½ cups mozzarella cheese, shredded

¼ cup ghee

2 quarts water

2 quarts chicken stock

Salt and black pepper, to taste

Fresh cilantro, for garnishing

Directions:

Put chicken, water and salt in a large pot and bring to a boil.

Reduce the heat to medium-low and cook for about 75 minutes.

Shred the meat off the bones using a fork and keep aside.

Put ghee, red onions and garlic in a large soup and cook over a medium heat.

Add chicken stock and bring to a boil over a high heat.

Add green beans and tomato to the pot and cook for about 15 minutes.

Add BBQ Sauce, shredded chicken, salt and black pepper to the pot.

Ladle the soup into serving bowls and top with shredded mozzarella cheese and cilantro to serve.

Nutrition: Calories: 449 Carbs: 7.1g Fats: 32.5g Proteins: 30.8g Sodium: 252mg Sugar: 4.7g

Mediterranean Garden Salad

Preparation Time: 5 minutes

Cooking Time: 10 minutes

Servings: 2

Ingredients:

6 cups mixed greens

2 cups cherry tomatoes, halved

1 medium red onion, sliced (1/2 cup)

3 TB. tahini paste

3 TB. fresh lemon juice

3 TB. balsamic vinegar

3 TB. plus 1 tsp. extra-virgin olive oil

3 TB. water

1/2 tsp. salt

1/2 tsp. fresh ground black pepper

1/2 cup pine nuts

Directions:

In a large bowl, add mixed greens, cherry tomatoes, and red onion.

In a small bowl, whisk together tahini paste, lemon juice, balsamic vinegar, 3 tablespoons extra-virgin olive oil, water, salt, and black pepper.

Preheat a small skillet over medium-low heat for 1 minute. Add remaining 1 teaspoon extra-virgin olive oil and pine nuts, and cook, stirring to toast evenly on all sides, for 4 minutes. Transfer pine nuts to a plate, and let cool for 2 minutes.

Pour dressing over vegetables, and toss to coat evenly. Top with toasted pine nuts, and serve immediately.

Nutrition: Calories 69, Fat 6.5 g, Fiber 2.6 g, Carbs 10.6 g, Protein 9.4 g

Buttery Millet

Preparation Time: 5 minutes

Cooking Time: 10 minutes

Servings: 2

Ingredients:

¼ cup mushrooms, sliced

¾ cup onion, diced

1 tablespoon olive oil

1 teaspoon salt

3 tablespoons milk

½ cup millet

1 cup of water

1 teaspoon butter

Directions:

Pour olive oil in the skillet and add the onion.

Add mushrooms and roast the vegetables for 10 minutes over the medium heat. Stir them from time to time.

Meanwhile, pour water in the pan.

Add millet and salt.

Cook the millet with the closed lid for 15 minutes over the medium heat.

Then add the cooked mushroom mixture in the millet.

Add milk and butter. Mix up the millet well.

Nutrition: :calories 198, fat 7.7, fiber 3.5, carbs 27.9, protein 4.7

Delicata Squash Soup

Preparation Time: 5 minutes

Cooking Time: 30 minutes

Servings: 2

Ingredients:

1½ cups beef bone broth

1 small onion, peeled and grated.

½ teaspoon sea salt

¼ teaspoon poultry seasoning

2 small Delicata Squash, chopped

2 garlic cloves, minced

2 tablespoons olive oil

¼ teaspoon black pepper

1 small lemon, juiced

5 tablespoons sour cream

Directions:

Put Delicata Squash and water in a medium pan and bring to a boil.

Reduce the heat and cook for about 20 minutes.

Drain and set aside.

Put olive oil, onions, garlic and poultry seasoning in a small sauce pan.

Cook for about 2 minutes and add broth.

Allow it to simmer for 5 minutes and remove from heat.

Whisk in the lemon juice and transfer the mixture in a blender.

Pulse until smooth and top with sour cream.

Nutrition: Calories: 109 Carbs: 4.9g Fats: 8.5g Proteins: 3g Sodium: 279mg Sugar: 2.4g

Parsley Couscous And Cherries Salad

Preparation Time: 5 minutes

Cooking Time: 0 minutes

Servings: 2

Ingredients:

2 cups hot water

1 cup couscous

½ cup walnuts, roasted and chopped

½ cup cherries, pitted

½ cup parsley, chopped

A pinch of sea salt and black pepper

1 tablespoon lime juice

2 tablespoons olive oil

Directions:

Put the couscous in a bowl, add the hot water, cover, leave aside for 10 minutes, fluff with a fork and transfer to a bowl.

Add the rest of the ingredients, toss and serve.

Nutrition: calories 200, fat 6.71, fiber 7.3, carbs 8.5, protein 5

Mint Quinoa

Preparation Time: 5 minutes

Cooking Time: 10 minutes

Servings: 2

Ingredients:

1 cup quinoa

1 ¼ cup water

4 teaspoons lemon juice

¼ teaspoon garlic clove, diced

5 tablespoons sesame oil

2 cucumbers, chopped

1/3 teaspoon ground black pepper

1/3 cup tomatoes, chopped

½ oz scallions, chopped

¼ teaspoon fresh mint, chopped

Directions:

Pour water in the pan. Add quinoa and boil it for 10 minutes.

Then close the lid and let it rest for 5 minutes more.

Meanwhile, in the mixing bowl mix up together lemon juice, diced garlic, sesame oil, cucumbers, ground black pepper, tomatoes, scallions, and fresh mint.

Then add cooked quinoa and carefully mix the side dish with the help of the spoon.

Store tabbouleh up to 2 days in the fridge.

Nutrition: :calories 168, fat 9.9, fiber 2, carbs 16.9, protein 3.6

Spicy Halibut Tomato Soup

Preparation Time: 5 minutes

Cooking Time: 60 minutes

Servings: 2

Ingredients:

2garliccloves, minced

1tablespoonolive oil

¼ cup fresh parsley, chopped

10anchoviescanned in oil, minced

6cupsvegetable broth

1teaspoonblack pepper

1poundhalibut fillets, chopped

3tomatoes, peeled and diced

1teaspoonsalt

1teaspoonred chili flakes

Directions:

Heat olive oil in a large stockpot over medium heat and add garlic and half of the parsley.

Add anchovies, tomatoes, vegetable broth, red chili flakes, salt and black pepper and bring to a boil.

Reduce the heat to medium-low and simmer for about 20 minutes.

Add halibut fillets and cook for about 10 minutes.

Dish out the halibut and shred into small pieces.

Mix back with the soup and garnish with the remaining fresh parsley to serve.

Nutrition: Calories: 170 Carbs: 3g Fats: 6.7g Proteins: 23.4g Sodium: 2103mg Sugar: 1.8g

Chicken salad

Preparation Time: 5 minutes

Cooking Time: 10 minutes

Servings: 2

Ingredients

1 cup buffalo sauce

1 tablespoon honey

1 tsp lime

1 tsp salt

1 tsp onion powder

1 tablespoon olive oil

1 cup salad dressing

Directions

In a bowl combine all ingredients together and mix well

Add dressing and serve

Farro salad

Preparation Time: 5 minutes

Cooking Time: 10 minutes

Servings: 2

Ingredients

1 cup farro

1 bay leaf

1 shallot

¼ cup olive oil

1 tablespoon apple cider vinegar

1 tsp honey

1 cup arugula

1 apple

¼ cup basil

¼ cup parsley

Directions

In a bowl combine all ingredients together and mix well

Add dressing and serve

Nutrition: Calories 69, Fat 6.5 g, Fiber 2.6 g, Carbs 10.6 g, Protein 9.4 g

Carrot salad

Preparation Time: 5 minutes

Cooking Time: 10 minutes

Servings: 2

Ingredients

1 lb. carrots

1 cup raisins

½ cup peanuts

½ cup cilantro

2 green onions

¼ cup olive oil

1 tablespoon honey

2 cloves garlic

1 tsp cumin

Directions

In a bowl combine all ingredients together and mix well

Add dressing and serve

Nutrition: Calories 69, Fat 6.5 g, Fiber 2.6 g, Carbs 10.6 g, Protein 9.4 g

Beets Steamed Edamame Salad

Preparation time: 15 minutes

Cooking time 5 minutes

Servings: 8

Ingredients:

2 bag of steamed edamame beans

White vinegar

20-24 oz. can of beets

4 teaspoon of olive oil of high quality

12 large organic carrots, cubed

6 corn on the cobs, corn cut off

Black pepper

1 pound of green beans cut in 1 inch segments

Directions

Wet a paper towel and wrapped the corn with the damp towel; place the wrapped corn in the microwave for 5 minutes.

Steam the entire ingredients (reserving corn and beets) in large steamer in this other; carrots cubes, green beans, and edamame beans on the top layer.

Mix beets together with the cooked corn and cooked vegetables.

Toss salad slightly with a few dashes of black pepper, white vinegar and olive oil.

Nutrition: Calories 317, Fat 36.5 g, Fiber 3.6 g, Carbs 17.6 g, Protein 17.4 g

Avocado Cilantro Chunky Salsa

Preparation time: 10 minutes

Cooking time 0 minutes

Servings: 6

Ingredients:

6 tbsp of chopped cilantro leaves

3 tbsp of avocado or macadamia nut oil

3 large diced ripe tomato

1 ½ finely diced spring onion

3 large diced avocado

Salt and pepper

6 tbsp of lime juice

Directions

Add the entire ingredients together in a bowl and carefully toss. Serve right away.

Nutrition: Calories 317, Fat 36.5 g, Fiber 3.6 g, Carbs 17.6 g, Protein 17.4 g

Potatoes Mixed Vegetables

Preparation time: 10 minutes

Cooking time 1 hour 20 minutes

Servings: 12

Ingredients:

12 thinly sliced medium tomatoes

2 tbsp of dried oregano

2 cup water

2 1/2 cups of tomato passata or tomato puree

1 cup of extra-virgin olive oil, plus more if needed

4 tbsp of finely chopped flat-leaf parsley

10 sliced into rounds small zucchini

2 thinly sliced large onion

24 cherry tomatoes

6 sliced garlic cloves

2 large eggplant, sliced lengthwise and cut into half round thick slices

Salt and fresh ground pepper

3 lbs (about 8 medium) potatoes cut into 1/2 inch cube

Directions

Heat up your oven to 425 F.

Pour about four tablespoons of olive oil in a saucepan over medium heat, cook the eggplant in hot oil in batches for about 5–7 minutes, (you can add more oil if needed) until the eggplants are golden and softened; Set aside in a bowl.

Add the sliced garlic cloves and sliced onion into the pan used in cooking eggplants, sauté until fragrant and softened, about 5 minutes. Set aside in the bowl containing the eggplants.

Add two cups of water, potato cubes, passata, zucchini and tomatoes to the bowl. Sprinkle on top with the chopped parsley leaf and oregano; Season with ground black pepper and salt. Mix very well to fully combine, then transfer to a broad ovenproof dish. Drizzle with oil.

Place in the preheated oven and bake for 30 minutes.

Reduce oven heat to 400 F and bake for 20–30 minutes extra, or until the vegetables are tender and top is brown. Let cool a bit before serving.

Nutrition: Calories 317, Fat 36.5 g, Fiber 3.6 g, Carbs 17.6 g, Protein 17.4 g

Toasted Mango Pepitas Kale Salad

Preparation time: 20 minutes

Cooking time 0 minutes

Servings 8

Ingredients:

4 tsps of honey

2 fresh mango, thinly diced (about 1 cup)

Freshly ground black pepper

4 full tbsp of toasted pepitas

Kosher salt

One lemon juice

2 large bunch of kale de-stalk and sliced into ribbons

1/2 cup of extra-virgin olive oil, plus more

Directions

Add the sliced kale into a large mixing bowl; add half the lemon juice and little salt.

Start working on the kale using your fingertips for five minutes, or until the kale leaves are tender and sweet.

Spread olive oil over the kale and work on the kale with your finger for few more minute. Set aside.

Blend the black pepper, honey with the remaining half lemon juice in a small bowl.

Steadily drip in 1/2 cup of olive oil while whisking until it forms a dressing. Season dressing with a pinch of salt.

Pour few dressing on the kale, and add the pepitas and mango. Toss together and serve.

Nutrition: Calories 317, Fat 36.5 g, Fiber 3.6 g, Carbs 17.6 g, Protein 17.4 g

Chickpea And Parsley Pumpkin Salad

Preparation time: 5 minutes

Cooking time 10 minutes

Servings: 6

Ingredients:

1 1/2 small thinly sliced red onion

1 1/2 handful parsley, chopped

1 1/2 diced avocado

1 1/2 tbsp of lemon juice

1 1/2 tsp of ground coriander

1 1/2 tsp of ground cumin

Salt and pepper, to season

3 tbsp of olive oil

1 1/2 cup of pumpkin, peeled and chopped into bite pieces

1 1/2 (21.5 oz) can of chickpeas, rinsed and drained

Directions

Season the pumpkin with a drizzle of olive oil, coriander and cumin on top.

Arrange seasoned pumpkin in an oven tray lined with parchment paper.

Roast until the pumpkin is lightly browned and soft.

2. Combine the salad ingredients into a bowl, and then drizzle in lemon juice.

Nutrition: Calories 317, Fat 36.5 g, Fiber 3.6 g, Carbs 17.6 g, Protein 17.4 g

White Bean Cherry Tomatoes Cucumber Salad

Preparation time: 10 minutes

Cooking time 10 minutes

Servings: 3

Ingredients:

1 ½ avocado, diced

Cherry tomatoes and chopped cucumbers

1 Cup of canned white beans, rinsed and drained

6 teaspoons of extra-virgin olive oil

3 tablespoon of red-wine vinegar

3/4 cup of crumbled feta cheese

3/4 cup of chopped red onion

Freshly ground pepper to taste

6 cups of mixed salad greens

3/4 teaspoon of kosher salt

Directions

Combine beans, veggies, avocado and greens in a medium bowl.

Season with salt and pepper.

Drizzle with vinegar and oil, combine by tossing then transfer into a large plate.

Nutrition: Calories 317, Fat 36.5 g, Fiber 3.6 g, Carbs 17.6 g, Protein 17.4 g

Arugula Cucumber Tuna Salad

Preparation time: 5 minutes

Cooking time 5 minutes

Servings: 4

Ingredients:

1 tsp of dried oregano

2 tbsp of lemon juice

4 tbsp of olive oil

12 oz canned of tuna, drained

2 handfuls of arugula leaves

1 sliced Lebanese cucumber

2 small coarsely grated zucchini

1 cup of cherry tomatoes, halved

Directions

In a medium mixing bowl, combine together all salad ingredients. Drizzle with lemon juice and olive oil. Enjoy!

Nutrition: Calories 317, Fat 36.5 g, Fiber 3.6 g, Carbs 17.6 g, Protein 17.4 g

Springtime Chicken Berries Salad

Preparation time: 5 minutes

Cooking time 5 minutes

Servings: 8

Ingredients:

Salad:

4 cups of quartered strawberries

2/3 cup of vertically sliced red onion

2 cup of fresh blueberries

24 oz of boneless, skinless, rotisserie chicken breast, sliced

8 cups of arugula

8 cups of torn romaine lettuce

Dressing:

2 tbsp of water

2/8 tsps of freshly ground black pepper

2/8 tsps of salt

4 tbsp of extra-virgin olive oil

4 tbsp of red wine vinegar

2 tbsp of low carb sweetener of your choice

Directions

In a large mixing bowl, combine together the blueberries, strawberries, arugula, romaine and onions. Toss gently to combine.

Combine together 2 tbsp of water, black pepper, red wine vinegar salt and sweetener in a small bowl. Fold in the olive oil, stirring often until well incorporated.

Arrange eight different plates and place up to 2 cups of chicken mixture on each. Drizzle with 4 teaspoons of the dressing.

Nutrition: Calories 317, Fat 36.5 g, Fiber 3.6 g, Carbs 17.6 g, Protein 17.4 g

Toaster Almond Spiralized Beet Salad

Preparation time: 15 minutes

Cooking time 15 minutes

Servings: 4

Ingredients:

1/8 teaspoon of ground pepper

1/8 cup of extra-virgin olive oil

1/4 teaspoon of freshly grated lemon zest

1 pounds beets (2 medium)

1/4 cup of (fresh) chopped flat-leaf parsley

1 tablespoons of lemon juice

1/4 cup of slivered almonds, toasted

1/4 teaspoon of salt

1/6 cup of minced shallot

Directions

Mix together the minced shallot, lemon juice, oil, salt, pepper and lemon zest into a small bowl. Mix gently to combine then set aside.

Peel the beets with a thin blade, then spiralize and cut into 3-inch lengths.

Arrange the spiralized beets into a large bowl. Sprinkle beets top with the dressing, toss gently to make sure salad is finely coated.

Add chopped parsley and almonds before serving. Toss to coat.

Nutrition: Calories 317, Fat 36.5 g, Fiber 3.6 g, Carbs 17.6 g, Protein 17.4 g

Apple Leeks Mascarpone Soup

Preparation time: 5 minutes

Cooking time 35 minutes

Servings: 3

Ingredients:

1/2 cup of chopped leeks

Salt and pepper

Nutmeg to taste

1 cored, peeled and diced apple

1.5 lbs of butternut squash, peeled and cubed

1/2 chopped medium onion

1 tbsp of unsalted butter

3 cups of chicken stock

For the Mascarpone Topping:

1 tablespoons of milk

1/4 teaspoon of cinnamon

1/4 cup of mascarpone cheese

Directions

Melt butter over medium heat in a large pot. Add apples, leeks, and onions. Cook about 8 minutes until soft and translucent.

Add chicken stock into the pot along with squash and cook until heated through, then simmer on low heat for about 20 to 25 minutes until squash is tender. Set aside.

Mascarpone topping: In the meantime, combine together the 3 last ingredients and stir until totally combined. Set aside.

Blend soup using an immersion blender or puree in a blender and transfer back to the pot.

Stir well and season the soup with pepper nutmeg and salt.

Pour soup into bowls and serve with a dollop of mascarpone topping in the middle.

Nutrition: Calories 317, Fat 36.5 g, Fiber 3.6 g, Carbs 17.6 g, Protein 17.4 g

Aminos Mushroom Soup

Preparation time: 10 minutes

Cooking time 35 minutes

Servings: 8

Ingredients:

4 dried bay leaves

Black pepper, freshly ground

4 tablespoons of tapioca flour

4 cups of unsweetened almond or cashew milk

4 cups of organic vegetable broth

2 tsp salt

40 stalks of fresh thyme, leaves removed

20 oz packages of sliced baby portobello mushroom

4 large diced white onions

20 oz packages of sliced white button mushroom

2 tablespoon of liquid aminos

Directions

Sweat the diced onions dry for about 5 to 7 minutes in a large non-stick saucepan over medium heat.

Shift the onions towards the sides of the saucepan, add mushrooms slices to the middle of the saucepan, and cook for 5 minutes without covering.

Mix both ingredients together, add in the thyme and keep cooking, about 10 minutes or more.

Add the liquid aminos, bay leaf and salt to the mushrooms onion mixture.

Mix the vegetable broth and tapioca starch in a small mixing bowl until no more lumps and well combined. Pour the mixture into the mushrooms and stir, then add almond milk.

Cook about 15 minutes, stirring once in a while until heated through. Adjust taste with freshly ground black pepper. You can add Parmesan cheese, cashew cheese if desired.

Nutrition: Calories 317, Fat 36.5 g, Fiber 3.6 g, Carbs 17.6 g, Protein 17.4 g

Detox-Liver Arugula And Broccoli Soup

Preparation time: 3 minutes

Cooking time 20 minutes

Servings: 4

Ingredients:

5 cups of water

2 cup of arugula leaves, packed

1/2 teaspoon of dried thyme

1/2 teaspoon of freshly ground black pepper

2 tablespoon olive oil

1/2 teaspoon of salt

1 lemon Juice

1 yellow or Spanish onion, roughly diced

2 clove of garlic, chopped

2 (about 4/6 pounds) head broccoli, cut into little florets

Directions

Heat 2 tablespoon of olive oil over medium in a large saucepan. Cook onion in the heated oil until soft and translucent.

Pour in chopped garlic and cook for 60 seconds, add broccoli and keep cooking for about 4 minutes more or until it is bright green. Add 1/2 teaspoon of freshly ground black pepper, salt, thyme and cups of water. Allow mixture to heat through, lower heat and cook with the lid on for about 8 minutes or until broccoli is tender.

Blend the soup in a blender or use an immersion blender. Add the arugula, blend until smooth. Serve with lemon juice.

Nutrition: Calories 352, Fat 22.5 g, Fiber 1.6 g, Carbs 7.6 g, Protein 10.4 g

Unique Lentil with KaleSoup

Preparation time: 10 minutes

Cook time 1 hour 10 minutes

Servings: 2

Ingredients

1/2 cup of wild rice

1/2 cup of steel cut oats or barley

1/2 cup of lentils (any will do)

4 cups of kale, chopped

1/2 cup of French lentils

8 cups of vegetarian broth

Directions

Cook the vegetarian broth in a soup pot over medium heat until heated through and add other ingredients, stir.

Simmer on low with the lid on for 45 minutes to 1 hour.

Add chopped kale, stir and simmer for 10 more minutes. Serve and enjoy.

Pasta Veggies Minestrone Soup

Preparation time: 15 minutes

Cooking time 40 minutes

Servings: 2-4

Ingredients:

1 tbsp basil, finely chopped or 1 tsp of dried basil

1 minced garlic cloves

14 ounce can of diced plum tomatoes

1/8 tsp of salt

1/8 cup of your preferred pasta

1/16 tsp black pepper, freshly ground

3/8 cup of diced celery

1/2 cup of cannellini beans

1.5 cups of water

1/2 cup of carrots, peeled and sliced

1 cups of diced zucchini

3/8 cup of chopped onion

1/2 tbsp of extra virgin olive oil

1/8 tsp of dried oregano

Directions

Heat-up a saucepan over medium heat.

Drizzle saucepan with olive oil and sauté the chopped onion, about 4 minutes, stirring periodically until browned a bit. Without the pasta, add in the rest ingredients and bring to a boil.

Reduce to low heat and simmer with the lid on for 25 minutes, stirring occasionally.

Add and cook pasta according to package instructions, about 10-12 minutes until pasta is al dente.

Nutrition: Calories 352, Fat 22.5 g, Fiber 1.6 g, Carbs 7.6 g, Protein 10.4 g

Pear Red Pepper Soup

Preparation time: 10 minutes

Cooking time 40 minutes

Servings: 4-5

Ingredients:

1 sliced shallots

1/4 tsp of dried crushed red pepper

1 (16-oz.) container of no-fat chicken broth

1/4 tsp of ground black pepper

Pinch of ground red pepper

1 peeled and sliced Anjou pears

1 tbsp of butter

1 1/2 large sliced red bell peppers

1 tsp of olive oil

1/8 tsp of salt

Garnishes (optional): fresh thinly sliced pears, chopped fresh chives, plain yogurt

1 sliced carrots

Directions

Melt the olive oil with 1 tablespoon of butter over medium heat in a Dutch oven; add bell pepper, carrots, shallots, and Anjou pears and sauté until tender, about 8 to 10 minutes.

Stir in chicken broth and all the peppers, add salt. Cook until heated through. Cover with a lid and simmer on low heat for 25 to 30 minutes. Allow cooling for 20 minutes.

In the bowl of a food processor, add and process soup in batches until smooth, scraping the sides down as necessary. Transfer back to Dutch oven to keep warm until you are ready to use. Garnish, if desired.

Nutrition: Calories 352, Fat 22.5 g, Fiber 1.6 g, Carbs 7.6 g, Protein 10.4 g

Low Heat Chicken Provençal

Preparation time: 5 minutes

Cooking time 8 hours

Servings: 8

Ingredients:

1/4 tsp of freshly ground black pepper

2 (16 oz each) can of cannellini beans, rinsed and drained

2 tsp of dried thyme

2 diced red pepper

2 diced yellow pepper

2 (14.5-oz each) can of petite diced tomatoes with basil, oregano and garlic, undrained

1/4 tsp of salt

4 tsp of dried basil

12 oz (skins removed) bone-in chicken breast halves

Directions

Arrange the chicken into a crock pot; add the rest ingredients into the pot.

Cook with the lid on for 8 hours on low-heat setting.

Nutrition: Calories 85, Fat 6.5 g, Fiber 0.6 g, Carbs 0.6 g, Protein 6.4 g

Danny's Tortellini Soup

Preparation time: 8 minutes

Cooking time 25 minutes

Servings: 3

Ingredients

1/2 peeled and diced potato

6-6 oz fresh tortellini or frozen (meat or cheese filled)

1 quarts of low sodium chicken stock

2 scallions

1/2 large can of crushed tomatoes (Spice the tomatoes with oregano and basil)

1 tbsp of olive oil

1 medium carrots, peeled and diced

1 small diced zucchini

Black pepper, to taste

1/4 teaspoon of salt

1 diced celery stalks

Directions

Heat 1 tablespoon of olive oil over medium in a large saucepan. Add in the scallions, diced potato, diced celery, carrots and diced zucchini.

Sauté the vegetables for 10 minutes over medium heat, stirring frequently until the vegetables are starting to soften. Add the tomatoes, chicken stock and salt. Flame heat up and bring to a low boil.

Add the tortellini and cook about two minutes, then simmer on low heat for 5 to 6 minutes more. Stir in the pepper.

Nutrition: Calories 85, Fat 6.5 g, Fiber 0.6 g, Carbs 0.6 g, Protein 6.4 g

Wellness Parsnip Soup

Preparation time: 10 minutes

Cooking time 20 minutes

Serves: 6

Ingredients:

3/4 cup of chopped pumpkin

Salt and pepper, to taste

1 1/2 tsps of ground cumin

7 1/2 cups of stock or broth

6 chopped medium parsnips

1 1/2 tbsp of dried oregano

1 1/2 tbsp of olive oil

4 1/2 crushed garlic cloves

1 1/2 finely chopped brown onion

3 chopped medium carrots

Directions

Heat 1 1/2 tablespoon of olive oil over medium heat in a large skillet. Sauté the onion and garlic in the pan for about 5 minutes until softened. Mix in the remaining ingredients, reserving only the broth or stock.

Cook and stir every now and then for 2 minutes. Add stock or broth and cook until soup is heated through. Simmer on low heat until the vegetables are tender. Puree the soup with an immersion blender, serve and enjoy.

Nutrition: Calories 85, Fat 6.5 g, Fiber 0.6 g, Carbs 0.6 g, Protein 6.4 g

Feel Good Chicken Soup

Preparation time: 10 minutes

Cooking time 10-15 minutes

Serves: 6

Ingredients:

3 large diced carrots

3 bay leaves

1 1/2 medium diced swede or turnip

3 sliced stalks celery

3 tsps of dried oregano

1 1/2 large sliced zucchini

3 tbsp of olive oil

7 1/2 cups of bone stock or broth

6 cups of leftover cooked chicken, shredded

1 1/2 cup of canned coconut cream

Salt and pepper

1 1/2 small diced brown onion

Directions

Add 3 tablespoons of olive oil in a large pot, sauté the vegetables until they are soft to your liking.

Add the remaining ingredients into the pot, reserving the coconut cream. When the vegetables are tender as desired, add in coconut cream and stir to combine.

Turn heat off, garnish with parsley.

Nutrition: Calories 85, Fat 6.5 g, Fiber 0.6 g, Carbs 0.6 g, Protein 6.4 g

Pork Soup

Preparation Time: 10 minutes

Cooking Time: 25 minutes

Servings: 2

Ingredients:

1 tablespoon avocado oil

1 onion, chopped

1 pound pork stew meat, cubed

4 cups of water

1 pound carrots, sliced

1 teaspoon tomato paste

Directions:

Heat up a pot with the oil over medium-high heat, add the onion and pork, and cook the ingredients for 5 minutes.

Add all remaining ingredients and cook the soup for 20 minutes.

Nutrition:

304 calories,

34.5g protein,

14.2g carbohydrates,

11.4g fat,

3.6g fiber,

98mg cholesterol,

155mg sodium,

Curry Soup

Preparation Time: 10 minutes

Cooking Time: 23 minutes

Servings: 2

Ingredients:

3 tablespoons olive oil

8 carrots, peeled and sliced

2 teaspoons curry paste

4 celery stalks, chopped

1 yellow onion, chopped

4 cups of water

Directions:

Heat up a pot with the oil and add onion, celery and carrots, stir and cook for 12 minutes.

Then add curry paste and water. Stir the soup well and cook it for 10 minutes more.

When all ingredients are soft, blend the soup until smooth and simmer it for 1 minute more.

Nutrition:

171 calories,

1.6g protein,

15.8g carbohydrates,

12g fat,

3.9g fiber,

0mg cholesterol,

106mg sodium,

Yellow Onion Soup

Preparation Time: 10 minutes

Cooking Time: 20 minutes

Servings: 2

Ingredients:

1 tablespoon avocado oil

1 yellow onion, chopped

1 teaspoon ginger, grated

1 pound zucchinis, chopped

4 cups low-sodium chicken broth

½ cup low-fat cream

1 teaspoon ground black pepper

Directions:

Heat up a pot with the oil over medium heat, add the onion and ginger, stir and cook for 5 minutes.

Add all remaining ingredients and simmer them over medium heat for 15 minutes.

Blend the cooked soup and ladle in the bowls.

Nutrition:

61 calories,

4.2g protein,

10.2g carbohydrates,

0.7g fat,

2.2g fiber,

1mg cholesterol,

101mg sodium,

8.4g fat,

18.5g fiber,

101mg cholesterol,

109mg sodium,

Garlic Soup

Preparation Time: 10 minutes

Cooking Time: 50 minutes

Servings: 2

Ingredients:

1 pound red kidney beans, cooked

8 cups of water

1 green bell pepper, chopped

1 tomato paste

1 yellow onion, chopped

1 teaspoon minced garlic

1 pound beef sirloin, cubed

1 teaspoon garlic powder

Directions:

Pour water in a pot and heat up over medium heat.

Add all ingredients and close the lid.

Simmer the soup for 45 minutes over the medium heat.

Nutrition:

620 calories,

60.9g protein,

75.8g carbohydrates,

Chapter 10: Desserts

Coconut Rhubarb Cream

Preparation Time: 1 hour

Cooking Time: 10 minutes

Servings: 4

Ingredients:

2 cups coconut cream

1 cup rhubarb, chopped

3 eggs, whisked

3 tablespoons coconut sugar

1 tablespoon lime juice

Directions:

In a small pan, combine the cream with the rhubarb and the other ingredients, whisk well, simmer over medium heat for 10 minutes, blend using an immersion blender, divide into bowls and keep in the fridge for 1 hour before serving.

Nutrition:

363calories

7.2g protein

17.3g carbohydrates

32g fat

65mg sodium

448g potassium

Honey-Cinnamon Grilled Plums

Preparation Time: 15 minutes

Cooking Time: 2 minutes

Servings: 4

Ingredients:

4 large plums, sliced in half and pitted

1 tablespoon olive oil

1 tablespoon honey

1 teaspoon ground cinnamon

2 cups vanilla bean frozen yogurt

Direction

Preheat the grill to medium heat.

Brush the plum halves with olive oil. Grill, flesh-side down, for 4 to 5 minutes, then flip and cook for another 4 to 5 minutes, until just tender.

In a small bowl, whisk together the honey and cinnamon.

Scoop the frozen yogurt into 4 bowls. Place 2 plum halves in each bowl and drizzle each with the cinnamon-honey mixture.

Nutrition

193 calories

8g fat

3g protein

30g carbohydrates

62mg sodium

192mg potassium

Raspberry Walnut Sorbet

Preparation Time: 5 minutes

Cooking Time: 0 minutes

Servings: 4

Ingredients:

2 cups fresh ripe raspberries

¼ cup chopped walnuts

1 teaspoon lemon juice

2 tablespoons organic agave nectar

Direction

In a food processor or blender, purée all ingredients together. Freeze in an ice cream maker. Alternately, spread fruit mixture onto a cookie sheet and place in freezer.

Every 20 minutes, scrape through fruit mixture with a spoon so that it doesn't freeze into a solid mass (this will keep it nice and light).

Nutrition

75 calories

4g fat

2g protein

9g carbohydrates

1mg sodium

18mg potassium

Chocolate Almond Pudding

Preparation Time: 5 minutes

Cooking Time: 15 minutes

Servings: 4

Ingredients:

2 tablespoons unsweetened cocoa powder

½ tablespoon arrowroot powder

1 cup evaporated skim milk

2 tablespoons agave nectar or brown rice syrup

1 teaspoon vanilla extract

4 tablespoons roasted slivered almonds

Direction

In a medium nonstick pan, whisk together the cocoa powder and arrowroot powder.

Over medium heat, add evaporated skim milk and agave nectar to cocoa powder mixture, and whisk to combine. Bring just to a simmer, whisking constantly to make sure it does not boil.

Cook 3 to 5 minutes, or until pudding is thick. Remove from heat. Stir in vanilla.

Allow to rest 30 minutes before serving or chill overnight. Spoon into four bowls. Top each bowl with 1 tablespoon of the almonds, and serve.

Nutrition

90 calories

3.6g fat

5.9g protein

11g carbohydrates

60mg sodium

101mg potassium

Figs with Honey-Chocolate Sauce

Preparation Time: 5 minutes

Cooking Time: 10 minutes

Servings: 4

Ingredients:

8 fresh or dried figs

¼ cup honey

2 tablespoons unsweetened cocoa powder

½ cup plain low-fat Greek yogurt

Direction

If using dried figs, place the figs in a small heat-proof bowl. Add boiling water to cover. Let rest in the hot water for 5 to 15 minutes; then drain before continuing.

Combine the honey and cocoa powder in a small bowl, and mix well to form a syrup.

Cut the figs in half and place cut side up. Drizzle with the syrup, top with a dollop of yogurt, and serve.

Nutrition

143 calories

0.7g fat

4g protein

35.2g carbohydrates

12mg sodium

48mg potassium

Lemon Ricotta Peaches

Preparation Time: 15 minutes

Cooking Time: 5 minutes

Servings: 4

Ingredients:

6 ripe peaches, pitted and thinly sliced

¼ cup water

2 tablespoons Sucanat, or other raw or brown sugar

1½ tablespoons lemon juice

1 cup low-fat ricotta

2 teaspoons lemon zest

Direction

In a heavy, medium-sized skillet, combine peaches, water, Sucanat, and lemon juice. Bring just to a simmer, stirring frequently. Remove from heat.

In a small bowl, combine ricotta and lemon zest. Mix well.

Divide peaches between four bowls. Top with ricotta and serve.

Nutrition

166 calories

5.3g fat

8g protein

26g carbohydrates

58mg sodium

118mg potassium

Rhubarb Compote

Preparation Time: 10 minutes

Cooking Time: 15 minutes

Servings: 4

Ingredients:

2 cups rhubarb, roughly chopped

3 tablespoons coconut sugar

1 teaspoon almond extract

2 cups of water

Directions:

In a pot, combine the rhubarb with the other ingredients, toss, bring to a boil over medium heat, cook for 15 minutes, divide into bowls and serve cold.

Nutrition:

52 calories

0.6g protein

11.9g carbohydrates

0.1g fat

6mg sodium

178g potassium

Vanilla Pumpkin Pudding

Preparation Time: 5 minutes

Cooking Time: 0 minutes

Servings: 6

Ingredients:

1½ cups fat-free vanilla yogurt

1 (20-ounce / 567-g) can plain pumpkin purée

½ teaspoon ground nutmeg

½ teaspoon ground cinnamon

1 vanilla bean

Direction

Combine yogurt, pumpkin purée, nutmeg, and cinnamon in a medium-sized mixing bowl. Scrape vanilla beans out of husk and into mixture. Mix well until all ingredients are combined. Chill until ready to serve.

Nutrition

95 calories

1.1g fat

4.1g protein

17g carbohydrates

38mg sodium

61mg potassium

Chocolate Truffles

Preparation Time: 15 minutes

Cooking Time: 0 minutes

Servings: 24

Ingredients:

For the truffles:

½ cup cacao powder

¼ cup chia seeds

¼ cup flaxseed meal

¼ cup maple syrup

1 cup flour

2 tablespoons almond milk

For the Coatings:

Cacao powder

Chia seeds

Flour

Shredded coconut, unsweetened

Directions:

Place all the fixing for the truffle in a blender; pulse until it is thoroughly blended; transfer contents to a bowl. Form into chocolate balls, then cover with the coating ingredients. Serve immediately.

Nutrition:

Calories 70

Sodium 2 mg

Fats 1 g

Carbohydrates 14 g

Fibers 2 g

Sugar 11 g

Proteins 1 g

Grilled Pineapple Strips

Preparation Time: 15 minutes

Cooking Time: 5 minutes

Servings: 6

Ingredients:

Vegetable oil

Dash of iodized salt

1 pineapple

1 tablespoon lime juice extract

1 tablespoon olive oil

1 tablespoon raw honey

3 tablespoons brown sugar

Directions:

Peel the pineapple, remove the eyes of the fruit, and discard the core. Slice lengthwise, forming six wedges. Mix the rest of the fixing in a bowl until blended.

Brush the coating mixture on the pineapple (reserve some for basting). Grease an oven or outdoor grill rack with vegetable oil.

Place the pineapple wedges on the grill rack and heat for a few minutes per side until golden brownish, basting it frequently with a reserved glaze. Serve on a platter.

Nutrition:

Calories 97

Fats 2 g

Carbohydrates 20 g

Sodium 2 mg

Sugar 17 g

Fibers 1 g

Proteins 1 g

Chocolate Chip Banana Muffin Top Cookies

Preparation Time: 15 minutes

Cooking Time: 15 minutes

Servings: 16

Ingredients:

1 cup quick oats

1 cup white whole-wheat flour

1/4 cup sugar

1 tablespoon sodium-free baking powder

1 teaspoon ground cinnamon

3 ripe medium bananas, mashed

4 tablespoons canola oil

1 tablespoon pure vanilla extract

3/4 cup chocolate chips

Directions:

Preheat oven to 350°F. Put aside a baking sheet with parchment paper. Measure the oats, flour, sugar, baking powder, and cinnamon into a mixing bowl and whisk. Put the rest of the fixing and stir just until combined.

Using a medium-sized ice cream scoop, scoop the batter onto the preparation ared baking sheet, leaving an inch or two between cookies. Bake within 15 minutes. Remove, then put on a wire rack to cool. Serve immediately.

Nutrition:

Calories: 150

Fat: 6 g

Protein: 2 g

Sodium: 0 mg

Fiber: 1 g

Carbohydrates: 23 g

Sugar: 10 g

Lemon Cookies

Preparation Time: 15 minutes

Cooking Time: 10 minutes

Servings: 36

Ingredients:

2 1/2 cups white whole-wheat flour

1 1/2 cups sugar

1 tablespoon sodium-free baking powder

3/4 cup canola oil

2 large lemons, juice, and grated zest

1 tablespoon pure vanilla extract

Directions:

Preheat oven to 350°F. Mix the flour, sugar, plus baking powder into a mixing bowl. Put the rest of the fixing and stir to form a stiff dough.

Drop by rounded tablespoons onto an ungreased baking sheet. Bake within 10 minutes. Remove, then let cool on sheet for a few minutes before transferring to a wire rack to cool fully. Serve immediately.

Nutrition:

Calories: 106

Fat: 5 g

Protein: 1 g

Sodium: 0 mg

Fiber: 0 g

Carbohydrates: 15 g

Sugar: 8 g

Peanut Butter Chocolate Chip Blondies

Preparation Time: 15 minutes

Cooking Time: 20 minutes

Servings: 24

Ingredients:

1/4 cup salt-free peanut butter

3/4 cup light brown sugar

1/2 cup unsweetened applesauce

1/4 cup canola oil

2 egg whites

1 tablespoon pure vanilla extract

2 teaspoons sodium-free baking powder

1 cup unbleached all-purpose flour

1/2 cup white whole-wheat flour

1/2 cup semisweet chocolate chips

Directions:

Preheat oven to 400°F. Oiled and flour a 9" × 13" baking pan and set aside. Measure the peanut butter, sugar, applesauce, oil, egg whites, and vanilla into a mixing bowl and stir well to combine.

Add the baking powder and mix. Gradually add in the flours, stirring well. Fold in the chocolate chips. Spread batter in preparation ared pan and smooth to even.

Bake within 20 minutes. Remove, then let it cool. Cool before cutting into bars and serving.

Nutrition:

Calories: 18

Fat: 5 g

Protein: 2 g

Sodium: 7 mg

Fiber: 1 g

Carbohydrates: 17 g

Sugar: 10 g

Ginger Snaps

Preparation Time: 15 minutes

Cooking Time: 10 minutes

Servings: 18

Ingredients:

4 tablespoons unsalted butter

1/2 cup light brown sugar

2 tablespoons molasses

1 egg white

21/2 teaspoons ground ginger

1/4 teaspoon ground allspice

1 teaspoon sodium-free baking soda

1/2 cup unbleached all-purpose flour

12 cup white whole-wheat flour

1 tablespoon sugar

Directions:

Warm oven to 375°F. Put aside a baking sheet with parchment paper. Put the butter, sugar, plus molasses into a mixing bowl and beat well.

Mix the egg white, ginger, and allspice. Mix in the baking soda, then put the flours, then beat.

Roll the dough into small balls. Put the balls on a preparation ared baking sheet and press down using a glass dipped in the tablespoon sugar.

Once the glass presses on the dough, it will moisten sufficiently to coat with sugar. Bake within 10 minutes. Let it cool, then serve.

Nutrition:

Calories: 81

Fat: 2 g

Protein: 1 g

Sodium: 6 mg

Fiber: 0 g

Carbohydrates: 14 g

Sugar: 8 g

Strawberries and Cream Cheese Crepes

Preparation Time: 10 minutes

Cooking Time: 10 minutes

Servings: 2

Ingredients:

4 tbsp cream cheese, softened

2 tbsp powdered sugar, sifted

2 tsp vanilla extract

2 pre-packaged crepes, each about 8 inches in diameter

8 strawberries, hulled and sliced

Directions:

Set the oven to heat at 325 degrees F. Grease a baking dish with cooking spray. Mix cream cheese with vanilla plus powdered sugar in a mixer. Spread the cream cheese mixture on each crepe and top it with 2 tablespoons strawberries.

Roll the crepes and place them in the baking dish. Bake them within 10 minutes until golden brown. Garnish as desired. Serve.

Nutrition:

Calories 144

Fat 4.9 g

Cholesterol 11 mg

Sodium 13 mg

Carbs 19.3 g

Fiber 1.9 g

Sugar 9.7 g

Protein 3.4 g

Apple & Berry Cobbler

Preparation Time: 10 minutes

Cooking Time: 40 minutes

Servings: 4

Ingredients:

Filling:

1 cup blueberries, fresh

2 cups apples, chopped

1 cup raspberries, fresh

2 tablespoons brown sugar

1 teaspoon lemon zest

2 teaspoon lemon juice, fresh

½ teaspoon ground cinnamon

1 ½ tablespoons corn starch

topping:

¾ cup whole wheat pastry flour

1 ½ tablespoon brown sugar

½ teaspoon vanilla extract, pure

¼ cup soy milk

¼ teaspoon sea salt, fine

1 egg white

Directions:

Turn your oven to 350, and get out six small ramekins. Grease them with cooking spray. Mix your lemon juice, lemon zest, blueberries, sugar, cinnamon, raspberries, and apples in a bowl. Stir in your cornstarch, mixing until it dissolves.

Beat your egg white in a different bowl, whisking it with sugar, vanilla, soy milk, and pastry flour. Divide your berry mixture between the ramekins and top with the vanilla topping. Put your ramekins on a baking sheet, baking for thirty minutes. The top should be golden brown before serving.

Nutrition:

Calories: 131

Fat: 0 g

Sodium: 14 mg

Carbs: 13.8 g

Fiber: 0 g

Sugar: 0 g

Protein: 7.2 g

Cream Cheese Cake

Preparation Time: 5 minutes

Cooking Time: 60 minutes

Servings: 2

Ingredients:

2 teaspoons cream cheese

1 cup Erythritol

2 egg whites

½ teaspoon lemon juice

½ teaspoon vanilla extract

2 strawberries, sliced

Directions:

Whisk the egg whites until you get soft peaks.

Keep whisking and gradually add Erythritol and lemon juice.

Whisk the egg whites till you get strong peak mass.

After this, mix up together cream cheese and vanilla extract.

Line the baking tray with baking paper.

With the help of the spoon make egg white nests in the tray.

Bake the egg white nests for 60 minutes at 205F.

When the "nests' are cooked, fill them with vanilla cream cheese and top with sliced strawberries.

Nutrition: :calories 36, fat 1.3, fiber 0.3, carbs 121.4, protein 3.9

Nutmeg Lemon Pudding

Preparation Time: 5 minutes

Cooking Time: 20 minutes

Servings: 2

Ingredients:

2 tablespoons lemon marmalade

4 eggs, whisked

2 tablespoons stevia

3 cups almond milk

4 allspice berries, crushed

¼ teaspoon nutmeg, grated

Directions:

In a bowl, mix the lemon marmalade with the eggs and the other ingredients and whisk well.

Divide the mix into ramekins, introduce in the oven and bake at 350 degrees F for 20 minutes.

Serve cold.

Nutrition: calories 220, fat 6.6, fiber 3.4, carbs 12.4, protein 3.4

Yogurt Panna Cotta With Fresh Berries

Preparation Time: 5 minutes

Cooking Time: 10 minutes

Servings: 2

Ingredients:

2 cups Greek yogurt

1 cup milk

1 cup heavy cream

2 teaspoons gelatin powder

4 tablespoons cold water

4 tablespoons honey

1 teaspoon vanilla extract

1 teaspoon lemon zest

1 pinch salt

2 cups mixed berries for serving

Directions:

Combine the milk and cream in a saucepan and heat them up.

Bloom the gelatin in cold water for 10 minutes.

Remove the milk off heat and stir in the gelatin until dissolved.

Add the vanilla, lemon zest and salt and allow to cool down.

Stir in the yogurt then pour the mixture into serving glasses.

When set, top with fresh berries and serve.

Nutrition: Per Serving:Calories:219 Fat:9.7g Protein:10.8g Carbohydrates:22.6g

Flourless Chocolate Cake

Preparation Time: 5 minutes

Cooking Time: 60 minutes

Servings: 2

Ingredients:

8 oz. dark chocolate, chopped

4 oz. butter, cubed

6 eggs, separated

1 teaspoon vanilla extract

1 pinch salt

4 tablespoons white sugar

Berries for serving

Directions:

Combine the chocolate and butter in a heatproof bowl and melt them together until smooth.

When smooth, remove off heat and place aside.

Separate the eggs.

Mix the egg yolks with the chocolate mixture.

Whip the egg whites with a pinch of salt until puffed up. Add the sugar and mix for a few more minutes until glossy and stiff.

Fold the meringue into the chocolate mixture then pour the batter in a 9-inch round cake pan lined with baking paper.

Bake in the preheated oven at 350F for 25 minutes.

Serve the cake chilled.

Nutrition: Per Serving:Calories:324 Fat:23.2g Protein:6.4g Carbohydrates:23.2g

Strawberry And Avocado Medley

Preparation Time: 5 minutes

Cooking Time: 10 minutes

Servings: 2

Ingredients:

2 cups strawberry, halved

1 avocado, pitted and sliced

2 tablespoons slivered almonds

Directions:

Place all Ingredients: in a mixing bowl.

Toss to combine.

Allow to chill in the fridge before serving.

Nutrition: Calories per serving: 107; Carbs: 9.9g; Protein: 1.6g; Fat: 7.8g

Creamy Mint Strawberry Mix

Preparation Time: 5 minutes

Cooking Time: 30 minutes

Servings: 2

Ingredients:

Cooking spray

¼ cup stevia

1 and ½ cup almond flour

1 teaspoon baking powder

1 cup almond milk

1 egg, whisked

2 cups strawberries, sliced

1 tablespoon mint, chopped

1 teaspoon lime zest, grated

½ cup whipping cream

Directions:

In a bowl, combine the almond with the strawberries, mint and the other ingredients except the cooking spray and whisk well.

Grease 6 ramekins with the cooking spray, pour the strawberry mix inside, introduce in the oven and bake at 350 degrees F for 30 minutes.

Cool down and serve.

Nutrition: calories 200, fat 6.3, fiber 2, carbs 6.5, protein 8

Creamy Pie

Preparation Time: 5 minutes

Cooking Time: 30 minutes

Servings: 2

Ingredients:

¼ cup lemon juice

1 cup cream

4 egg yolks

4 tablespoons Erythritol

1 tablespoon cornstarch

1 teaspoon vanilla extract

3 tablespoons butter

6 oz wheat flour, whole grain

Directions:

Mix up together wheat flour and butter and knead the soft dough.

Put the dough in the round cake mold and flatten it in the shape of pie crust.

Bake it for 15 minutes at 365F.

Meanwhile, make the lemon filling: Mix up together cream, egg yolks, and lemon juice. When the liquid is smooth, start to heat it up over the medium heat. Stir it constantly.

When the liquid is hot, add vanilla extract, cornstarch, and Erythritol. Whisk well until smooth.

Brin the lemon filling to boil and remove it from the heat.

Cool it to the room temperature.

Cook the pie crust to the room temperature.

Pour the lemon filling over the pie crust, flatten it well and leave to cool in the fridge for 25 minutes.

Nutrition: :calories 225, fat 11.4, fiber 0.8, carbs 34.8, protein 5.2

Watermelon Ice Cream

Preparation Time: 5 minutes

Cooking Time: 10 minutes

Servings: 2

Ingredients:

8 oz watermelon

1 tablespoon gelatin powder

Directions:

Make the juice from the watermelon with the help of the fruit juicer.

Combine together 5 tablespoons of watermelon juice and 1 tablespoon of gelatin powder. Stir it and leave for 5 minutes.

Then preheat the watermelon juice until warm, add gelatin mixture and heat it up over the medium heat until gelatin is dissolved.

Then remove the liquid from the heat and pout it in the silicone molds.

Freeze the jelly for 30 minutes in the freezer or for 4 hours in the fridge.

Nutrition: :calories 46, fat 0.2, fiber 0.4, carbs 8.5, protein 3.7

Hazelnut Pudding

Preparation Time: 5 minutes

Cooking Time: 40 minutes

Servings: 2

Ingredients:

2 and ¼ cups almond flour

3 tablespoons hazelnuts, chopped

5 eggs, whisked

1 cup stevia

1 and 1/3 cups Greek yogurt

1 teaspoon baking powder

1 teaspoon vanilla extract

Directions:

In a bowl, combine the flour with the hazelnuts and the other ingredients, whisk well, and pour into a cake pan lined with parchment paper,

Introduce in the oven at 350 degrees F, bake for 30 minutes, cool down, slice and serve.

Nutrition: calories 178, fat 8.4, fiber 8.2, carbs 11.5, protein 1.4

Cheesecakes

Preparation Time: 5 minutes

Cooking Time: 10 minutes

Servings: 2

Ingredients:

4 cups shredded phyllo (kataifi dough)

1/2 cup butter, melted

12 oz. cream cheese

1 cup Greek yogurt

3/4 cup confectioners' sugar

1 TB. vanilla extract

2 TB. orange blossom water

1 TB. orange zest

2 large eggs

1 cup coconut flakes

Directions:

Preheat the oven to 450ºF.

In a large bowl, and using your hands, combine shredded phyllo and melted butter, working the two together and breaking up phyllo shreds as you work.

Using a 12-cup muffin tin, add 1/3 cup shredded phyllo mixture to each tin, and press down to form crust on the bottom of the cup. Bake crusts for 8 minutes, remove from the oven, and set aside.

In a large bowl, and using an electric mixer on low speed, blend cream cheese and Greek yogurt for 1 minute.

Add confectioners' sugar, vanilla extract, orange blossom water, and orange zest, and blend 1 minute.

Add eggs, and blend for about 30 seconds or just until eggs are incorporated.

Lightly coat the sides of each muffin tin with cooking spray.

Pour about 1/3 cup cream cheese mixture over crust in each tin. Do not overflow.

Bake for 12 minutes.

Spread shredded coconut on a baking sheet, and place in the oven with cheesecakes to toast for 4 or 5 minutes or until golden brown. Remove from the oven, and set aside.

Remove cheesecakes from the oven, and cool for 1 hour on the countertop.

Place the tin in the refrigerator, and cool for 1 more hour.

To serve, dip a sharp knife in warm water and then run it along the sides of cheesecakes to loosen from the tin. Gently remove cheesecakes and place on a serving plate.

Sprinkle with toasted coconut flakes, and serve.

Melon Cucumber Smoothie

Preparation Time: 5 minutes

Cooking Time: 5 minutes

Servings: 2

Ingredients:

½ cucumber

2 slices of melon

2 tablespoons lemon juice

1 pear, peeled and sliced

3 fresh mint leaves

½ cup almond milk

Directions:

Place all Ingredients: in a blender.

Blend until smooth.

Pour in a glass container and allow to chill in the fridge for at least 30 minutes.

Nutrition: Calories per serving: 253; Carbs: 59.3g; Protein: 5.7g; Fat: 2.1g

Fruit Medley

Preparation Time: 5 minutes

Cooking Time: 10 minutes

Servings: 7

Ingredients:

4 fuyu persimmons, sliced into wedges

1 ½ cups grapes, halved

8 mint leaves, chopped

1 tablespoon lemon juice

1 tablespoon honey

½ cups almond, toasted and chopped

Directions:

Combine all Ingredients: in a bowl.

Toss then chill before serving.

Nutrition: Calories per serving:159; Carbs: 32g; Protein: 3g; Fat: 4g

White Wine Grapefruit Poached Peaches

Preparation Time: 5 minutes

Cooking Time: 40 minutes

Servings: 2

Ingredients:

4 peaches

2 cups white wine

1 grapefruit, peeled and juiced

¼ cup white sugar

1 cinnamon stick

1 star anise

1 cardamom pod

1 cup Greek yogurt for serving

Directions:

Combine the wine, grapefruit, sugar and spices in a saucepan.

Bring to a boil then place the peaches in the hot syrup.

Lower the heat and cover with a lid. Cook for 15 minutes then allow to cool down.

Carefully peel the peaches and place them in a small serving bowl.

Top with yogurt and serve right away.

Nutrition: Per Serving:Calories:157 Fat:0.9g Protein:4.2g Carbohydrates:20.4g

Cinnamon Stuffed Peaches

Preparation Time: 5 minutes

Cooking Time: 5 minutes

Servings: 2

Ingredients:

4 peaches, pitted, halved

2 tablespoons ricotta cheese

2 tablespoons of liquid honey

¾ cup of water

½ teaspoon vanilla extract

¾ teaspoon ground cinnamon

1 tablespoon almonds, sliced

¾ teaspoon saffron

Directions:

Pour water in the saucepan and bring to boil.

Add vanilla extract, saffron, ground cinnamon, and liquid honey.

Cook the liquid until the honey is melted.

Then remove it from the heat.

Put the halved peaches in the hot honey liquid.

Meanwhile, make the filling: mix up together ricotta cheese, vanilla extract, and sliced almonds.

Remove the peaches from honey liquid and arrange in the plate.

Fill 4 peach halves with ricotta filling and cover them with remaining peach halves.

Sprinkle the cooked dessert with liquid honey mixture gently.

Nutrition: :calories 113, fat 1.8, fiber 2.8, carbs 23.9, protein 2.7

Eggless Farina Cake (namoura)

Preparation Time: 5 minutes

Cooking Time: 40 minutes

Servings: 2

Ingredients:

2 cups farina

1/2 cup semolina

1/2 cup all-purpose flour

1 TB. baking powder

1 tsp. active dry yeast

1/2 cup sugar

1/2 cup plain Greek yogurt

1 cup whole milk

3/4 cup butter, melted

1/4 cup water

2 TB. tahini paste

15 almonds

2 cups Simple Syrup (recipe in Chapter 21)

Directions:

In a large bowl, combine farina, semolina, all-purpose flour, baking powder, yeast, sugar, Greek yogurt, whole milk, butter, and water. Set aside for 15 minutes.

Preheat the oven to 375ºF.

Spread tahini paste evenly in the bottom of a 9×13-inch baking pan, and pour in cake batter. Arrange almonds on top of batter, about where each slice will be. Bake for 45 minutes or until golden brown.

Remove cake from the oven, and using a toothpick, poke holes throughout cake for Simple Syrup to seep into. Pour syrup over cake, and let cake sit for 1 hour to absorb syrup.

Cool cake completely before cutting and serving.

Nutrition: Calories 85, Fat 6.5 g, Fiber 0.6 g, Carbs 0.6 g, Protein 6.4 g

Mixed Berry Sorbet

Preparation Time: 5 minutes

Cooking Time: 10 minutes

Servings: 2

Ingredients:

2 cups water

½ cup white sugar

2 cups mixed berries

1 tablespoon lemon juice

2 tablespoons honey

1 teaspoon lemon zest

1 mint sprig

Directions:

Combine the water, sugar, berries, lemon juice, honey and lemon zest in a saucepan.

Bring to a boil and cook on low heat for 5 minutes.

Add the mint sprig and remove off heat. Allow to infuse for 10 minutes then remove the mint.

Pour the syrup into a blender and puree until smooth and creamy.

Pour the smooth syrup into an airtight container and freeze for at least 2 hours.

Serve the sorbet chilled.

Nutrition: Per Serving:Calories:84 Fat:0.1g Protein:0.4g Carbohydrates:21.3g

Almonds And Oats Pudding

Preparation Time: 5 minutes

Cooking Time: 10 minutes

Servings: 2

Ingredients:

1 tablespoon lemon juice

Zest of 1 lime

1 and ½ cups almond milk

1 teaspoon almond extract

½ cup oats

2 tablespoons stevia

½ cup silver almonds, chopped

Directions:

In a pan, combine the almond milk with the lime zest and the other ingredients, whisk, bring to a simmer and cook over medium heat for 15 minutes.

Divide the mix into bowls and serve cold.

Nutrition: calories 174, fat 12.1, fiber 3.2, carbs 3.9, protein 4.8

Banana And Berries Trifle

Preparation Time: 5 minutes

Cooking Time: 10 minutes

Servings: 2

Ingredients:

8 oz biscuits, chopped

¼ cup strawberries, chopped

1 banana, chopped

1 peach, chopped

½ mango, chopped

1 cup grapes, chopped

1 tablespoon liquid honey

1 cup of orange juice

½ cup Plain yogurt

¼ cup cream cheese

1 teaspoon coconut flakes

Directions:

Bring the orange juice to boil and remove it from the heat.

Add liquid honey and stir until it is dissolved.

Cool the liquid to the room temperature.

Add chopped banana, peach, mango, grapes, and strawberries. Shake the fruits gently and leave to soak the orange juice for 15 minutes.

Meanwhile, with the help of the hand mixer mix up together Plain yogurt and cream cheese.

Then separate the chopped biscuits, yogurt mixture, and fruits on 4 parts.

Place the first part of biscuits in the big serving glass in one layer.

Spread it with yogurt mixture and add fruits.

Repeat the same steps till you use all ingredients.

Top the trifle with coconut flakes.

Nutrition: :calories 164, fat 6.2, fiber 1.3, carbs 24.8, protein 3.2

Chocolate Rice

Preparation Time: 5 minutes

Cooking Time: 20 minutes

Servings: 2

Ingredients:

1 cup of rice

1 tbsp cocoa powder

2 tbsp maple syrup

2 cups almond milk

Directions:

Add all ingredients into the inner pot of instant pot and stir well.

Seal pot with lid and cook on high for 20 minutes.

Once done, allow to release pressure naturally for 10 minutes then release remaining using quick release. Remove lid.

Stir and serve.

Nutrition: Calories 474 Fat 29.1 g Carbohydrates 51.1 g Sugar 10 g Protein 6.3 g Cholesterol 0 mg

Lemon And Semolina Cookies

Preparation Time: 5 minutes

Cooking Time: 20 minutes

Servings: 2

Ingredients:

½ teaspoon lemon zest, grated

4 tablespoons Erythritol

4 tablespoons semolina

2 tablespoons olive oil

8 tablespoons wheat flour, whole grain

1 teaspoon vanilla extract

½ teaspoon ground clove

3 tablespoons coconut oil

¼ teaspoon baking powder

¼ cup of water

Directions:

Make the dough: in the mixing bowl combine together lemon zest, semolina, olive oil, wheat flour, vanilla extract, ground clove, coconut oil, and baking powder.

Knead the soft dough.

Make the small cookies in the shape of walnuts and press them gently with the help of the fork.

Line the baking tray with the baking paper.

Place the cookies in the tray and bake them for 20 minutes at 375F.

Meanwhile, bring the water to boil.

Add Erythritol and simmer the liquid for 2 minutes over the medium heat. Cool it.

Pour the cooled sweet water over the hot baked cookies and leave them for 10 minutes.

When the cookies soak all liquid, transfer them in the serving plates.

Nutrition: :calories 165, fat 11.7, fiber 0.6, carbs 23.7, protein 2

Strawberry Sorbet

Preparation Time: 5 minutes

Cooking Time: 20 minutes

Servings: 2

Ingredients:

1 cup strawberries, chopped

1 tablespoon of liquid honey

2 tablespoons water

1 tablespoon lemon juice

Directions:

Preheat the water and liquid honey until you get homogenous liquid.

Blend the strawberries until smooth and combine them with honey liquid and lemon juice.

Transfer the strawberry mixture in the ice cream maker and churn it for 20 minutes or until the sorbet is thick.

Scoop the cooked sorbet in the ice cream cups.

Nutrition: :calories 57, fat 0.3, fiber 1.5, carbs 14.3, protein 0.6

Halva (halawa)

Preparation Time: 5 minutes

Cooking Time: 10 minutes

Servings: 2

Ingredients:

11/2 cups honey

11/2 cups tahini paste

1 cup pistachios, coarsely chopped

Directions:

Pour honey into a saucepan, set over low heat, and bring to 240ºF.

In another saucepan over low heat, bring tahini paste to 120ºF.

In a bowl, whisk together heated honey and tahini paste until smooth. Fold in pistachios.

Line a loaf pan with parchment paper and spray with cooking spray. Pour tahini mixture into the loaf pan, and refrigerate for 2 days to set.

Cut halva into bite-size pieces, and serve.

Nutrition: Calories 85, Fat 6.5 g, Fiber 0.6 g, Carbs 0.6 g, Protein 6.4 g

Semolina Cake

Preparation Time: 5 minutes

Cooking Time: 20 minutes

Servings: 6

Ingredients:

½ cup wheat flour, whole grain

½ cup semolina

1 teaspoon baking powder

½ cup Plain yogurt

1 teaspoon vanilla extract

4 tablespoons Erythritol

1 teaspoon lemon rind

2 tablespoons olive oil

1 tablespoon almond flakes

4 teaspoons liquid honey

½ cup of orange juice

Directions:

Mix up together wheat flour, semolina, baking powder, Plain yogurt, vanilla extract, Erythritol, and olive oil.

Then add lemon rind and mix up the ingredients until smooth.

Transfer the mixture in the non-sticky cake mold, sprinkle with almond flakes, and bake for 30 minutes at 365F.

Meanwhile, bring the orange juice to boil.

Add liquid honey and stir until dissolved.

When the cake is cooked, pour the hot orange juice mixture over it and let it rest for at least 10 minutes.

Cut the cake into the servings.

Nutrition: :calories 179, fat 6.1, fiber 1.1, carbs 36.3, protein 4.5

Shredded Phyllo And Sweet Cheese Pie (knafe)

Preparation Time: 5 minutes

Cooking Time: 30 minutes

Servings: 2

Ingredients:

1 lb. pkg. shredded phyllo (kataifi dough)

1 cup butter, melted

1/2 cup whole milk

2 TB. semolina flour

1 lb. ricotta cheese

2 cups mozzarella cheese, shredded

2 TB. sugar

1 cup Simple Syrup (recipe later in this chapter)

Directions:

1 cup Simple Syrup (recipe later in this chapter)

In a food processor fitted with a chopping blade, pulse shredded phyllo and butter 10 times. Transfer mixture to a bowl.

In a small saucepan over low heat, warm whole milk.

Stir in semolina flour, and cook for 1 minute.

Rinse the food processor, and to it, add ricotta cheese, mozzarella cheese, sugar, and semolina mixture. Blend for 1 minute.

Preheat the oven to 375ºF.

In a 9-inch-round baking dish, add 1/2 of shredded phyllo mixture, and press down to compress. Add cheese mixture, and spread out evenly. Add rest of shredded phyllo mixture, spread evenly, and gently press down. Bake for 40 minutes or until golden brown.

Let pie rest for 10 minutes before serving with Simple Syrup drizzled over top.

Nutrition: Calories 85, Fat 6.5 g, Fiber 0.6 g, Carbs 0.6 g, Protein 6.4 g

Lemon Pear Compote

Preparation Time: 5 minutes

Cooking Time: 10 minutes

Servings: 2

Ingredients:

3 cups pears, cored and cut into chunks

1 tsp vanilla

1 tsp liquid stevia

1 tbsp lemon zest, grated

2 tbsp lemon juice

Directions:

Add all ingredients into the inner pot of instant pot and stir well.

Seal pot with lid and cook on high for 15 minutes.

Once done, allow to release pressure naturally for 10 minutes then release remaining using quick release. Remove lid.

Stir and serve.

Nutrition: Calories 50 Fat 0.2 g Carbohydrates 12.7 g Sugar 8.1 g Protein 0.4 g Cholesterol 0 mg

Cinnamon Pear Jam

Preparation Time: 5 minutes

Cooking Time: 10 minutes

Servings: 2

Ingredients:

8 pears, cored and cut into quarters

1 tsp cinnamon

1/4 cup apple juice

2 apples, peeled, cored and diced

Directions:

Add all ingredients into the inner pot of instant pot and stir well.

Seal pot with lid and cook on high for 4 minutes.

Once done, allow to release pressure naturally. Remove lid.

Blend pear apple mixture using an immersion blender until smooth.

Serve and enjoy.

Nutrition: Calories 103 Fat 0.3 g Carbohydrates 27.1 g Sugar 18 g Protein 0.6 g Cholesterol 0 mg

Apple And Walnut Salad

Preparation Time: 5 minutes

Cooking Time: 5 minutes

Servings: 2

Ingredients:

Juice from ½ orange

Zest from ½ orange, grated

2 tablespoons honey

1 tablespoon olive oil

4 medium Gala apples, cubed

8 dried apricots, chopped

¼ cup walnuts, toasted and chopped

Directions:

In a small bowl, whisk together the orange juice, zest, honey, and olive oil. Set aside.

In a larger bowl, toss the apples, apricots, and walnuts.

Drizzle with the vinaigrette and toss to coat all Ingredients.

Serve chilled.

Nutrition: Calories per serving: 178; Carbs: 30g; Protein: 1g; Fat: 6g

Banana Kale Smoothie

Preparation Time: 5 minutes

Cooking Time: 10 minutes

Servings: 2

Ingredients:

2 cups kale leaves

1 cup almond milk

½ cup crushed ice

1 banana, peeled

1 apple, peeled and cored

A dash of cinnamon

Directions:

Place all Ingredients: in a blender.

Blend until smooth.

Pour in a glass container and allow to chill in the fridge for at least 30 minutes.

Nutrition: Calories per serving: 165; Carbs: 32.1g; Protein: 2.3g; Fat: 4.2g

Phyllo Custard Pockets (shaabiyat)

Preparation Time: 5 minutes

Cooking Time: 10 minutes

Servings: 2

Ingredients:

8 phyllo sheets

1/2 cup butter, melted

21/4 cups Ashta Custard (recipe later in this chapter)

1 cup Simple Syrup (recipe later in this chapter)

1/2 cup pistachios, ground

Directions:

Preheat the oven to 450ºF.

Lay out a sheet of phyllo dough, brush with butter, and layer another sheet of phyllo dough on top. Cut sheets into 3 equal-size columns, each about 3 or 4 inches wide.

Place 3 tablespoons Ashta Custard at one end of each column, and fold the bottom-right corner up and over custard. Pull up bottom-left corner, and repeat folding each corner up to the opposite corner, forming a triangle as you fold.

Place triangle pockets on a baking sheet, brush with butter, and bake for 10 minutes or until golden brown.

Serve warm or cold, drizzled with Simple Syrup and sprinkled with pistachios.

Nutrition: Calories 85, Fat 6.5 g, Fiber 0.6 g, Carbs 0.6 g, Protein 6.4 g

Chocolate Baklava

Preparation Time: 5 minutes

Cooking Time: 35minutes

Servings: 2

Ingredients:

24 sheets (14 x 9-inch) frozen whole-wheat phyllo (filo) dough, thawed

1/8 teaspoon salt

1/3 cup toasted walnuts, chopped coarsely

1/3 cup almonds, blanched toasted, chopped coarsely

1/2 teaspoon ground cinnamon

1/2 cup water

1/2 cup hazelnuts, toasted, chopped coarsely

1/2 cup pistachios, roasted, chopped coarsely

3/4 cup honey

1/2 cup of butter, melted

1 cup chocolate-hazelnut spread (I used Nutella)

1 piece (3-inch) cinnamon stick

Cooking spray

Directions:

Into medium-sized saucepan, combine the water, honey, and the cinnamon stick; stir until the honey is dissolved. Increase the heat/flame to medium; continue cooking for about 10 minutes without stirring. A candy thermometer should read 230F. Remove the saucepan from the heat and then keep warm. Remove and discard the cinnamon stick.

Preheat the oven to 350F.

Put the chocolate-hazelnut spread into microwavable bowl; microwave the spread for about 30 seconds on HIGH or until the spread is melted.

In a bowl, combine the hazelnuts, pistachios, almonds, walnuts, ground cinnamon, and the salt.

Lightly grease with the cooking spray a 9x13-inch ceramic or glass baking dish.

Put 1 sheet lengthwise into the bottom of the preparation ared baking dish, extending the ends of the sheet over the edges of the dish. Lightly brush the sheet with the butter. Repeat the process with 5 sheets phyllo and a light brush of butter. Drizzle 1/3 cup of the melted chocolate-hazelnut spread over the buttered phyllo sheets. Sprinkle about 1/3 of the nut mixture (1/2 cup) over the spread. Repeat the process, layering phyllo sheet, brush of butter, spread, and with nut mixture. For the last, nut mixture top layer, top with 6 phyllo sheets, pressing each phyllo gently into the dish and brushing each sheet with butter.

Slice the layers into 24 portions by making 3 cuts lengthwise and then 5 cuts crosswise with a sharp knife; bake for about 35 minutes at 350F or until the phyllo sheets are golden. Remove the dish from the oven, drizzle the honey sauce over the baklava. Pace the dish on a wire rack and let cool. Cover and store the baklavas at normal room temperature if not serving right away.

Nutrition: :238 Cal, 13.4 g total fat (4.3 g sat. fat, 5.6 g mono fat, 2 g poly fat), 4 g protein, 27.8 g total carbs., 1.6 g fiber, 10 mg chol., 1.3 mg iron, 148 mg sodium, and 29 mg calcium.

Apricot Rosemary Muffins

Preparation Time: 5 minutes

Cooking Time: 60 minutes

Servings: 2

Ingredients:

2 eggs

1/3 cup white sugar

1 teaspoon vanilla extract

1 cup buttermilk

¼ cup olive oil

1 ½ cups all-purpose flour

¼ teaspoon salt

1 teaspoon baking powder

¼ teaspoon baking soda

4 apricots, pitted and diced

1 teaspoon dried rosemary

Directions:

Combine the eggs, sugar and vanilla in a bowl and mix until double in volume.

Stir in the oil and buttermilk and mix well.

Fold in the flour, salt, baking powder and baking soda then add the apricots and rosemary and mix gently.

Spoon the batter in a muffin tin lined with muffin papers and bake in the preheated oven at 350F for 20-25 minutes or until the muffins pass the toothpick test.

Serve the muffins chilled.

Nutrition: Per Serving:Calories:140 Fat:5.4g Protein:3.4g Carbohydrates:20.1g

Blueberry Yogurt Mousse

Preparation Time: 5 minutes

Cooking Time: 0 minutes

Servings: 2

Ingredients:

2 cups Greek yogurt

¼ cup stevia

¾ cup heavy cream

2 cups blueberries

Directions:

In a blender, combine the yogurt with the other ingredients, pulse well, divide into cups and keep in the fridge for 30 minutes before serving.

Nutrition: calories 141, fat 4.7, fiber 4.7, carbs 8.3, protein 0.8

Pistachio Cheesecake

Preparation Time: 5 minutes

Cooking Time: 10 minutes

Servings: 2

Ingredients:

½ cup pistachio, chopped

4 teaspoons butter, softened

4 teaspoon Erythritol

2 cups cream cheese

½ cup cream, whipped

Directions:

Mix up together pistachios, butter, and Erythritol.

Put the mixture in the baking mold and bake for 10 minutes at 355F.

Meanwhile, whisk together cream cheese and whipped cream.

When the pistachio mixture is baked, chill it well.

After this, transfer the pistachio mixture in the round cake mold and flatten in one layer.

Then put the cream cheese mixture over the pistachio mixture, flatten the surface until smooth.

Cool the cheesecake in the fridge for 1 hour before serving.

Nutrition: :calories 332, fat 33, fiber 0.5, carbs 7.4, protein 7

Almond Citrus Muffins

Preparation Time: 5 minutes

Cooking Time: 10 minutes

Servings: 2

Ingredients:

2 eggs, beaten

1 ½ cup whole wheat flour

½ cup almond meal

1 teaspoon vanilla extract

1 tablespoon butter, softened

1 teaspoon orange zest, grated

1 tablespoon orange juice

¾ cup Erythritol

1 oz orange pulp

1 teaspoon baking powder

½ teaspoon lime zest, grated

Cooking spray

Directions:

Make the muffin batter: combine together almond meal, eggs, whole wheat flour, vanilla extract, butter, orange zest, orange juice, and orange pulp.

Add lime zest and baking powder.

Then add Erythritol.

With the help of the hand mixer mix up the ingredients.

When the mixture is soft and smooth, it is done.

Spray the muffin molds with cooking spray from inside and preheat the oven to 365F.

Fill ½ part of every muffin mold with muffin batter and transfer them in the oven.

Cook the muffins for 30 minutes.

Then check if the muffins are cooked by piercing them with a toothpick (if it is dry, the muffins are cooked; if it is not dry, bake the muffins for 5-7 minutes more.)

Nutrition: :calories 204, fat 7.7, fiber 1.9, carbs 57.1, protein 6.8

Mediterranean Bread Pudding (aish El Saraya)

Preparation Time: 5 minutes

Cooking Time: 10 minutes

Servings: 2

Ingredients:

8 slices white bread, crust removed

1 cup sugar

1/2 cup water

1 TB. fresh lemon juice

2 cups Simple Syrup (recipe later in this chapter)

4 cups Ashta Custard (recipe later in this chapter)

1/2 cup coconut flakes, toasted

1/2 cup pistachios, ground

1 strawberry, sliced

Directions:

Preheat the oven to 450ºF.

Place slices of bread on a baking sheet, and toast for 10 minutes or until bread is golden brown and dry.

In a small saucepan over medium-low heat, combine sugar, water, and lemon juice. Simmer for 5 to 7 minutes or until sugar reaches a dark golden brown color.

Carefully pour hot dark brown syrup into an 8×8-inch baking dish, shifting the dish from side to side to spread syrup around bottom of dish.

Place 4 slices of bread on top of brown syrup. Pour 1 cup of Simple Syrup over bread, spread 2 cups Ashta Custard over bread, and add another layer of 4 slices of bread. Pour remaining 1 cup Simple Syrup over bread, and spread remaining 2 cups Ashta Custard over top bread layer.

Cover the dish with plastic wrap, and refrigerate for 4 hours.

Decorate top of dish with toasted coconut, pistachios, and strawberry slices, and serve.

Nutrition: Calories 85, Fat 6.5 g, Fiber 0.6 g, Carbs 0.6 g, Protein 6.4 g

Cinnamon Apple Rice Pudding

Preparation Time: 5 minutes

Cooking Time: 10 minutes

Servings: 2

Ingredients:

1 cup of rice

1 tsp vanilla

1/4 apple, peeled and chopped

1/2 cup water

1 1/2 cup almond milk

1 tsp cinnamon

1 cinnamon stick

Directions:

Add all ingredients into the instant pot and stir well.

Seal pot with lid and cook on high for 15 minutes.

Once done, release pressure using quick release. Remove lid.

Stir and serve.

Nutrition: Calories 206 Fat 11.5 g Carbohydrates 23.7 g Sugar 2.7 g Protein 3 g Cholesterol 0 mg

Custard-filled Pancakes (atayef)

Preparation Time: 5 minutes

Cooking Time: 10 minutes

Servings: 2

Ingredients:

1 cup all-purpose flour

1/2 cup whole-wheat flour

1 cup whole milk

1/2 cup water

1 tsp. active dry yeast

1 tsp. baking powder

1/2 tsp. salt

2 TB. sugar

2 cups Ashta Custard

1/2 cup ground pistachios

1 cup Simple Syrup)

Directions:

In a large bowl, whisk together all-purpose flour, whole-wheat flour, whole milk, water, yeast, baking powder, salt, and sugar. Set aside for 30 minutes.

Preheat a nonstick griddle over low heat.

Spoon 3 tablespoons batter onto the griddle, and cook pancake for about 30 seconds or until bubbles form along entire top of pancake. Do not flip over pancake. You're only browning the bottom.

Transfer pancake to a plate, and let cool while cooking remaining pancakes. Do not overlap the pancakes while letting them cool.

Form pancake into a pocket by folding pancake into a half-moon, and pinch together the edges, but only halfway up.

Spoon Ashta Custard into a piping bag or a zipper-lock plastic bag, snip off the corner, and squeeze about 2 tablespoons custard into each pancake pocket. Sprinkle custard with pistachios.

Serve pancakes chilled with Simple Syrup drizzled on top.

Nutrition: Calories 85, Fat 6.5 g, Fiber 0.6 g, Carbs 0.6 g, Protein 6.4 g

Pomegranate Granita With Lychee

Preparation Time: 5 minutes

Cooking Time: 5 minutes

Servings: 2

Ingredients:

500 millimeters pomegranate juice, organic and sugar-free

1 cup water

½ cup lychee syrup

2 tablespoons lemon juice

4 mint leaves

1 cup fresh lychees, pitted and sliced

Directions:

Place all Ingredients: in a large pitcher.

Place inside the fridge to cool before serving.

Nutrition: Calories per serving: 96; Carbs: 23.8g; Protein: 0.4g; Fat: 0.4g

Lime Grapes And Apples

Preparation Time: 5 minutes

Cooking Time: 25 minutes

Servings: 2

Ingredients:

½ cup red grapes

2 apples

1 teaspoon lime juice

1 teaspoon Erythritol

3 tablespoons water

Directions:

Line the baking tray with baking paper.

Then cut the apples on the halves and remove the seeds with the help of the scooper.

Cut the apple halves on 2 parts more.

Arrange all fruits in the tray in one layer, drizzle with water, and bake for 20 minutes at 375F.

Flip the fruits on another side after 10 minutes of cooking.

Then remove them from the oven and sprinkle with lime juice and Erythritol.

Return the fruits back in the oven and bake for 5 minutes more.

Serve the cooked dessert hot or warm.

Nutrition: :calories 142, fat 0.4, fiber 5.7, carbs 40.1, protein 0.9

Mediterranean Baked Apples

Preparation Time: 5 minutes

Cooking Time: 20 minutes

Servings: 2

Ingredients:

1.5 pounds apples, peeled and sliced

Juice from ½ lemon

A dash of cinnamon

Directions:

Preheat the oven to 250F.

Line a baking sheet with parchment paper then set aside.

In a medium bowl, apples with lemon juice and cinnamon.

Place the apples on the parchment paper-lined baking sheet.

Bake for 25 minutes until crisp.

Nutrition: Calories per serving: 90; Carbs: 23.9g; Protein: 0.5g; Fat: 0.3g

Honey Cream

Preparation Time: 5 minutes

Cooking Time: 10 minutes

Servings: 2

Ingredients:

½ cup cream

¼ cup milk

2 teaspoons honey

1 teaspoon vanilla extract

1 tablespoons gelatin

2 tablespoons orange juice

Directions:

Mix up together milk and gelatin and leave it for 5 minutes.

Meanwhile, pour cream in the saucepan and bring it to boil.

Add honey and vanilla extract.

Remove the cream from the heat and stir well until honey is dissolved.

After this, add gelatin mixture (milk+gelatin) and mix it up until gelatin is dissolved.

After this, place 1 tablespoon of orange juice in every serving glass.

Add the cream mixture over the orange juice.

Refrigerate the pannacotta for 30-50 minutes in the fridge or until it is solid.

Nutrition: :calories 100, fat 4, fiber 0, carbs 11, protein 4.6

Dragon Fruit, Pear, And Spinach Salad

Preparation Time: 5 minutes

Cooking Time: 3 minutes

Servings: 2

Ingredients:

5 ounces spinach leaves, torn

1 dragon fruit, peeled then cubed

2 pears, peeled then cubed

10 ounces organic goat cheese

1 cup pecan, halves

6 ounces blackberries

6 ounces raspberries

8 tablespoons olive oil

8 tablespoons red wine vinegar

1 tablespoon poppy seeds

Directions:

In a mixing bowl, combine all Ingredients: except for the poppy seeds.

Place inside the fridge and allow to chill before serving.

Sprinkle with poppy seeds on top before serving.

Nutrition: Calories per serving:321; Carbs: 27.2g; Protein: 3.3g; Fat: 3.1g

Kataifi

Preparation Time: 5 minutes

Cooking Time: 10 minutes

Servings: 2

Ingredients:

1 kilogram almonds, blanched and then chopped

1 teaspoon cinnamon

1/4 kilogram kataifi phyllo

2 eggs

4 tablespoons sugar

400 g butter

1 1/2 kilograms sugar

1 lemon rind

1 teaspoon lemon juice

5 cups water

Directions:

Preheat the oven to 170C.

Put the sugar, eggs, cinnamon, and the almonds in a bowl.

With your fingers, open the kataifi pastry gently. Lay it on a piece of marble and wood. Put 1 tablespoon of the almond mixture in one end and then roll the pastry into a log or a cylinder. Make sure you fold the pastry a little tight so the filling is enclosed securely. Repeat the process with the remaining pastry and almond mixture.

Melt the butter and put into a baking dish.

Brush the kataifi rolls with the melted butter, covering all the sides.

Place into baking sheets and bake for about 30 minutes.

Meanwhile, preparation are the syrup.

Except for the lemon juice, cook the rest of the syrup ingredients for about 5-10 minutes. Add the lemon juice and let cook for a few minutes until the syrup is slightly thick.

After baking the kataifi, pour the syrup over the still warm rolls.

Cover the pastry with a clean towel. Let cool as the kataifi absorbs the syrup.

Nutrition: :1085 cal., 83.3 total fat (24.6 g sat. fat), 119 mg chol., 248 mg sodium, 759 mg pot., 76.6 g total carbs., 12.7 g fiber, 59.1 g sugar, and 22.6 g protein.

Walnuts Kataifi

Preparation Time: 5 minutes

Cooking Time: 50 minutes

Servings: 2

Ingredients:

7 oz kataifi dough

1/3 cup walnuts, chopped

½ teaspoon ground cinnamon

¾ teaspoon vanilla extract

4 tablespoons butter, melted

¼ teaspoon ground clove

1/3 cup water

3 tablespoons honey

Directions:

For the filling: mix up together walnuts, ground cinnamon, and vanilla extract. Add ground clove and blend the mixture until smooth.

Make the kataifi dough: grease the casserole mold with butter and place ½ part of kataifi dough.

Then sprinkle the filling over the kataifi dough.

After this, sprinkle the filling with 1 tablespoon of melted butter.

Sprinkle the filling with remaining kataifi dough.

Make the roll from ½ part of kataifi dough and cut it.

Gently arrange the kataifi roll in the tray.

Repeat the same steps with remaining dough. In the end, you should get 2 kataifi rolls.

Preheat the oven to 355F and place the tray with kataifi rolls inside.

Bake the dessert for 50 minutes or until it is crispy.

Meanwhile, make the syrup: bring the water to boil.

Add honey and heat it up until the honey is dissolved.

When the kataifi rolls are cooked, pour the hot syrup over the hot kataifi rolls.

Cut every kataifi roll on 2 pieces.

Serve the dessert with remaining syrup.

Nutrition: :calories 120, fat 1.5, fiber 0, carbs 22, protein 3

Cinnamon Tea

Preparation Time: 5 minutes

Cooking Time: 10 minutes

Servings: 2

Ingredients:

6 cups water

1 (3-in.) cinnamon stick

6 TB. Ahmad Tea, Ceylon tea, or your favorite

3 TB. sugar

Directions:

In a teapot over low heat, bring water and cinnamon stick to a simmer for 30 minutes. Remove cinnamon stick.

Stir in Ahmad tea and sugar, and simmer for 2 minutes.

Remove from heat, and let sit for 10 minutes.

Strain tea into tea cups, and serve warm.

Nutrition: Calories 85, Fat 6.5 g, Fiber 0.6 g, Carbs 0.6 g, Protein 6.4 g

Biscotti

Preparation Time: 5 minutes

Cooking Time: 10 minutes

Servings: 2

Ingredients:

2 eggs

1 cups whole-wheat flour

1 cup all-purpose flour

3/4 cup parmesan cheese, grated

2 teaspoons baking powder

2 tablespoons sugar

1/4 cup sun-dried tomato, finely chopped

1/4 cup Kalamata olive, finely chopped

1/3 cup olive oil

1/2 teaspoon salt

1/2 teaspoon black pepper, cracked

1 teaspoon dried oregano (preferably Greek)

1 teaspoon dried basil

Directions:

Into a large-sized bowl, beat the eggs and the sugar together. Pour in the olive; beat until smooth.

In another bowl, combine the flours, baking powder, pepper, salt, oregano, and basil. Stir the flour mix into the egg mixture, stirring until blended.

Stir in the cheese, tomatoes, and olives; stirring until thoroughly combined.

Divide the dough into 2 portions; shape each into 10-inch long logs. Place the logs into a parchment-lined cookie sheet; flatten the log tops slightly.

Bake for about 30 minutes in a preheated 375F oven or until the logs are pale golden and not quite firm to the touch.

Remove from the oven; let cool on the baking sheet for 3 minutes. Transfer the logs into a cutting board; slice each log into 1/2-inch diagonal slices using a serrated knife.

Place the biscotti slices on the baking sheet, return into the 325F oven, and bake for about 20 to 25 minutes until dry and firm. Flip the slices halfway through baking. Remove from the oven, transfer on a wire rack and let cool.

Nutrition: :731.6 Cal, 36.5 g total fat (9 g sat. fat), 146 mg chol., 1238.4 mg sodium, 77.8 g carb., 3.5 g fiber, 10.7 g sugar, and 23.3 g protein.

Tiny Orange Cardamom Cookies

Preparation Time: 5 minutes

Cooking Time: 12 minutes

Servings: 2

Ingredients:

1/2 cup whole-wheat flour

1/2 cup all-purpose flour

1 large egg

1 tablespoon sesame seeds, toasted, optional (salted roasted pistachios, chopped)

1 teaspoon orange zest

1 teaspoon vanilla extract

1/2 cup butter, softened

1/2 cup sugar

1/4 teaspoon ground cardamom

Directions:

Preheat the oven to 375F.

In a medium bowl, blend the orange zest and the sugar thoroughly, and then blend in the cardamom. Add the butter and with a mixer, beat until the mixture is fluffy and light. Beat in the egg and the vanilla into the mixture. With the mixer on low speed, mix in the flours into the mixture.

Line 3 baking sheets with parchment paper. Using a level teaspoon measure, drop batter of the cookie mixture onto the sheets. Top each cookie with a pinch of sesame seeds or nuts, if desired; bake for 1bout 10-12 minutes or until the cookies are brown at the edges and crisp. When baked, transfer the cookies on a cooling rack and let them cool completely.

Nutrition: :113 Cal, 1.4 g protein, 6.5 g total fat (3.8 g sat. fat) 12 g total carbs., 0.3 g fiber, 46 mg sodium, and 29 mg chol.

Mixed Fruit Bowl

Preparation Time: 5 minutes

Cooking Time: 10 minutes

Servings: 2

Ingredients

½ C. fresh strawberries, hulled and sliced

½ C. fresh blueberries

½ C. fresh blackberries

½ C. fresh cherries, pitted and halved

1 tbsp. fresh lemon juice

1 tbsp. organic honey

2 tbsp. almonds, chopped

Directions

In a large bowl, add fruit, lemon juice and honey and gently toss to coat well.

Place fruit mixture in 2 serving bowls.

Top with almonds and serve.

Nutrition: Calories 85, Fat 6.5 g, Fiber 0.6 g, Carbs 0.6 g, Protein 6.4 g

Spinach & Fruit Treat

Preparation Time: 5 minutes

Cooking Time: 10 minutes

Servings: 2

Ingredients

1¼ C. fresh spinach

2 frozen ripe bananas, peeled and sliced

¾ C. frozen mango chunks

¼ C. frozen pineapple chunks

1 tbsp. unsweetened almond milk

1 tsp. organic vanilla extract

Directions

In a food processor, add all ingredients and pulse until smooth and creamy.

Serve immediately.

Nutrition: Calories 85, Fat 6.5 g, Fiber 0.6 g, Carbs 0.6 g, Protein 6.4 g

Cherry Ice Cream

Preparation Time: 5 minutes

Cooking Time: 10 minutes

Servings: 2

Ingredients

2 C. fresh cherries, pitted

1 small avocado, peeled, pitted and chopped

10 dates, pitted and chopped

¼ C. cashews, soaked for 30 minutes and drained

1¾ C. unsweetened almond milk

2/3 C. water

1 tbsp. fresh lemon juice

1 tbsp. fresh beet juice

6 fresh cherries, pitted and chopped finely

½ C. fresh whole cherries

Directions

In a blender, add all ingredients except chopped and whole cherries and pulse until creamy and smooth.

Transfer into a bowl and stir in chopped cherries.

Now, transfer into an ice cream maker and process according to manufacturer's directions.

Transfer into an airtight container and freeze for at least 4-5 hours.

Top with fresh whole cherries and serve.

Nutrition: Calories 85, Fat 6.5 g, Fiber 0.6 g, Carbs 0.6 g, Protein 6.4 g

Tofu & Berries Pudding

Preparation Time: 5 minutes

Cooking Time: 10 minutes

Servings: 2

Ingredients

1 C. fresh strawberries, hulled and sliced

1/3 C. fresh blackberries

1/3 C. fresh blueberries

12-oz. silken tofu, drained and pressed

2 scoops unsweetened protein powder

1 tsp. organic vanilla extract

1 tsp. applesauce

1 tsp. pumpkin pie spice

Directions

In a food processor, add all ingredients and pulse until smooth and creamy.

Transfer into a large serving bowl and refrigerate to chill before serving.

Nutrition: Calories 85, Fat 6.5 g, Fiber 0.6 g, Carbs 0.6 g, Protein 6.4 g

Bean & Walnut Mousse

Preparation Time: 5 minutes

Cooking Time: 10 minutes

Servings: 2

Ingredients

½ C. unsweetened almond milk

1 C. cooked black beans

4 Medjool dates, pitted and chopped

½ C. walnuts, chopped

2 tbsp. cacao powder

1 tsp. organic vanilla extract

2 tbsp. fresh raspberries

4 fresh mint leaves

Directions

In a food processor, add all ingredients and pulse until smooth and creamy.

Transfer into serving bowls and refrigerate to chill before serving.

Garnish with raspberries and mint leaves and serve.

Nutrition: Calories 85, Fat 6.5 g, Fiber 0.6 g, Carbs 0.6 g, Protein 6.4 g

Egg Custard

Preparation Time: 5 minutes

Cooking Time: 10 minutes

Servings: 2

Ingredients

5 organic eggs

Salt, to taste

½ C. organic honey

20-oz. unsweetened almond milk

¼ tsp. ground ginger

¼ tsp. ground cinnamon

¼ tsp. ground nutmeg

¼ tsp. ground cardamom

1/8 tsp. ground clove

1/8 tsp. ground allspice

Directions

Preheat the oven to 325 degrees F. Grease 8 small ramekins.

In a bowl, add eggs and salt and beat well.

Through a fine mesh sieve, strain the eggs into a bowl by moving the sieve in a circle.

Add the honey in eggs and stir to combine.

Add almond milk and spices and beat until well combined.

Transfer the mixture into preparation ared ramekins.

Arrange the ramekins in a large baking dish.

Add hot water in the baking dish about 2-inch high around the ramekins.

Bake for about 30-40 minutes or until a toothpick inserted in the center comes out clean.

Serve warm.

Nutrition: Calories 85, Fat 6.5 g, Fiber 0.6 g, Carbs 0.6 g, Protein 6.4 g

Apple Crisp

Preparation Time: 5 minutes

Cooking Time: 10 minutes

Servings: 2

Ingredients

For Filling

2 large apples, peeled, cored and chopped

2 tbsp. fresh apple juice

2 tbsp. water

¼ tsp. ground cinnamon

For Topping

½ C. quick rolled oats

¼ C. unsweetened coconut flakes

2 tbsp. walnuts, chopped

½ tsp. ground cinnamon

¼ C. water

Directions

Preheat the oven to 300 degrees F.

In a large baking dish, place all filling ingredients and gently mix.

In a bowl, mix together all topping ingredients.

Spread the topping over filling mixture evenly.

Bake for about 20 minutes or until top becomes golden brown.

Nutrition: Calories 185, Fat 13.5 g, Fiber 0.6 g, Carbs 2.6 g, Protein 15.4 g

Peach Crumble

Preparation Time: 5 minutes

Cooking Time: 10 minutes

Servings: 2

Ingredients

¾ C. old-fashioned oats

¼ C. whole wheat flour

1 tsp. ground cinnamon, divided

2 tbsp. coconut oil, softened

2 tbsp. agave nectar

4 extra-large peaches, pitted and chopped

2 tbsp. cornstarch

1½ tsp. organic almond extract

Directions

Preheat the oven to 350 degrees F.

In a bowl, mix together oats, flour and ¾ tsp. of the cinnamon.

Add coconut oil and agave nectar and mix until well combined.

In another bowl, add peaches, cornstarch, remaining cinnamon and almond extract and mix until well combined.

In the bottom of a 2-quart baking dish, place the peach mixture evenly and sprinkle with the oats mixture.

Bake for about 35-45 minutes, or until the oat mixture becomes golden brown and crunchy.

Remove from the oven and keep onto a wire rack to cool completely.

Nutrition: Calories 185, Fat 13.5 g, Fiber 0.6 g, Carbs 2.6 g, Protein 15.4 g

Black Bean Brownies

Preparation Time: 5 minutes

Cooking Time: 10 minutes

Servings: 2

Ingredients

2 C. cooked black beans

12 Medjool dates, pitted and chopped

2 tbsp. almond butter

2 tbsp. quick rolled oats

2 tsp. organic vanilla extract

¼ C. cacao powder

1 tbsp. ground cinnamon

Directions

Preheat the oven to 350 degrees F. Line a large baking dish with parchment paper.

In a food processor, add all ingredients except cacao and cinnamon and pulse until well combined and smooth.

Transfer the mixture into a large bowl.

Stir in cacao powder and cinnamon.

Now, transfer the mixture into preparation ared baking dish and with the back of a spatula, smooth the mixture evenly.

Bake for about 30 minutes.

Remove from oven and keep aside to cool.

With a sharp knife cut into 12 equal sized brownies and serve.

Nutrition: Calories 185, Fat 13.5 g, Fiber 0.6 g, Carbs 2.6 g, Protein 15.4 g

Chickpeas Almond Fudge

Preparation Time: 5 minutes

Cooking Time: 10 minutes

Servings: 2

Ingredients

2 C. cooked chickpeas

8 Medjool dates, pitted and chopped

½ C. unsweetened almond milk

½ C. almond butter

1 tsp. organic vanilla extract

2 tbsp. cacao powder

Directions

Line a large baking dish with parchment paper and keep aside.

In a food processor, add all ingredients except cacao and cinnamon and pulse until smooth.

Transfer the mixture into a large bowl and stir in the cacao powder.

Now, transfer the mixture into preparation ared baking dish and with the back of a spatula, smooth the top surface.

Freeze for at least 4-5 hours or until set completely.

Cut into desired sized squares and serve.

Nutrition: Calories 185, Fat 13.5 g, Fiber 0.6 g, Carbs 2.6 g, Protein 15.4 g

Mixed Dried Fruit Oatmeal Cookies

Preparation Time: 10 minutes

Cooking Time: 20 minutes

Servings: 20

Ingredients:

1 1/3 cups uncooked old-fashioned oats or quick-cooking rolled oats

1 cup whole-wheat flour

1 teaspoon baking powder

1 teaspoon ground cinnamon

¼ teaspoon ground mace

½ cup loosely packed brown sugar

1/3 cup plain low-fat yogurt

2 tablespoons canola oil

1 egg

1 teaspoon vanilla extract

½ cup mixed dried fruit

½ cup dark chocolate chips

Direction

Preheat oven to 350ºF (180ºC). Line two baking sheets with baking mats or parchment paper.

In a medium bowl, stir together oats, flour, baking powder, cinnamon, mace, and sugar.

In a large bowl, stir together yogurt, oil, egg, and vanilla. Add flour mixture to yogurt mixture. Using a spatula, mix until just combined. Stir in dried fruit and chocolate chips.

Using a tablespoon, drop cookie dough onto baking sheet about 2 inches apart.

Bake 10 to 12 minutes, until lightly browned. Remove from oven and cool on a wire rack.

Nutrition

79 calories

3g fat

2g protein

12g carbohydrates

3mg sodium

91mg potassium

Cinnamon Sugar Apple Cake

Preparation Time: 15 minutes

Cooking Time: 20 minutes

Servings: 6

Ingredients:

1¾ cups granulated sugar

3 teaspoons ground cinnamon

1½ cups all-purpose flour

1½ teaspoons baking powder

½ teaspoon ground ginger

¼ teaspoon ground nutmeg

¼ teaspoon ground mace

½ cup (4 ounces / 113 g) low-fat cream cheese

1/3 cup unsweetened applesauce

2 tablespoons canola oil

1 teaspoon vanilla extract

2 egg whites

3 Fuji apples, peeled and chopped into 1-inch pieces

Cooking spray

Direction

Preheat oven to 350ºF (180ºC). Spray an 8-inch springform pan or four mini springform pans with cooking spray.

In a small bowl, mix ¼ cup of the sugar with 2 teaspoons of the cinnamon. Set aside.

In a medium bowl, combine flour, baking powder, ginger, nutmeg, mace, and remaining teaspoon cinnamon. Set aside.

In the bowl of a stand mixer fitted with the paddle attachment, beat 1½ cups sugar, cream cheese, applesauce, canola oil, and vanilla extract until well blended, about 4 minutes. Add egg whites to batter and continue beating until incorporated. Add flour mixture to batter, ¼ cup at a time, mixing until well incorporated.

In another small bowl, mix the apples with 3 tablespoons of the cinnamon sugar mixture. Gently stir the apple-cinnamon mixture into the batter.

Pour the batter into the pan or pans, and sprinkle with the remaining cinnamon sugar.

Bake for 20 minutes, or until a toothpick inserted in the center comes out clean. Individual pans will cook more quickly; check after 12 minutes.

Nutrition

340 calories

12g fat

4g protein

57g carbohydrates

136mg sodium

261mg potassium

Peanut Butter Oatmeal Chocolate Chip Cookies

Preparation Time: 15 minutes

Cooking Time: 12 minutes

Servings: 12

Ingredients:

1½ cups natural creamy peanut butter

½ cup dark brown sugar

2 large eggs

1 cup old-fashioned rolled oats

1 teaspoon baking soda

½ teaspoon kosher or sea salt

½ cup dark chocolate chips

Direction

Preheat the oven to 350ºF (180ºC). Line a baking sheet with parchment paper.

In the bowl of a stand mixer fitted with the paddle attachment, whip the peanut butter until very smooth. Continue beating and add the brown sugar, then one egg at a time, until fluffy. Beat in the oats, baking soda, and salt until combined. Fold in the dark chocolate chips.

Use a small cookie scoop or teaspoon and place globs of the cookie dough on the baking sheet, about 2 inches apart. Bake for 8 to 10 minutes depending on your preferred level of doneness.

Nutrition

153 calories

10g fat

4.1g protein

12g carbohydrates

130mg sodium

217mg potassium

Peach Crumble Muffins

Preparation Time: 25 minutes

Cooking Time: 25 minutes

Servings: 6

Ingredients:

Crumble:

2 tablespoons dark brown sugar

1 tablespoon honey

1 teaspoon ground cinnamon

2 tablespoons canola oil

½ cup old-fashioned rolled oats

Peach Muffins:

1¾ cups whole-wheat flour or whole-wheat pastry flour

1 teaspoon baking powder

1 teaspoon baking soda

1 teaspoon ground cinnamon

½ teaspoon ground ginger

½ teaspoon kosher or sea salt

¼ cup canola oil

¼ cup dark brown sugar

2 large eggs

1½ teaspoons vanilla extract

¼ cup plain nonfat Greek yogurt

3 peaches, diced (about 1½ cups)

Direction

Preheat the oven to 425ºF (220ºC). Line a 12-cup muffin tin with muffin liners and coat with cooking spray.

Make the Crumble

In a small bowl, mix together the brown sugar, honey, cinnamon, canola oil, and oats until combined. Set aside.

Make the Muffins

In a large bowl, whisk together the flour, baking powder, baking soda, cinnamon, ginger, and salt.

In another bowl, use a hand mixer to beat together the canola oil, brown sugar, and one egg at a time, until fluffy. Beat in the vanilla extract and yogurt. Slowly add the flour mixture to the bowl and whisk until the ingredients are just combined. Fold in the diced peaches with a spatula.

Fill each muffin well with batter about three-quarters of the way full. Spoon the crumble mixture on top of each. Bake for 5 to 6 minutes, then reduce the oven temperature to 350ºF (180ºC) and bake for 15 to 18 additional minutes, until a toothpick inserted into the center comes out clean. Let slightly cool before removing from the muffin tin.

Once completely cooled, store in a sealed plastic bag in the refrigerator for up to 5 days or freeze for up to 2 months.

Nutrition

188 calories

8g fat

4g protein

26g carbohydrates

215mg sodium

301mg potassium

Cinnamon Baked Apples with Walnuts

Preparation Time: 10 minutes

Cooking Time: 25 minutes

Servings: 4

Ingredients:

4 firm apples, such as Cortland or Granny Smith, peeled and cored

3 teaspoons light brown sugar

½ teaspoon cinnamon

½ teaspoon cardamom

1 cup unsweetened apple cider

1 cup unsweetened orange juice

1 tablespoon cornstarch

2 tablespoons cold water

2 tablespoons chopped black walnuts

Direction

Preheat oven to 350ºF (180ºC).

Place apples in a lined baking pan, and sprinkle with brown sugar, cinnamon, and cardamom.

Pour cider and orange juice into the dish and bake for 20 to 25 minutes. Remove apples to 4 dessert dishes and set aside.

Pour baking juices into a small saucepan, and heat on medium heat to a low simmer. In a separate bowl, mix cornstarch and water, then whisk into pan. Continue stirring until thickened, then spoon over each apple. Sprinkle chopped walnuts over each portion and serve warm.

Nutrition: Calories 185, Fat 13.5 g, Fiber 0.6 g, Carbs 2.6 g, Protein 15.4 g

Conclusion

Liver disease is not a life sentence and it can actually be managed to the point where you enjoy all aspects of your life.

The early manifestations of an unfortunate liver are awful breath, bulging, heartburn, abrupt weight reduction, and untimely turning gray of hair. Nonetheless, numerous greasy liver patients don't give indications and side effects until it's past the point of no return. That is the reason you ought to be additional wary and improves your eating routine and way of life. Here are a few food sources and an eating routine arrangement that can shield you from greasy liver. On the whole, we should see how the liver and body capacities are influenced in the event that you have fatty liver.

Being pro-active is important. Don't wait until it's too late. Remember you only have one liver. Start with baby steps and take things slowly. Again you can achieve a healthy liver by following the tips and preventive measures shared in this book so don't wait another day to get started. I wish you all the best and ever improving health!

Made in the USA
Monee, IL
24 August 2022